Physical Education and Sport

Physical Education and Sport

Editor: Edward Osborne

Callisto Reference
www.callistoreference.com

Callisto Reference,
118-35 Queens Blvd., Suite 400,
Forest Hills, NY 11375, USA

Visit us on the World Wide Web at:
www.callistoreference.com

ISBN: 978-1-64116-634-8 (Hardback)

Cataloging-in-Publication Data

Physical education and sport / edited by Edward Osborne.
p. cm.
Includes bibliographical references and index.
ISBN 978-1-64116-634-8
1. Physical education and training. 2. Sports. 3. Food. 4. Dietetics. I. Osborne, Edward.
GV206 .P49 2022
613.7--dc23

Table of Contents

Preface

The component of school education which focuses on psychomotor learning through movement exploration and play is known as physical education. It also seeks to impart knowledge regarding the health benefits of regular exercise and balanced diet as well as the risks associated with inactivity and poor diet. The system of activities which are based on physical athleticism or physical dexterity fall under the category of sports. They are generally used to maintain and improve physical abilities and skills. Sports are generally governed by a set of rules which exist to ensure fair competition and allow consistent adjudication of a winner. Some of the associated fields of study related to sports are sports engineering and sports science. It presents these complex subjects in the most comprehensible and easy to understand language. The various advancements in the fields of physical education and sport are glanced at and their applications as well as ramifications are looked at in detail. This book will help the readers in keeping pace with the rapid changes in these fields.

All of the data presented henceforth, was collaborated in the wake of recent advancements in the field. The aim of this book is to present the diversified developments from across the globe in a comprehensible manner. The opinions expressed in each chapter belong solely to the contributing authors. Their interpretations of the topics are the integral part of this book, which I have carefully compiled for a better understanding of the readers.

At the end, I would like to thank all those who dedicated their time and efforts for the successful completion of this book. I also wish to convey my gratitude towards my friends and family who supported me at every step.

Editor

1

CRITERIA OF EFFECTIVENESS OF STUDENTS' PHYSICAL EDUCATION SYSTEM IN HIGHER EDUCATIONAL ESTABLISHMENTS

Anikieiev D.M.
Institute of Penal Service

Abstract. *Purpose:* to work out criteria, permitting assessment of physical education in higher educational establishments. *Material:* theoretical analysis and generalization of scientific methodic literature and documents; method of experts' assessments. As experts, 26 professors and associate Professors of higher educational establishments of different profile were invited (13 doctors of science and 13 candidates of science). *Results:* we have generalized the data about effectiveness criteria of physical education, present in program normative documents. We have presented criteria, permitting to quantitatively assess the correspondence of physical education, in higher educational establishments, results to its purposes and tasks. *Conclusions:* the most acceptable method of physical education quality control is regular monitoring of indicators of students' physical condition. Individual target of every student shall be indicators of academic trainings' quality. Analysis of optional lessons' attendance is also very important indicators of quality of students' physical condition.
Key words: physical, fitness, health, expertise, optional, student.

Introduction

In the most general case effectiveness is the level of correspondence of any functioning results to the set task. Risk is a possibility of failure in this functioning [1]. Criterion (from Greek kriterion – mean for judgment) – is a sign, on the base of which assessment, determination and classification of something; measure of assessment [4]. Thus, criteria of effectiveness of physical education are understood by us as measures of correspondence of physical education results to the set tasks.

In Article 26 of Law of Ukraine "On physical culture and sports" (adopted in 2009) it is noted: "physical culture in educational sphere shall be targeted at ensuring students and pupils' physical health, complex approach to formation of mental and physical abilities of a personality, perfection of physical and psychological fitness for active life, professional functioning on the base of individual approach, priority of health related orientations, wide usage of different forms and means of physical education and mass sports, continuous character of this process during all life" [10].

Academic program for Ukrainian higher educational establishments of 3rd–4th levels of accreditation [14] defines nine criteria of effectiveness of graduate's physical education and not all of them can be put in the base of exact control methods and assessment of physical education quality. As on to-day there are no clearly determined effectiveness criteria for physical education in higher educational establishments. Decree of the Cabinet of Ministers, dt. November 5, 2008, №992 cancelled tests for assessment of population's physical fitness. Time and practice show that with positive character of intentions, State system of tests was not perfect. For example, Yu. Vykhliayev et al. [5] think that except actually important motor qualities of such tests (for example, endurance and strength) they also include not very important for human life qualities (jumping ability, quickness, dexterity, flexibility and swimming). It makes the system bulky and devaluates importance of first two qualities – endurance and strength. So the authors developed alternative methodic of assessment of physical condition.

The use of its application is confirmed by V. Samoshkin13], who determined satisfactory correlation coefficients (from 0.27 to 0.63) between level of cardio-respiratory system's functional potentials and students' physical fitness. The author confirmed existence of direct connection between health condition and physical fitness. From point of view of V. Samoshkin [13], it is also important to consider student's motor regiment.

The system of tests and normative shall strictly correspond to targets, tasks and content of physical education. It shall meet age and gender peculiarities of people, health condition. The system shall not require extreme physical loads. A.T. Litvin offer base (in assessment of physical education effectiveness) on criteria, grouped in six blocks: body constitution, condition of most important functional systems, weekly volume of energy consumption due to motor functioning, weekly scope and correlation of different kinds of motor functioning, indicators of strength, coordination and flexibility; morbidity [12].

Alongside with it, variety of opinions in respect to criteria of physical education effectiveness requires to conduct additional researches and analyze existing publications.

Purpose, tasks of the work, material and methods

The purpose of the research is to work out criteria, permitting assessment of physical education in higher educational establishments.

We used the following methods of the research in compliance with tasks and purpose of our work: theoretical analysis and generalization of scientific-research literature and documents, method of experts' assessments. Analysis of official documents was fulfilled by methodic, which is sufficiently completely described inA special literature [6, 7]. In the research we used the following kinds of experts' assessments: method of preference and method of direct assessment [7].

As experts, 26 professors and associate Professors of higher educational establishments of different profile were invited (13 doctors of science and 13 candidates of science).

Results

Analysis of physical education and sports in Ukrainian higher educational establishments showed that just higher school is the last stage of future specialists' training for independent activity. It imposes great responsibility for students' health and physical fitness on pedagogic staff [8].

In official documents, regulating students' physical education there is no clear formulation of its tasks and aims. That is why for determination of priorities in physical education in HEEs experts were given the task: "Rank the tasks to be solved by physical education in HEE by their importance". Results of expertise by method of preference (after reducing quantity of experts by Delfa's method) are given in table 1.

Table 1. Results of experts' questioning about importance of tasks to be solved by HEE physical education (W = 0,82, n = 21)

Object of expertise: ranking of tasks to be solved by HEE physical education	Rank
Formation of motivation – value attitude to physical culture, demand in regular practicing of physical exercises and sports	1
Formation of system of knowledge about physical culture and healthy life style	3
Strengthening of health, promoting of correct formation and comprehensive development of organism prophylaxis of diseases, ensuring of high physical condition, workability for all period of studying	2
Acquiring of motor skills' fund, general and professionally-applied physical fitness	4
Preparation for State or departmental tests and normative of physical fitness at level of requirements of educational-qualification characteristics and educational-professional programs for certain specialists	5

One of the most important problems of construction of HEE physical education technology is to form student's interested attitude to discipline, to awaken interest to building healthy body, to form own health in the widest sense [3]. Only if a student understands real possibility of such influence on own organism it becomes possible to effectively solve separate motor tasks, which are the components of every academic training [9].

That is why one of questionnaire's items implied definition of the most acceptable methods of physical education quality control in HEE. Results are given in table 2.

Table 2. Results of experts' questioning about the most acceptable methods of physical education quality control in HEE (W=0,789, n=24)

Object of expertise: the most acceptable method of physical education quality control in HEE.	Rank
Testing of physical fitness	2
Regular monitoring of physical condition indicators, changes of which is individual target of a student	1
Analysis of optional trainings' attendance on senior years of studying (after finishing of compulsory trainings)	3
Monitoring of theoretical knowledge on physical culture and healthy life style	4
Other methods	5

Considering modern students' low motivation for practicing physical exercises we organized experts' assessment of methods of students' motivation for physical culture. The results are given in table 3.

Table 3. Results of experts' questioning about methods of students' motivation for physical culture (W=0,738, n =23)

Object of expertise: methods of students' motivation for physical culture	Rank
Semester physical education test	2
Current physical education testing	3
Regular monitoring of physical condition indicators, changes of which is individual target of a student	1
Every year State testing of physical fitness	4
Other methods	5

Thus, regular monitoring of physical condition indicators (as individual target of a student) is, at the same time, the most acceptable methods of physical education quality control and motivation of students for trainings. Just achievement of individual target is a powerful factor, stimulating further activity. Any activity is regulated and controlled owing to feedback. If results grow, motivation for activity increases. That is why testing of results creates strong positive emotional feeling and gives new impulse for self-perfection [11, 15]. Though, choice of physical condition indicators to be improved in physical education process – is an open question. With it, it is necessary to base on our questioning of students [2]. Physical condition indicators can be divided into 2 groups:

1. Indicators, connected with good appearance (fat percentage, correlation of muscular and fat tissues and so on);
2. Indicators, connected with strengthening of health (functional indicators of cardio-respiratory systems, muscular skeletal apparatus and etc.).

It should also be noted that it is important to correctly choose physical condition indicators. Positive changes of these indicators will facilitate solution the main task in HEEs: formation of students' motivation-value attitude to physical culture, demand in regular practicing of physical exercises and sports.

Discussion

Results of our researches confirmed the data of other authors about importance of physical education quality control and correct choice of physical condition indicators of students [16–20, 23–26].

When composing academic plan on physical education it is necessary to consider that physical fitness and health can not be preserved for future usage. Regular motor functioning is important target for students. Students shall feel advantages of healthy life style already in the process of studying. After graduation advantages, acquired with physical exercises, will quickly disappear. Thus, academic plan shall form students' responsibility for their way of life [21, 22].

Unfortunately, nowadays there appears danger tendency to refuse compulsory physical education lessons in HEEs for saving money, required for maintenance of sport facilities. These actions are provoked by the following:

- Order of Ministry of education and science, dt. January 26, 2015, № 47 "On formation of curriculums for 2015/2016 academic year";
- Letter of MES of Ukraine, dt. 13.03.2015 № 1 / 9–126.

In this letter it is noted: "Physical culture trainings in sport circles can be organized both as optional (i.e. they are not included in curriculums and have no final control)". It contradicts to Cl.26, it. 4 and it. 17 of Law of Ukraine "On higher education". In these documents it is noted: "Administrators of higher educational establishments are obliged to create favorable conditions for proper motor functioning of students".

That is why analysis of optional trainings' attendance we consider to be very important indicator of physical education quality at HEEs in spite of the fact that it takes only third position be results of expertise. Its correspondence to the task, which id the most important in HEEs: formation of motivation-value attitude to physical culture, demand in regular sports' and physical exercises' practicing, attracts attention. Optional trainings can be paid but in reasonable limits. A share of the earned money can be directed for financial incentives of instructors.

Conclusions

The most acceptable method of physical education quality control in HEEs is regular monitoring of students' physical condition indicators. Indicators of trainings' quality shall be individual target of every student. Alongside with it, analysis of optional trainings' attendance we consider to be an important indicators of physical education quality at HEE.

Acknowledgement

The problem of the work corresponds to topic 3.1 "Perfection of program-normative principles of physical education in educational establishments" of combine plan of SRW in sphere of physical culture and sports for 2011–2015.

Conflict of interests

The author declares that there is no conflict of interests.

References:

1. Alekseev VV. *Razrabotka logiko-veroiatnostnykh modelej, metodov i algoritmov dlia upravleniia riskom i effektivnost'iu v strukturno-slozhnykh sistemakh. Cand. Diss.* [Development of logical-probabilistic models for control of risks and effectiveness in structurally-complex systems. Cand. Diss.]. Sankt Petersburg; 2009. (in Russian)
2. Anikieiev DM. Analiz sposobu zhittia suchasnoi students'koi molodi [Analysis of modern students' life style]. *Moloda sportivna nauka Ukraini*. 2010;2:10–14. (in Ukrainian)
3. Antonova TV. *Pedagogicheskie usloviia valeologicheskogo samorazvitiia studenta v processe fizicheskogo vospitaniia. Cand. Diss.* [Pedagogic conditions of student's valuelogic self-development in physical education process. Cand. Diss.]. Cheboksary; 2005. (in Russian)
4. *Bol'shoj Enciklopedicheskij Slovar'* [Large Encyclopedic Dictionary]. Available at: http://slovari.299.ru/enc.php (accessed 23.07.2015)
5. Vikhliaiev Iu, Sichov S, Shcherbachenko V. Ocinka fizichnoi pidgotovlenosti studentiv [Assessment of students' physical fitness]. *Vseukrains'ka naukova praktichna konferenciia, Kiiv, 1988. "Students'kij fizkul'turno-sportivnij rukh v Ukraini na porozi XXI stolittia" Kiiv, 1998.* [All-Ukrainian scientific-practical conference, Kyiv, 1988. "Students' physical culture – sports movement in Ukraine on the eve of 21st century", Kyiv, 1988]. Kiev; 1998. p. 111. (in Ukrainian)
6. Godik MA. *Sportivnaia metrologiia* [Sport metrology]. Moscow: Physical Culture and Sport; 1988. (in Russian)
7. Denisova LV. *Izmereniia i metody matematicheskoj statistiki v fizicheskom vospitanii i sporte* [Measurements and methods of mathematical statistic in physical education and sports]. Kiev: Olympic Literature; 2008. (in Russian)
8. Dolzhenko LP. *Fizicheskaia podgotovlennost' i funkcional'nye osobennosti studentov s razlichnym urovnem fizicheskogo zdorov'ia. Cand. Diss.* [Physical fitness and functional characteristics of students with different level of health. Cand. Diss.]. Kiev; 2006. (in Russian)
9. Durkin PK, Lebedeva MP. K probleme vospitaniia lichnoj fizicheskoj kul'tury u shkol'nikov i studentov [On the problem of cultivation of pupils' and students' personal physical culture]. *Fizicheskaia kul'tura: vospitanie, obrazovanie, trenirovka*. 2000;2:50–53. (in Russian)
10. Zakon Ukraini "Pro fizichnu kul'turu i sport" [Law of Ukraine: "On physical culture and sports"] *Oficijnij visnik Ukraini,* 2009;97:30 (in Ukrainian)
11. Korolins'ka SV. *Klubna forma organizacii fizichnogo vikhovannia u vishchikh navchal'nikh zakladakh. Cand. Diss.* [Cub form of physical education organization in higher educational establishments. Cand. Diss.]. Lviv; 2007. (in Ukrainian)
12. Litvin AT. *Istoricheskie predposylki i teoretiko-metodologicheskie osnovy sovremennoj sistemy fizicheskogo vospitaniia. Cand. Diss.* [Historical pre-conditions and theoretical-methodological principles of modern system of physical education. Cand. Diss.], Kiev, 2007. (in Russian)
13. Samoshkin VV. Vzaiemozv'iazok funkcional'nogo rezervu kardiorespiratornoi sistemi ta fizichnoi pidgotovlenosti studentiv [Interconnection of cardio-respiratory systems' functional reserve and students' physical fitness]. *Vseukrains'ka naukova praktichna konferenciia "Aktual'ni problemi fizichnogo vikhovannia u vuzi", Donec'k. 1998* [All-Ukrainian scientific-practical conference "Actual problems of physical education in HEE, Donetsk, 1998.]. Donetsk; 1998. (in Ukrainian)
14. *Fizichne vikhovannia, navchal'na programa dlia vishchikh navchal'nikh zakladiv Ukraini 3–4 rivniv akreditacii* [Physical education, academic program for higher educational establishments of Ukraine of 3rd-4th accreditation levels]. Kiev; 2003. (in Ukrainian)
15. Forrester S. Student attitude toward sports and fitness activities after graduation. Scott Forrester, Christopher Arterberry, Bob Barcelona. *Recreational Sports Journal*, 2006;30:87–99.
16. Iermakova TS. Education of children in Polish family in a context of forming health culture. *Pedagogics, psychology, medical-biological problems of physical training and sports,* 2014;11:17–22. http://dx.doi.org/10.15561/18189172.2014.1104
17. Iermakova TS. The peculiarities of work of the european network of health promoting schools (comparative analysis). *Pedagogics, psychology, medical-biological problems of physical training and sports*, 2013;10:93–96. http://dx.doi.org/10.6084/m9.figshare.775339

18. Kolokoltsev MM, Cieslicka Miroslawa, Muszkieta Radoslaw. Optimization of physical training of students of high school with regard to quantitative features muscular components of their bodies. *Physical Education of Students*. 2015;1:22–30. http://dx.doi.org/10.15561/20755279.2015.0104
19. Kozina ZL, Iermakov SS. Analysis of students' nervous system's typological properties, in aspect of response to extreme situation, with the help of multi-dimensional analysis. *Physical Education of Students*. 2015;3:10–19. http://dx.doi.org/10.15561/20755279.2015.0302
20. Michael Chia, Marcus Lee. Relationship between quality of life and resilience among sport-active Singaporean youth. *Physical Education of Students*. 2015;2:29–36. http://dx.doi.org/10.15561/20755279.2015.0205
21. *PE4life: developing and promoting quality physical education*. Champaign: Human Kinetics, 2007;XXIV.
22. *Physical Education for Lifelong Fitness: the Physical Best Teacher's Guide*. Champaign: Human Kinetics; 1999.
23. Prosvirina LN, Kolokoltsev MM, Kolchanova MA, Cieslicka Miroslawa, Stankiewicz Blazej. The characteristic of the engine qualities of the students of technical institute of III functional health group (special medical group). *Physical Education of Students*. 2015;1:43–49. http://dx.doi.org/10.15561/20755279.2015.0107
24. Rovnaya OA, Podrigalo LV, Iermakov SS, Prusik Krzysztof, Cieślicka Mirosława. Morphological and functional features of synchronous swimming sportswomen of high qualification. *Pedagogics, psychology, medical-biological problems of physical training and sports*, 2014;4:45–49. http://dx.doi.org/10.6084/m9.figshare.951916
25. Żukowska Hanna, Szark-Eckardt Mirosława, Muszkieta Radosław, Iermakova TS. Characteristics of body posture in the sagittal plane and fitness of first-form pupils from rural areas. *Pedagogics, psychology, medical-biological problems of physical training and sports,* 2014;7:50–60. http://dx.doi.org/10.6084/m9.figshare.1015583
26. Yermakova TS. Individualization of forming health culture in schoolchildren of Polish schools. *Pedagogics, psychology, medical-biological problems of physical training and sports*. 2015;1:29–33. http://dx.doi.org/10.15561/18189172.2015.0106

2

SPORT AND MENTAL HEALTH LEVEL AMONG UNIVERSITY STUDENTS

Kenioua Mouloud[1*], Boumasjed Abd Elkader [2]
[1] Institute of physical education and sport, Ouargla University, Algeria
[2] Institute of physical education and sport, Mostaganem University, Algeria

Abstract. *Purpose:* study of mental health level of university student, athletes and non-athletes. *Material:* The tested group consisted of 160 male and female undergraduates from Ouargla University, Algeria; 80 students-athletes from Institute of Physical Education and Sports and 80 students-non-athletes from Department of Psychology, English and Mathematics. In the study we used health mental scale, adapted by Diab (2006) to Arab version scale, formed from five dimensions (Competence and self-confidence, Capacity for social interaction, Emotional maturity, Freedom from neurotic symptoms, self rating and aspects of natural deficiencies). *Results:* the findings indicated that university students have high level of mental health. And the mean of the responses of students-athletes group by mental health scale reached (M = 32.40), with standard deviation (STD =5.83), while the mean of the responses of students-non athletes group by mental health scale has reached (M=27.47), with standard deviation (STD=7.88). T-value, required to know significance of differences between means of students-athletes and students-non athletes has reached (T=4.51), (DF=185, $p < 0.01$). So there are significant statistical differences between student athletes and non-athletes in their responses by mental health scale in favor of the student athletes. *Conclusion*: sports are beneficial in respect to mental health among university students and emphasizing the importance of the mental health of university students through its integration in the various recreational and competitive activities. Future qualitative research, covering multi-variables' tests on mental health and others psychological characteristics could be performed in sports area.
Key words: mental health, sports, university students.

Introduction

Although it has been known for some time that physical exercises are good for physical health, it is within the past decade, that it has become commonplace to read in magazines and health newsletters that exercises can also be valuable in promoting sound psychological health. This optimistic appraisal has attracted a great deal of attention among public. However, for the most part, scientific community has been much more cautions in offering such unsubstantiated endorsement. Until recent time, assessment of the research literature on psychological outcomes associated with exercise, such as reduced anxiety and depression, current state have been equivocal. (Landers & Arent, 2001)

Ninety-five percents of college counseling center directors said that the number of students with significant psychological problems is of growing concern in their centers or campus, according to the latest Association for University and College Counseling Center Directors survey of counseling center directors. Seventy percents of directors believe that the number of students with severe psychological problems in their campuses has increased in the past year (Directors report that 21 % of counseling center students had severe mental health problems, while another 40 % had mild mental health problems). (AUCCCD, 2013)

People have regular tendency to do so, because it gives them an enormous sense of well-being. They feel more energetic throughout the day, sleep better at night, have sharper memory, and feel more relaxed and positive about themselves and their lives. And it's also powerful medicine for many common mental health challenges. Most previous researches do conclude that sports, physical activity and exercises do have beneficial effects on general mental health. Within higher education environment, it is surprising that little research has explored the potential benefits of sports in a cohort of individuals who are at risk of mental health problems, i.e., university students. Of the few studies that have been conducted, Van Raalte et al. (2015) referred that viewing the www.SupportForSport.org site resulted in enhanced mental health referral knowledge and efficacy relative to a control group. Results suggest that tailored on-line programming can affect outcomes for student-athletes across geographic region and resource availability levels. Tyson et al. (2010) conducted a study on physical activity and mental health in student population. Results indicated that significant differences were observed between the low, medium and high exercise groups on the mental health scales, indicating better mental health for those, who engaged in more intensive exercises' practicing. Whilst Ahmadi et al. (2002) reported that engaging in body building and swimming reduced scores on the beck Depression Inventory in female students, other searcher Toskovic (2001) found that students engaging in dynamic Taekwondo also reported lower levels of depression than in control group.

The purpose of study

Taking into account the evidence to suggest that sports are beneficial for mental health, and that university students are at elevated risk of such problems, the following study sought to investigate the impact of sports on mental health level among university students.

For the purpose of this study, the research study questions were as follows:

SQ1. What's the level of health mental among university students?

SQ2. Are there significant differences in the level of mental health between student athletesand non-athletes?

The Hypotheses

HY1. There is high level of mental health among university students.

HY2. There are significant differences in the level of mental health between student athletes and non-athletes.

Material and methods

Participants

The sample of study consisted of 160 male and female undergraduates students from Ouargla University Algeria; 80 students' athletes from Institute of Physical Education and Sports and 80 students' non-athletes from Department of Psychology, English and Mathematics (figure.1). Participants were selected randomly.

Institute (department)	**Student athletes**	**Student non-athletes**		
class	**Institute of physical educational**	**Psychology**	**English**	**Mathematics**
The first	20	7	7	6
The second	30	10	10	10
The third	30	10	10	10
Total	80	80		

Figure.1. Distribution the members of sample

Tool

In this study, Scale of Mental Health was used to collect data. adapted by Diab (2006) to Arab version, scale formed from five dimensions (Competence and self-confidence, Capacity for social interaction, Emotional maturity, Freedom from neurotic symptoms, self-rating and aspects of natural deficiencies).

To ensure the psychometric properties of the scale, it has been applied on 30 students; as the value of validity scale (T= 7.91) level of significance (0.01). The reliability was done, the value of Cronbach's alpha coefficient equal to (0.67) and the value of Spearman- Brown coefficient equal to (0.87).

Data analysis

Data analysis was carried out with the help of statistical packet for social sciences (SPSS) 20.00 software program. The results were presented as descriptive statistics. Regarding the correct tool, there is in front of each item estimate balance consists of one degree, where the "no" give (0) and "Yes" to give (1).

Results

In this section, the findings obtained from the data analysis related Sports and mental health level among university students are given in detail. Findings concerning the level of mental health among university students are shown in table 1.

Table 1. Distribution percentages for members of sample on the mental health scale

Level of mental health	**Repetition**	**percentage**
High level	136	85%
Low level	24	15%
Total	160	100%

In table 1, the number of students with high mental health has reached (s= 136), percentage (85%). While the number of students with low mental health has reached (s=24), percentage (15%). Thus, we can conclude that the level of mental health among students is high.

In table 2, mean values of students-athletes group's responses by mental health scale has reached (M = 32.40), with standard deviation (STD =5.83), while the mean values of students-non athletes group's responses by mental health scale has reached (M=27.47), with standard deviation (STD=7.88). T –value (to know significance of differences between means of group student athletes and group students' athletes) has reached (T=4.51), (DF=185, p <0.01). So, there are significant statistical differences between students-athletes and non-athletes in their responses by mental health scale in favor of students-athletes.

Table 2. Significance of differences in the mental health level of the tested sample

Sample	N	M	Std	T Calculated	DF	Sing
Student-athletes	80	32.40	5.83	4.51	158	yes
Student –non athletes	80	27.47	7.88			
0.01						

Discussion

The study, which was carried out in order to determine the level of mental health among students, revealed some important information, findings, and results. As results of this study, it was concluded that the students in university had high level of mental health.

This study differs from most previous studies, except the work of Samin (2012), who showed that there was high personal compatibility among university students. This difference exists due to nature of the mentioned studies' goals as well as different characteristics of the samples in their sex, age, and cultural/social background. Based on the above, and the result of our findings of the first hypothesis, it is clear that there are factors helping students, such as social conditions, stable economic and situations, making them to feel self-importance as well as enabling them to cope with the psychological effects of life difficulties that might pass out during the study. These factors contribute to the sharp rise in the degree of psychological and social compatibility, and represent a kind of moral support, stimulating students' abilities to cope with various difficulties. Ganellen et al. (1984) referred that these factors mitigate the impact pressure on the individual, and strengthen psychological sources, and increase individual's sense of value and importance.

Basing on results we concluded that there were significant differences between students-athletes and students-non athletes in level of mental health. Perhaps sports activities affect the various aspects of personality and growth, and also develop some life needs of students, thus influencing on their behavior and personality. For example, opportunity for social interaction (Crone et al.2005), psycho-social, such as positive emotional experiences (Carless and Douglass, 2004; Carless & Sparkes, 2008; Crone, 2007), sense of achievement (Fogarty and Happell,2005) and improvements in general mental wellbeing (Laforge et al., 2002), are positively influenced on by sport activity as well as moderate depression (Craft, 2005; Craft & Perna, 2004) and anxiety (Biddle & Mutrie, 2001). Sports activity promotes self-confidence Larry (1983) referred that physical exercises let college men to be more satisfied, more outgoing, sociable and confident.

Conclusion

Finally, there is high level of mental health among university students in University Ouargla, and there are significant differences between students-athletes and students-non athletes. Thus, sports have potential to be of benefit for mental health of university students and emphasize importance of the mental health of university students through its integration in the various recreational and competitive activities.

Future qualitative research, covering multi-variables' tests on mental health and others psychological characteristics could be performed in sports area.

References

Ahmadi J, Samavat F, Sayyad M, & Ghanizadeh A. Various types of exercise and scores on the Beck Depression Inventory. *Psychological Reports*, 2002; 90(3): 821–822.

AUCCCD. College students' mental health is a growing concern, survey finds. *Monitor on psychology*, 2013;44(6): 13-20.

Biddle SJH, & Mutrie N. Psychology of physical activity: Determinants, well-being and interventions. London: Routledge; 2001.

Carless D, & Douglas K. A golf programme for people with severe and enduring mental illness. *Journal of Mental Health Promotion,* 2004;*3*(4): 26–39.

Carless D, & Sparkes A. Narrative, identity and mental health: How men with serious mental illness restory their lives through sport and exercise. *Psychology of Sport and Exercise*, 2008; 9(5): 576–594.

Craft LL. Exercise and clinical depression: Examining two psychological mechanisms. *Psychology of Sport and Exercise*, 2005;6(2): 151–171.

Craft LL, & Perna FM. The benefits of exercise for the clinically depressed. Primary Care Companion, *Journal of Clinical Psychiatry*, 2004; 6: 104–111.

Crone D. Walking back to health: A qualitative investigation into service user's experiences of a walking project. *Issues in Mental Health Nursing*, 2007;28(2): 167–183.

Crone D, Smith A, & Gough B. 'I feel totally alive, totally happy and totally at one': A psycho-social explanation of the physical activity and mental health relationship from the experiences of participants on exercise referral schemes. *Health Education Research*, 2005; 20(5): 600–611.

Diab AAM. *Social Support as a Mediating Factor between Stressful Events and Mental Health for Palestinian Adolescents.* Unpublished master thesis. Psychology Department University of Gaza. Palestine; 2006.

Fogarty M, & Happell B. Exploring the benefits of an exercise program for people with schizophrenia:A qualitative study. *Issues in Mental Health Nursing*, 2005; 26, 341–351.

Ganellen R. Hardiness and Social Support as Moderators of the Effect of Life Stress. *Journal of Personality and Psychology,* 1984;47(1): 156-163.

Laforge RG, Rossi JS, Prochaska JO, Velicer WF, Levesque DA, & McHorney CA. Stage ofexercise and health related quality of life. *Journal of Preventive Medicine,* 2002;28(4): 349–360.

Landers MD, & Arent MS. physical activity and mental health. In: RN Singer, HA Hausenblas and CM Janelle. (Ed). *Handbook of sport psychology*. John Wiley and Sons: New York;2001.

Larry AT. Muscular Strength and Mental Health. *Journal of Personality and Social Psychology*, 1983;45(6): 1355-1360.

Samin ZB. Personal compatibility and its relationship of Exercise among university students. *Journal of College of Basic Education*, 2012;74:100-115.

Toskovic N. Alterations in selected measures of mood with a single bout of dynamic Taekwondo exercise in college-age students. *Perceptual and Motor Skills*, 2001; 92(3): 1031–1038.

Tyson P, Wilson K, Crone D, Brailsford R, & Laws K. Physical activity and mental health in a student population. *Journal of Mental Health.* 2010;1:1-8.

Van Raalte LJ, Cornelius EA, Andrews S, Diehl SN, & Brewer WB. Mental Health Referral for Student-Athletes: Web-Based Education and Training. *Journal of Clinical Sport Psychology*, 2015; 9: 197-212. doi:10.1123/jcsp.2015-0011

3

SOMATIC ASPECTS OF SPORTS CHAMPIONSHIP IN TAEKWON-DO ITF

Jagiello W,[1] Kozina Zh.L.[2], Jagiello Marina[1]
[1]University of Physical Education and Sport, Gdansk, Poland
[2]Kharkov National Pedagogical University, Ukraine

Abstract. *The purpose* of the study is to answer a basic question: which somatic characteristics of taekwon-do ITF athletes correlate the most with their sports level and experience training. *Material:* Representatives of the Polish taekwon-do ITF national team (n=21) took part in the study. The subjects' age was in the range of 18.51–32.22 years (24.5±4.1), and their training experience 8.4–22.4 years (13.6±3,4). *Results:* Measurements of 20 basic somatic characteristics were taken. It was determined that correlations with the sports level and training experience were non-homogeneous and diverse due to the represented weight category. *Conclusions:* correlations of somatic indices with sports level and training experience among Polish representatives in taekwon-do are heterogeneous and largely dependent on weight category.
Keywords: taekwon-do, ITF, body, composition, sports, championship.

Introduction

Modern sport theorists and practitioners' research clearly indicates correlations between athletes' somatic composition and the represented by them sports discipline [7, 8, 11, 16].

In most cyclical disciplines of sport and team sports games, morphological indicators constitute the basic criterion for recruitment and selection. In many cases, they define the efficiency of the competitive activity and, what is directly connected with this, the level of sports championship [1, 6, 10, 17].

However, the problem is much more complex in speed-strength sports with a complicated coordination structure and a large range of body weight. Taekwon-do ITF undoubtedly meets these conditions [3, 18, 20].

Therefore, the purpose of the research is to answer a basic question: which somatic characteristics of taekwon-do ITF athletes correlate with the sports level and training experience to the greatest extent.

Material and methods

The study involved taekwon-do ITF athletes (n=21). Among them 14 were representatives of Poland in senior category. The remaining subjects represented a high sports level. The subjects' age ranged between 18.51 and 32.22 years (24.5±4.1), body weight varied within 62.70–100 kg (75.3±10.3), and the body height 167.0–195 cm (179.6±8.3). The sports level was determined on the basis of experts' opinions (coaches of the Polish national team in Taekwon-do ITF) by means of ranking.

The training experience varied between 8.4 and 22.4 years (13.6±3.4) and was significantly varied (V%=24.8). Anthropometric measurements were taken during the Polish national team camp trainings (Spala – Central Sport Centre, February 29–March 5, 2012) and during Seniors and Juniors Polish Cup competitions (Klobuck, 2-4 February 2012).

Anthropometric measurements were taken in accordance with the adopted rules [4], using standard instruments. In addition, five indicators were calculated: slenderness, Rohrer's, Quetelet's II. Manouvrier's, and the shoulder-pelvis index.

The total body fat in percentage from body weight was calculated according to Brożek and Keks's equation [2]. The density of body, on the basis of measurements of subcutaneous fat, was calculated by Piechaczek's anticipating equation [19]. Measurements of total of 20 basic somatic characteristics were made.

The results of the study were then subjected to basic statistical analysis by calculating the arithmetic mean (X), the standard deviation (±SD), the coefficient of variation (V%) and the level of correlations (r).

Results

Correlations of somatic characteristics with training experience (TE) and sports level (SL) among taekwon-do athletes show a varied character (Tab. 1).

Taking into account mean value of all the correlations, they are slightly higher in relation to the training experience than to the sports level (0.439 and 0.370, respectively), and they represent an average level. However, if to consider weight categories. mean value of correlations between somatic characteristics and the sports level is the greatest in the hyper-weight category (r=0.462) and the light-weight one (r=0.440), and the weakest one in the middle-weight category (r=0.232). Level of correlations with the training experience is slightly higher. In hyper-weight category it amounts to 0.506, in light-weight one 0.506, and it is the lowest in the middle-weight category (r=0.372).

Table 1

Correlations of somatic characteristics with the training experience (TE) and the sports level (SL) among taekwon-do athletes, different weight categories

Somatic characteristics	Weight categories							
	<63 kg, n=5		<7 l kg, n=6		<80 kg, n=6		>80 kg, n=4	
	TE	SL	TE	SL	TE	SL	TE	SL
body mass	0.137	-0.635	-0.357	0.131	-0.305	-0.217	0.771	-0.636
body height	-0.560	0.354	-0.307	-0.138	0.256	-0.375	0.607	-0.735
sitting body height	0.100	0.694	-0.322	-0.174	-0.352	-0.131	0.608	-0.513
length of upper extremity	-0.424	-0.150	-0.281	-0.390	-0.220	-0.221	-0.097	-0.689
length of lower extremity	-0.730	0.131	-0.715	-0.561	0.721	-0.627	-0.332	0.148
pelvic width	0.415	0.920	-0.236	0.298	0.298	0.202	0.875	-0.322
shoulders width	-0.607	-0.009	-0.493	-0.058	-0.388	0.255	0.759	0.053
elbow width	-0.161	0.446	-0.173	0.325	-0.100	0.217	-0.143	0.775
knee width	0.741	0.394	0.440	0.202	-0.077	0.749	0.409	0.408
forearm perimeter	-0.564	-0.433	0.474	-0.217	0.731	-0.727	0.466	-0.078
shank perimeter	0.381	0.683	-0.333	-0.652	0.420	-0.802	0.199	0.366
body density	-0.217	0.488	0.377	-0.060	0.770	-0.216	-0.664	0.610
fat %	0.217	-0.489	-0.374	0.063	-0.770	0.215	0.665	-0.610
active tissue %	-0.217	0.489	0.374	-0.063	0.770	-0.215	-0.665	0.610
body surface	-0.588	0.310	-0.313	-0.134	0.210	-0.374	0.835	-0.727
slenderness index	-0.551	0.366	-0.304	-0.139	0.272	-0.375	-0.433	0.243
Rohrer's index	0.531	-0.376	0.283	0.147	-0.268	0.382	0.411	-0.233
BMI index	0.531	-0.379	0.286	0.146	-0.277	0.380	0.545	-0.375
Manouvrier's index	-0.685	-0.430	0.294	0.199	0.624	-0.213	-.,318	-0.293
Shoulder-pelvis index	0.732	0.630	0.707	0.553	0.640	-0.034	0.318	-0.812

High level of correlations between somatic characteristics with the sports level in the light-weight category was recorded with reference to the pelvis width (r=0.92). In middle-weight category no correlations at high level were noted. In heavy-weight category high correlations of the sports level became apparent with the shank perimeter (r= -0.80), knee width (r=0.75), and forearm perimeter (r= -0.73). In hyper-weight category 4 correlations were revealed at a high level: with the shoulder-pelvis index (r =-0.81), elbow width (r=0.78), body height (r= -0.74) and body surface (r= -0.74). The structure of correlations between somatic characteristics and sports level is varied depending on the weight category (Figure 1).

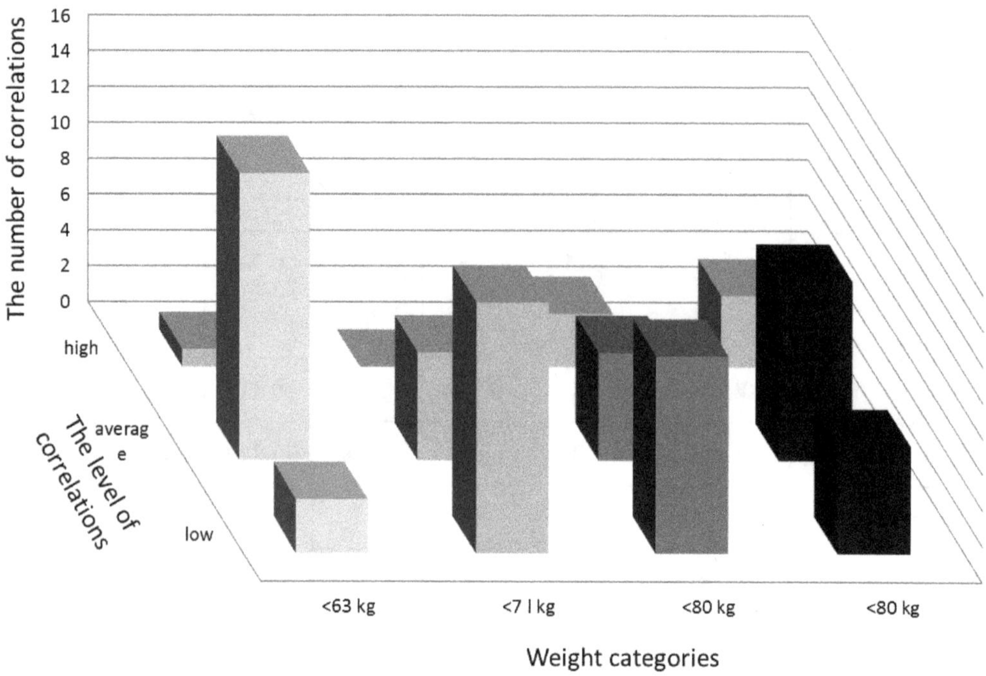

Fig. 1. The structure of correlations between somatic characteristics and the sports level among highly qualified taekwon-do ITF athletes.

The high level of correlations between somatic characteristics and the training experience in the light-weight category was revealed in relation to the knee width (r=0.74) and the length of the lower extremity and the shoulder-pelvis index (r=0.73). In the middle-weight category, high correlations were reported with reference to the length of the lower extremity (r= -0.72) and the shoulder-pelvis index (r=0.71). In the heavyweight category 5 correlations were revealed at a high level: with the body density, and the directly related fat content and the active body weight (-0.77; and 0.77, respectively), with the forearm perimeter (0.73) and the length of the lower extremity (0.72). In hyper-weight category 4 correlations were recorded at a high level: with the pelvic width index (r=0.88), the body surface (r=0.84), the body mass (r=0.77) and the shoulders width (r=0.76).

The structure of correlations between somatic characteristics and the training experience is again varied, depending on weight categories (Figure 2).

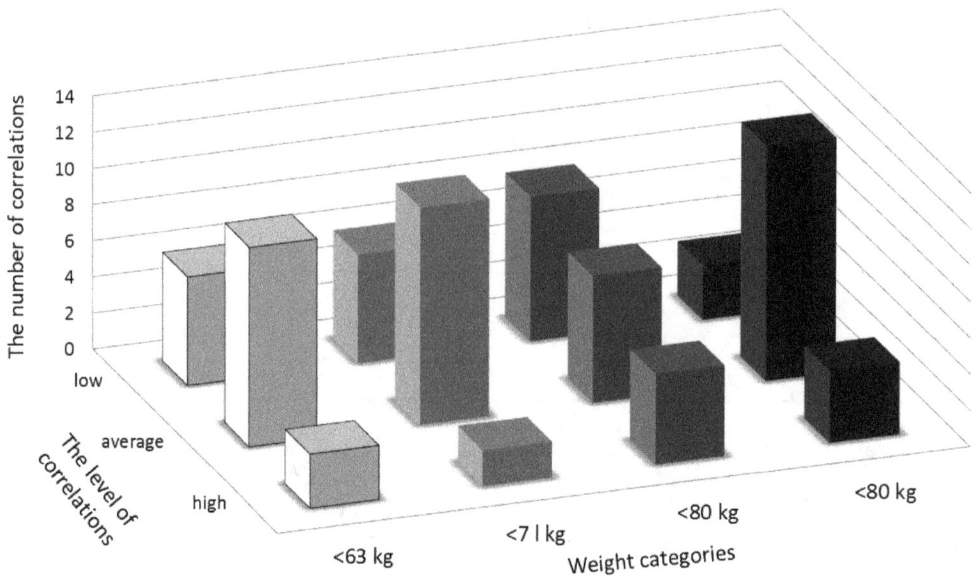

Fig. 2. The structure of correlations between somatic characteristics and the training experience among highly qualified taekwon-do ITF athletes.

Discussion

The study results clearly indicate that the problem of constitutional aspects of taekwon-do ITF athletes' sports championship is a complex scientific issue. In research on Polish male and female representatives in wrestling [12, 13], the authors state that with an increase in body mass also the number and the level of correlations between somatic characteristics and the sports level and training experience increases. Just as in this study, a slightly higher level of correlations is observed with training experience than with the sports level.

A study of Polish representatives in modern pentathlon [9] showed that among women anthropometric indices correlate with the training experience to a greater extent than with sports level. On the other hand, males' sports level is more closely associated with their somatic composition.

An interesting study was conducted with a group of women practicing fencing [5]. A high correlation between body composition and the sports experience was reported only in relation to one somatic index – Manouvrier's index. As to sports level, correlations at high level were revealed with three somatic characteristics: body weight, forearm perimeter and upper extremity length.

The study, which was conducted at the European Championships in tennis [14] revealed an important trend. Along with increase in tennis players' sports level, a reduction in the athletes' body massiveness indices was reported. Hence, the authors conclude that tennis players' slim body build can predispose them to achieving better sports results. Also study of Polish tennis representatives [6] showed that somatic indices have larger impact on men's sports level than on women's. A correlation between tennis players' body composition and their training experience is high with reference to two indices: elbow width and forearm perimeter. Only knee width highly correlates with their sports level. Among men only pelvis width correlates with training experience at high level. In turn, as many as six indices correlate with sports level: body height, upper extremity length, forearm and shank perimeter, body weight and its surface. The authors conclude that the structure of the correlations between somatic indices and sports level and training experience in tennis has a dimorphic character.

Taking into account overall index of correlation of somatic characteristics among Polish representatives in taekwon-do ITF with their training experience and sport level, as in most of analysed researches, a higher correlation was noted with the training experience than with sports level. In all analysed weight categories, mean value of correlations of somatic characteristics with sports level was lower than in relation to training experience.

Shank perimeter highly correlates with sports level in all weight categories (apart from the hyper-weight one) –mean value of correlation index for all categories amounts to 0.63, just as shoulder-pelvis index (apart from the heavyweight category) – 0.51.

High correlation with training experience was reported for lower extremity length (apart from the hyper-weight category) – the mean value of the correlation index was 0.62, for the shoulder-pelvis index (apart from the hyper-weight category) – the mean value of the correlation index was 0.60; for the shoulder width (apart from the heavyweight category) and for the forearm perimeter – the mean value of the correlation index was 0.56.

The results of the conducted studies and literature analysis give grounds to believe that the problem of somatic aspects of sports championship is a very complex and ambiguous issue. A sport discipline (the nature of effort) and the weight categories, in which a bout takes place has an impact on the structure and level of correlations.

Conclusions

1. Correlations of somatic indices with sports level and training experience among Polish representatives in taekwon-do are heterogeneous and largely dependent on weight category.

2. Shank perimeter (apart from the hyper-weight category) and shoulder-pelvic index (apart from the heavy weight category) highly correlate with sports level in all weight categories.

3. Lower extremity length (apart from hyper-weight category), shoulder-pelvis index (apart from hyper-weight category), shoulder width (apart from heavy weight category) and forearm perimeter highly correlate with training experience.

References

1. Baxter-Jones ADG, Helms P, Maffulli N, Baines-Preece JC. Growth and development of male gymnasts, swimmers, soccer and tennis players: a longitudinal stady. *Annals of Human Biology*, 1995;5:381-394.
2. Brożek J, Keys A. The evaluation of leanness fatness in man. Norm and interrelationships. *Brit. J. Nutr.* 1949;5:194-206.
3. Bujak Z. *Physical development and physical fitness of people practice taekwon-do*. Warsaw; 2000.
4. Drozdowski Z. Anthropometry in physical education. *Textbooks*, 1998;24:54-60.
5. Jagiełło M, Jagiełło W. Somatic Aspects of Sports Mastery in Female Competitors of the Polish National Fencing Team. *Pedagogics, psychology, medical-biological problems of physical training and sports.* 2008;7:160-162.

6. Jagiełło M, Jagiełło W. Constitutional aspects of sports mastery in tennis. *Physical education of students*, 2009;1:73-76.
7. Jagiełło W. Differentiation of the body build in judo competitors of the men's Polish national team. *Archives of Budo*, 2013;9(2):117-123.
8. Jagiełło W, Jagiełło M. Internal proportions of body build of the Polish representatives in tennis. *Pedagogics, psychology, medical-biological problems of physical training and sports*. 2006;5:141-145.
9. Jagiełło W, Jagiełło M. Constitutional aspects of sports mastery in modern pentathlon *Pedagogics, psychology, medical-biological problems of physical training and sports*. 2009;11:154-157.
10. Jagiełło W, Jagiełło M, Kozina ZhL. Type of structure of men body engaged baseball. *Physical education of students,* 2012;6:140-143.
11. Jagiełło W., Kalina R., Korobielnikow G. Morphological diversification of female judo athletes. *Archives of Budo,* 2007, Vol. 3:27-34.
12. Jagiełło W, Kruszewski A. Somatic aspects of sports mastery of Polish representatives in wrestling. *Pedagogics, psychology, medical-biological problems of physical training and sports*. 2008;7:160-162.
13. Jagiełło W, Kruszewski A. Morphological Diversification of Competitors Training Greko-Roman Style of Wrestling. *Archives of Budo*, 2009;5:147-153.
14. Jagiełło M, Tkaczuk W, Jagiełło W. Somatic aspects of sports mastery female tennis players. *Physical training of students of creative specialties.* 2003;2:3-10.
15. Jagiełło W, Wołowicz J. Body Composition in Junior Polish Representatives in Judo. *Pedagogics, psychology, medical-biological problems of physical training and sports*. 2009;12:196-201.
16. Leake CN, Carter JE. Comparison of body composition and somatotype of trained female triathletes. *Journal of Sports Sciences*, 1991;9(2):125-135.
17. Litwiniuk S. *Taekwon-do ITF as a form of physical activity and sport discipline*. Biala Podlaska: IWFiS; 2000.
18. Piechaczek H. Determination of total fat densitometry and anthropometric methods. *Materials and work Anthropological*, 1975;89:3-48.
19. Saczuk J, Wilczewski A. *Assessing body composition taekwondo athletes*. Warsaw; 2002.

4

COMPARATIVE ANALYSIS OF COMPETITIVE STATE ANXIETY AMONG TEAM SPORT AND INDIVIDUAL SPORT ATHLETES IN IRAN

Hossein Soltani*[1], Zahra Hojati[2], Seyed Reza Attarzadeh Hossini[3]

[1]Young Researchers and Elite Club, Torbat-e Heydarieh Branch, Islamic Azad University, Torbat-e Heydarieh, Iran.

[2]Department of Physical Education and Sport Sciences, Birjand Branch, Islamic Azad University, Birjand, Iran.

[3]Sport Physiology Faculty of Physical Education and Sport Sciences, Ferdowsi University of Mashhad, Mashhad, IR Iran

Abstract. *Purpose:* With respect to the fact that every sport field has its own special nature, the aim of present study was to compare competitive state anxiety among team sport and individual sport athletes in Iran. *Material:* The statistic sample included 120 male athletes, 60 athletes in individual sports (wrestling, taekwondo and karate) and 60 athletes in team sports (futsal, volleyball and basketball). The research instrument employed was the Persian version of the Competitive State Anxiety Inventory-2. This inventory was distributed among the subjects about 30 minutes before the first competition. Finally by one-way ANOVA data was analyzed. *Results:* The results indicated that the mean score of somatic anxiety and cognitive anxiety among individual sport athletes was significantly higher than that of team sport athletes ($p<0.05$). The levels of self-confidence of individual sports athletes was higher than that of team sports athletes, but the difference was not significant ($p >0.05$). *Conclusion:* It seems the being part of a team alleviates some of the pressure experienced by those who compete alone. It seems the individual sport athletes may be more exposed to evaluation and more engaged in their own skills and abilities than team sport athletes given that responsibility for performance is not distributed across several performers.
Keywords: competitive, state anxiety, cognitive anxiety, somatic anxiety, team sports, individual sports.

Introduction

Competitive anxiety is one of the most thoroughly examined topics in sport psychology literature. This is mainly due to the perceived detrimental effects anxiety has on performance, creating the negative view most individuals hold of this concept. Anxiety is defined as feelings of nervousness and tension caused by the environment or surrounding expectation that is related to 'arousal'. These demands are usually stressful, indicating to the athletes a perception of imbalance between the demand given and their abilities to fulfill the demand [1]. Dealing with competitive state anxiety is a main task for coaches because players and sport teams could not perform when they are under stress. Players could not perform their best as they usually could because of anxiety. Consequently, their performance is affected during the competition and they seldom achieve victory [2].

State anxiety is generally regarded as an unpleasant emotional reaction related to stressful situations, in which the arousal component is one inherent element [3]. An important distinction between arousal and anxiety is that anxiety involves interpretation of the situation as threatening, whereas arousal is unrelated to any such interpretations [4]. Moreover, anxiety has been suggested as a better predictor of the performance outcome than arousal when the tasks are of a more complex nature and contain a higher cognitive load [5].

Multidimensional theory was developed by [6]. The multidimensional theory proposed that anxiety three subscales cognitive anxiety, somatic anxiety and self-confidence. Cognitive anxiety is defined as "the mental component of anxiety and is caused by negative expectations about success or by negative self-evaluation". Second element of anxiety is somatic anxiety that "refers to the physiological and affective elements of the anxiety experience that develop directly from autonomic arousal" [6]. Martens et al. have suggested that somatic anxiety should affect performance in a curvilinear fashion, with both lower and higher levels of somatic anxiety being detrimental to performance. "It is likely to reach its peak at the onset of competition and dissipate once the contest begins". Therefore, somatic anxiety, due to its time course, is thought to have less of an influence on performance than doe's cognitive anxiety [6]. A third element of competitive state anxiety discussed by Martens et al. is self-confidence. This encompasses the athlete's global perceptions of confidence. Although not originally proposed as a subcomponent of anxiety, Martens et al. have since included self-confidence in their study of the anxiety/performance relationship. They have proposed a positive linear relationship between self-confidence and performance [6].

The findings of various research works regarding competitive state anxiety in athletes have had contradictory results. Pigozzi, showed the skill level of athletes is an important factor for control of competitive state anxiety [7]. The research [8] confirmed that elite athletes have lower levels of competitive state anxiety than non-elite athletes. The studies [9], [10] showed that the kind of sport, nature of sport (individual sport or team sport) and gender of athletes are affecting factors on their performance.

Howard compared the levels of cognitive State anxiety, Somatic state anxiety, and competitive trait anxiety for varsity athletes between team sports and individual sports. Results showed that Competitive State Anxiety scores for team sports and it was significantly higher than that of individual sport athletes [11]. Mohsenpour studied state anxiety among male athletes of individual and team sports and concluded that there was no significant difference between somatic factor of group and individual examinable items but athletes of major group obtained lower cognitive grades than individual athletes [12].

According to [13] anxiety levels before and during competition are not clear due to conflicting findings, various athletes have reported different levels of anxiety from much to low. Behzadi, Adem reported significant difference in levels of competitive state anxiety among team sports and individual sports athletes [14], [15]. In contrast, [16], [17] have not reported significant difference in high, moderate or low level of anxiety. It seems that the levels of competitive state anxiety in team and individual sport athletes are not clear. With respect to the fact that every sport field has its own special nature, and also the results of most of the researches done are not in accordance with each other, therefore lack of a comprehensive theory in this field made the author to take action and compare competitive state anxiety among team sport and individual sport athletes in Iran.

Material and Methods

A. Participants

The statistical population used in this study contained team sports (volleyball, basketball, futsal) and individual sports (thaekwondo, karate, and wrestling) in Iran. Samples were male volleyball, basketball, futsal, taekwondo, karate, and wrestling team players who had competed in the leagues and super leagues competition of Iran in 2012 year. The total number of subjects was 120 male athletes consisted of 60 athletes in individual sports and 60 athletes in team sports who participated in competitions of leagues and super leagues of Iran.

B. Measures

1. Demographic Questionnaire

Participants were asked to indicate their age, training experience, and skill level.

2. Competitive State Anxiety Inventory-2 (CSAI-2)

This measurement tool is often used in research studies in order to estimate the participants' cognitive and somatic types of anxieties, as well as their self-confidence [6]. The test requires the subjects to choose the answer that corresponds with how they feel now, right now. Cognitive anxiety items are numbers 1, 4, 7, 10, 13, 16, 19, 22, and 25. Somatic anxiety items are numbers 2, 5, 8, 11, 14 (reverse), 17, 20, 23, and 26. Self-confidence items are numbers 3, 6, 9, 12, 15, 18, 21, 24, and 27. Scoring of the CSAI-2 was achieved by the following way. Persons rated how they were feeling right at that moment by circling one of the presented answers. The four-presented answers included not at all (1), somewhat (2), moderately so (3) and very much so (4). The final scores for each subscale range from 9 to 36, with 9 indicating low anxiety/confidence and 36 indicating high anxiety/confidence [6]. The validity of this questionnaire was confirmed by professors and the reliability was measured by Cronbach's Alpha ("=0.89). In addition, internal reliability of this questionnaire was reported by Peter, 2007 as 85.75, and 0.83 respectively [18].

C. Procedures

At first, the researcher visited coaches from the various teams that had been selected and explained the nature of the study and in the second stage explained the study to the athletes and distributed materials containing a letter describing the study and informed consent forms. At the third stage, Personal Information Questionnaire and state Competitive Anxiety Inventory (CSAI-2) for both elite and non-elite players were administered to the subjects within 30 minutes prior to the start of the competition and the nature of study was described at the top of the questionnaire to the subjects. Each questionnaire took approximately 5 minutes to complete.

D. Statistical Analysis

In order to calculate measures of central tendency and variability measures descriptive statistics was utilized. At first *Levene's test* checked homogeneity of variances between sets of scores. After making sure of variances homogeneity, One way analysis of variance was conducted for between group's comparisons, then the hypotheses were examined at $P<0.05$.

Results

Table 1 shows that the amount of Levene Statistic of somatic anxiety, cognitive anxiety and self-confidence are 0.172, 0.390 and 0.645 respectively. The obtained "P" value is 0.679, 0.533 and 0.423 respectively ($P>0.05$). Therefore, team sport and individual sport athletes are homogenous in term of studied variable.

Table 2 shows the scores of cognitive anxiety, somatic anxiety, and self-confidence in team and individual sport athletes.

The one-way ANOVA results indicated that means of cognitive anxiety in team and individual sport athletes are 17.23 and 15.96 respectively. The standard deviations of cognitive anxiety in team and individual sport athletes are 4.45 and 4.05 respectively. The obtained "F" is 5.302 and "P" value is 0.022 . The one-way ANOVA results indicated that team sport athletes had significantly lower levels of cognitive anxiety compared with individual sport athletes (P<0.05).

The one-way ANOVA results indicated that means of somatic anxiety in team and individual sport athletes are 15.74 and 14.49 respectively. The standard deviations of somatic anxiety in team and individual sport athletes are 4.20 and 4.12 respectively. The obtained "F" is 5.41 and "P" value is 0.021. The one-way ANOVA results indicated that team sport athletes had significantly lower levels of somatic anxiety compared with individual sport athletes (P<0.05).

The one-way ANOVA results indicated that means of self-confidence in team and individual sport athletes are 26.90 and 26.08 respectively. The standard deviations of self-confidence in team and individual sport athletes are 3.56 and 3.91 respectively. The obtained "F" is 2.11 and "P" value is 0.148. The one-way ANOVA results indicated that there was no significant difference between the scores of self- confidence among team sport and individual sport athletes in Iran (P>0.05).

Table 1. Levene's Homogeneity Test

Variables	Groups	Levene Statistic	Sig.
Cognitive Anxiety	Team game and Individual game Players	.390	0.533
Somatic Anxiety	Team game and Individual game Players	.172	0.679
State Self Confidence	Team game and Individual game Players	0.645	0.423

Table 2. Mean Values and One- Way ANOVA of Cognitive Anxiety, Somatic Anxiety and Self-Confidence between Team Sport and Individual Sport Athletes in Iran (N=120)

Variables	Groups	N	M±SD	F	Sig.
Cognitive anxiety	Individual Sport Athletes	60	17.23 ± 4.45	5.302	0.022
	Team Sport Athletes	60	15.96 ± 4.05		
Somatic Anxiety	Individual sport Athletes	60	15.74 ± 4.20	5.41	0.021
	Team Sport Athletes	60	14.49 ± 4.12		
Self-Confidence	Individual Sport Athletes	60	26.90± 3.56	2.11	0.148
	Team Sport Athletes	60	26.08± 3.91		

Discussion

One-way ANOVA results indicated that the scores of cognitive anxiety among individual sport athletes was higher than team game athletes scores and there was a significant difference in cognitive anxiety between individual game athletes and team game athletes in Iran (p<0.05). It may be due to the fact that fear of failure is a stronger predictor of cognitive anxiety for individual sport athletes than for team sport athletes given the potential accountability for failure placed on individual sport athletes. Athletes who participate in individual sports have also been found to experience more anxiety than those who play team sports [19]. For athletes in high-contact sports and martial arts such as karate, thaekwondo and wrestling the possibility of getting hurt can also be a source of anxiety. It seems that in individual sports, the athletes are more engaged in their own skills and abilities, while in team sports such as volleyball, basketball, and futsal, they are affected by their team members and their performance will depend on the performance of the group. The role assigned to the athlete in team sports may not correspond to their inner role. An additional factor that causes cognitive anxiety is the expectation of success. Some athletes rise to the challenge imposed by public expectation while others can choke. The trick is to become sufficiently 'psyched-up' without becoming 'psyched-out' [19].

One-way ANOVA results indicated that is a significant difference in somatic anxiety between team sport athletes and individual sport athletes in Iran (P<0.000). It seems that athletes who participate in individual sports have been found to experience more anxiety than those who play team sports. Common sense suggests that being part of a team alleviates some of the pressure experienced by those who compete alone [20]. This finding is consistent with predictions that competitive situations elicit both cognitive and somatic anxiety. An alternative explanation is that the physiological arousal demands of the specific sports tested confounded the individual team comparison. Thaekwondo, karate and wrestling (individual sports) and volleyball, basketball and futsal (team sports) used in this comparison; seem to demand moderate arousal levels for optimal performance. Thus, the significant difference in somatic anxiety between individual and team games may simply reflect the differential arousal demands of the sport chosen for comparison rather than significant differences between these sport types [11, 15, 21]. In addition, Martin and Hall research demonstrated that Skaters experienced grater somatic and cognitive anxiety prior to an individual competitive event than prior to a team competition. Maybe this is because of a diffusion of responsibility that occurs in the team framework but not in an individual framework [22]. Researches comparing athletes competing in team sports with those competing in individual sports have found that athletes competing in individual sports reported significantly higher somatic anxiety than team sports athletes. This finding is supported by Simon 1977, Howard and Zeng 2003, Adem et al. 2010.

One-way ANOVA results indicated that mean difference of self-confidence in individual sport athletes and team sport athletes were not significant ($p>0.05$). It may be related to nature of these sports because in team sports a diffusion of responsibility occurs in the team framework that can decrease competitive state anxiety and increase sate self-confidence and on the other hand in individual sports athletes are forced to stand alone, to fight alone, and to perform alone. Decisions must be made by the athletes in the moment. If the athletes fail, it is on his/her on shoulders, and if s/he succeeds, that too is his/her success alone.

This makes a strong feeling of self-confidence and self-reliance. It instills the knowledge that one is capable of acting alone against challenging circumstances. On the other hand, in team sports a diffusion of responsibility occurs in the team framework that can decrease anxiety and improve self-confidence. So while team sports offer a lot of benefits to athletes in terms of teamwork and sportsmanship, individual sports should not be overlooked. It seems athletes of team and individual sports used effective coping strategies to manage anxiety before getting out of hand. Additionally, exposing athletes to psychological training programs from an early age is probable to have a very positive influence on their levels of self-confidence, which may be transferred into their adult sporting careers [23].

Conclusion:

The present study found that the team game athletes experience lower levels of competitive state anxiety than individual games athletes. In conclusion, individual games athletes are more prone to feel the effects of anxiety on performance than team games athletes.

Furthermore individual sports athletes may be more exposed the evaluation than team sport athletes given that responsibility for performance is not distributed across several performer. In other word in individual sports, the athlete is more engaged in their own skills and abilities, while in team sports such as volleyball, basketball and futsal, they are affected by their team members and their performance will depend on the performance of the group. The role assigned to the athlete in team sports may not correspond to their inner role. Therefore it is suggested that coaches and athletic authorities of participating teams in sport leagues employ sport psychologist to teach and prepare comprehensive planning to develop psychological skills and suitable strategies for coping competitive anxiety specific non elite athletes and individual games athletes and also help them to eliminate negative thoughts and focus on the positive outcomes and not on the chances of failure by the help of sport psychologists.

Conflict of interests

The authors declare that there is no conflict of interests.

References

1. Gould D, Greenleaf C, & Krane V. *Advances in sport Psychology.* (2nd Ed.). s.l.: Champaign, IL: Human Kinetics; 2002.
2. Patsiaouras A, Papanikolaou Z, Haritonidis K, Nikolaidis D, Keramidas P. The use of the person-centered approach for the reduction of the state-trait anxiety in volleyball players. *Journal of Sport Psychology* 2008;10(2):24-30.
3. Woodman T, & Hardy L. *Handbook of sport psychology*, John Wiley & Sons; 2011.
4. Hammermeister J, & Burton D. Stress, Appraisal, and Coping Revisited: Examining the Antecedents of Competitive State Anxiety with Endurance Athletes. *Sport Psychologist,* 2001;15(1):66-90. doi:10.1123/tsp.15.1.66
5. Arent, S. M., & Landers, D.M. *Arousal, anxiety, and performance: A reexamination of the inverted-U hypothesis.* Res Q Exerc Sport. 2003;74(4):436-44. doi: 10.1080/02701367.2003.10609113
6. Martens R, Burton D, Vealey RS, Bump LA, & Smith DE. *Competitive anxiety in sport.* Champaign, IL: Human Kinetics; 1990.
7. Pigozzi F. Role of exercise stress test in master athletes. *British Journal of Sports Medicine*. 2005;39(8):527–531. doi:10.1136/bjsm.2004.014340
8. Soltani, H. Comparative Analysis of Competitive State Anxiety among Elite and Non-Elite karate Athletes in Iran. *Advances in Environmental Biology,* 2013;7(7):1244-1248.
9. Grossbard JR, Smith RE, Smoll FL, Cumming SP. Competitive anxiety in young athletes: Differentiating somatic anxiety, worry, and concentration disruption. *Anxiety, Stress & Coping.* 2009;22(2):153–166. doi:10.1080/10615800802020643
10. Cristina, A. Anxiety and performance in table tennis players. *Journal of Sport Psychology*, 2004;24:185-204.
11. Howard, z. a. The Differences between Anxiety and self– confidence between Team and Individual sports college varsity Athletes. *International Sports Journal*, 2003;7(1):28-33.
12. Mohsenpour F. *Studying and comparing of competitive state anxiety of men athletes in individual and group majors of championship contests of institutions in Khuzestan province.* [PhD thesis]. Shahid Chamran University of Ahvaz; 2003.

13. Mellalieu SD. *A competitive anxiety review: recent directions in sport psychology research.* New York: Nova Science Publishers; 2006.
14. Behzadi F, Mohammadpour A, Hedayatikatooli A, & Nourallahi H. A Description and Comparison of Personality Traits of Competitive Individual and Team Athletes. *Annals of Biological Research*, 2012;3:36-40.
15. Adem, C. Comparison of pre and post-game state and trait anxiety levels of individual and team athletes. *Journal of Human Sciences,* 2010;7(1):193-206.
16. Passand F. *Studying and comparing of the amount of the competitive state anxiety in individual and team majors of women participating in the second students' sports Olympiad across the country* [M thesis]. Tarbiat Moalem University: Iran; 1997.
17. Perry J.D. and Williams, J. M. Relationship of intensity and direction of competitive trait anxiety to skill level and gender in tennis. *Sport Psychologist*, 1998;12:169-179.
18. Terry Peter C, Munro Angus. Mood and anxiety scores predict winning and losing performances in tennis. In: *43rd Australian Psychological Society Annual Conference (APS 2008): Psychology Leading Change*, 23-27 Sep 2008, Hobart, Australia; 2008.
19. Flowers R, & Brown C. Effects of sport context and birth order on state anxiety. *Journal of Sport Behavior*, 2002;25:41-56.
20. Arlin C. *Guide. Sports and Performance Anxiety.* 2010.
21. Simon JA, & Martens R. S.C.A.T. as a predictor of A-states in varying competitive situations. In: D. M. Landers & R. W. Christina (Eds.), *Psychology of Motor Behaviour and Sport (Vol. 2),* Human Kinetics: Champaign, IL; 1977, p. 146-156.
22. Ahmed, Shamshad. *Psychological basis of physical education.* India: Gayan books; 2005.
23. Mamassis, G. D. The effects of mental training program on juniors pre competitive anxiety, self-confidence and tennis performance. *Asian Social Science*, 2004;10(18):90-95.

5

MECHANISMS OF ADAPTATION TO INTENSIVE LOADS OF 400 METERS' HURDLES RUNNERS AT STAGE OF INITIAL BASIC TRAINING

Rovniy A.S., Lastochkin V.M.
Kharkov State Academy of Physical Culture
Sumy State A.S.Makarenko Pedagogical University

Abstract. *Purpose:* is study of adaptation mechanisms of 400 meter' hurdles-runners to intensive physical loads. *Material:* in the research 13 - 400 meters' hurdles-runners and 13 - 400 meters' runners participated. *Results:* it was found that physiological cost of sportsmen's special workability has fragmentary character. We presented results of physiological and bio-chemical adaptation mechanisms to dozed work. The received results have no confident distinctions and can not objectively characterize mechanisms of sportsmen's special workability. We did not detect definite differences in indicators of mechanisms, ensuring sportsmen's special workability under dozed loads. We found, that level of anaerobic glycolysis is an objective criterion of 400 meter' hurdles-runners' special workability. It was shown that for determination of functional potentials for such kind of functioning it is necessary to apply special loads. *Conclusions:* the received results deepen information about mechanisms of adaptation to specific competition functioning. Correct approaches to processing and analysis of the research's results permit to more specifically determine sportsmen's functional potentials in different kinds of competition functioning.
Key words: adaptation, anaerobic glycolysis, lactate, specific, non-specific, distance.

Introduction

The problem of adaptation to physical loads is one of the main in system of training in different kinds of sports. Alongside with specific character of adaptation in every kind of sports, there are some general principles and laws [3, 18]. Physical loads' duration and intensity are important factors of sportsmen's adaptation to them as well as individual sensitivity to anaerobic hypoxic impacts [3, 19].

Sport achievements in 400 meters hurdles are not sufficient in Ukraine. That is why registration of adaptation responses in process of sportsmen's training is one of main factors of management of training process [1, 4].

Analysis of literature data witnesses that to large extent aspects of sportsmen's organism's adaptation to physical loads in running smooth distances have been studied rather in detail [12, 14, 20]. Comparative characteristic of adaptation responses of 400 meters hurdles-runners under different training loads will facilitate optimization of training process. Just this fact preconditioned the topicality of the given research.

Purpose, tasks of the work, material and methods of the research

The purpose of our work was studying of 400 meter' hurdles-runners' mechanisms of adaptation to intensive physical loads.

The tasks:

- To determine optimal scopes of training loads for 400 meters' hurdles-runners on the base of physiological and bio-chemical reactions;
- To determine the most adequate combination of load and rest in process of training of 400 meters' hurdles-runners;

Material and methods of the research: in the research 13 - 400 meters' hurdles-runners and 13 - 400 meters' runners participated. Sportsmen fulfilled work on treadmill with constant angle of elevation of 3°. The sportsmen endured load with step-by-step increasing of intensity: from 2.5 m.p.sec. to 0.5 m.p.sec. (transition – every 2 minutes and further – up to the end). Determination of maximal oxygen consumption (MOC) was carried out by automatic gas analyzer "Backman" with computer data registration. Before and after loads the tested underwent blood sampling from finger for determination of acid-base balance (pH) and concentration of lactate (HL).

Results of the research

Analysis of mean group values showed that during work on treadmill ventilation of sportsmen's lungs increases sharply in comparison with rest state (more than 10 times) (see table 1). Increase of lungs' ventilation results from increase of oxygen consumption during work. It is witnessed by coefficient of correlation: between MOC and lung ventilation (r=0.65); MOC and carbon dioxide (CO_2) accumulation (r=0.54).

Table 1

Indicators of maximal physiological and bio-chemical reactions of 400 meters hurdles-runners before and after work on treadmill

Before load	After load
Indicators (M±m)	Indicators (M±m)
HBR 62.3±0.47	HBR 198.9±9.0
PCO_2 (mm) 39.43±0.58	PCO_2 (mm) 42.35±1.37
PO_2 (mm.merc.col) 70.53±1.98	PO_2 (mm.merc.col) 80.76±1.38
pH (conv.un.) 7.38±0.02	pH (conv.un.) 7.12±0.03
HL (mol p.l) 2.7±0.13	HL (mol p.l) 11.6±0.84
LV (l.p.min.) 12.78±0.31	LV (l.p.min) 134.4±6.87

Notes: * Work up to the end lasted in average 8-14 min.; * MOC with such work– 68.77±1.64 ml.p.kg.p.min. HBR – heart beats rate; LV - lung ventilation; PCO_2 – partial pressure of carbon dioxide; PO_2 – partial pressure of oxygen; pH – homeostasis (acid-base balance); HL – lactate.

We determined the state of homeostasis and differences in it as well as differences in character of HL removal from blood in rest period. In some sportsmen lactate quickly diffused from muscles to blood and was quickly removed from blood. But there were cases when lactated diffused only by 10th minute of rest.

Quantity of lactate in blood by 20th minute of rest is confidently connected with maximal pH level (r=0.540), reserves of buffer bases (r=0.580), value of oxygen O_2 supply (r=0.590).

Having determined general regularities of physiological and bio-chemical parameters' dynamic under load on treadmill we made attempt to compare adaptation reserves of 400 meters' runners and 400 meters' hurdles-runners (see table 2).

Table 2

Comparative characteristic of physiological and biochemical indicators, taken in process of work on treadmill, of 400 meters runners and 400 meters' hurdles-runners.

In rest						After load						
HBR	LV	HL	pH	PCO_2	PO_2	HBR	LV	MOC	pH	HL	PCO_2	PO_2
400 meters' hurdles-runners												
61.0	12.5	1.44	7.37	39.7	69.8	187.8	140.7	69.2	7.11	13.36	42.24	73.7
400 meters' runners												
62.4	11.56	1.74	7.39	39.8	69.8	205.4	132.4	67.8	7.13	13.14	46.22	84.54

Analysis of results witnesses that differences between indicators of functional reactions and physical workability of both groups' sportsmen in laboratory conditions are statistically unconfident (p>005). We found that duration of work on treadmill is confidently connected with oxidation process of re-synthesis of adenosine triphosphate (ATP): with MOC r=0.580. It is known that in 400 meters' run and 400 meters hurdles high role is played by anaerobic glycolysis. Lactate concentration can change from 18 to 27-30 mmol p.l. Therefore functional distinction and functional reserves can not be open to full extent in laboratory conditions (work on treadmill of 400 meters' runners and 400 meters' hurdles-runners).

That is why we made an attempt to compare assessment of sportsmen's competition functioning in specific and non-specific conditions. Wee studied functional condition of 7 the strongest 400 meters' hurdles-runners. During one day the sportsmen fulfilled two competition loads: in the morning they ran 400 meters' distance as hurdles-runners; after 3 hours they ran 400 meters' smooth distance. The competitions were of selective character.

These competitions were conducted against the background of ordinary training process (there were no fasting days before competitions). That is why in blood we observed significant values of lactate (2.97±0.14 and 3.13±0.24 mmol p.l.). This fact points at finishing of recreational process.

Mean indicator of time of 400 meters' hurdles was 52.39±0.46; of 400 meters of smooth run – 49.83±0.38 sec. (differences are confident p<0.01).

Analysis of HBR response to specific and non-specific loads did not show statistically confident differences (p>0.05) (see table 3).

Table 3

Influence of specific and non-specific competition loads on functional and bio-chemical indicators of 400 meters' hurdles-runners

Indicators	400 meters' hurdles		400 meters' run	
	In rest	After load	In rest	After load
HBR	84.0±1.20	197.0±9.1	71.0±0.41	184.0±3.1
Lactate (mmol p.l.)	2.77±0.31	16.93±1.36	3.13±0.49	19.39±0.78
Glucose (mmol p.l.)	7.09±0.74	5.77±0.33	4.57±0.48	6.37±0.71

Confident distinctions were observed when combining bio-chemical reactions to certain load. Different speed of run influenced differently on intensity of anaerobic glycolysis. Its indicator was level of lactate after work. As we can see this indicator is confidently higher with 400 meter' "smooth" run.

Increase of glucose in blood under less loads witnesses about mobilization of carbohydrate reserves of liver [4]. With fulfillment of two competition loads we observed glucose concentration in both cases. But its dynamic (rest-work-recreation) is ambiguous (see table 3).

Analysis of metabolic responses with fulfillment of two competition loads showed that sportsmen with high result on both distances did not differ significantly by functional responses. On the base of results of the research we can assume that the most promising for 400 meters' hurdles are sportsmen with high level of anaerobic glycolysis in "smooth" 400 meters' run.

Discussion

In process of training and competition functioning there appear changes of functional systems, which significantly increase special workability. Presence of objective information about levels of sportsmen's fitness permits to determine strong and weak sides of sportsmen's fitness. As a result it is possible to optimize training process [3, 4, 9, 10, 11].

In kinds of sports with complex coordination against the background of speed-power endurance combination of anaerobic abilities with motor coordination is of great importance. Especially it is important in hurdles. Analysis of literature data witnesses that most of researches are devoted to different problems of sportsmen's training in "smooth" run. These researches dealt with development of hypoxic potentials [6, 11, 13].

The existing researches (A.L. Novikova, I.N. Soroka, 1994) recommend significant increasing of physical fitness [5]. S.V. Biriuk (2001) pays special attention to formation of run rhythm in hurdles on initial stage [1]. Chi Dunlin recommends to pay special attention to speed-power and coordination training [9, 10].

However, fundamental researches [2, 5, 15, 16, 17] show that in kinds of sports of sub maximal intensity study of oxygen demand and work's fulfillment energy cost as well as organism's adaptation potentials are of great importance.

However, with usage of dozed loads it is impossible to exactly restore advantages of sportsmen of different run specializations (L.G. Kharitonova, 1991; A.S. Rovniy, V.A. Rovniy 2009) [7, 8]. It is confirmed in our researches. We also affirm that for determination of functional potentials for certain kind of activity it is necessary to apply special loads.

Thus, the received results deepen information about specific features of mechanisms of adaptation to specific competition functioning. Correct approaches to processing and analysis of results of the research permit to more specifically determine sportsmen's functional potentials in different kinds of competition functioning.

Conclusions

Determination of promising sportsmen in laboratory conditions does not reflect actual special workability. Level of anaerobic glycolysis is a limiting factor of special workability of 400 meters' hurdles-runners. The received results permit to say that application of the mentioned in this paper methods of research give objective information about special workability indicators and makes possible to prognosticate level of sport achievements.

Conflict of interests

The authors declare that there is no conflict of interests.

Reference

1. Biriuk SV. *Formuvannia ritmu bigu z bar'ierami u khlopciv 13-15 rokiv na pochatku sportivnoi specializacii. Cand. Diss.* [Formation of 13-15 years old boys' run rhythm in hurdles at the beginning of sport specialization. Cand. Diss.], Mikolaiv; 2001. (in Ukrainian)
2. Volkov NI, Biriuk SV, Savel'ev IA. Kislorodnyj zapros i energicheskaia stoimost' napriazhennoj myshechnoj deiatel'nosti [Oxygen demand and energy cost of tensed muscular functioning]. *Fiziologiia cheloveka,* 2002;28(4): 80-93. (in Russian)
3. Krivoshchekov SG, Divert GM, Divert VE. Rasshirenie funkcional'nogo diapazona reakcij dykhaniia i gazoobmena pri povtornykh gipoksicheskikh vozdejstviiakh [Expanding of functional range of gas metabolism and respiratory responses under repeated hypoxic impacts]. *Fiziologiia cheloveka,* 2005;31(3):100-107. (in Russian)
4. Mishchenko VS, Lysenko EN, Vinogradov VE. *Reaktivnye svojstva kardiorespiratornoj sistemy kak otrazhenie adaptacii k napriazhennoj fizicheskoj trenirovke v sporte* [Responsive characteristics of cardio-respiratory system as reflection of adaptation to intensive physical training in sports]. Kiev; 2007. (in Russian)
5. Novikov AL, Soroka IN. *Trenirovka v bege na 400 m s bar'erami (muzhchiny)* [Training in 400 meters hurdles (male)], Minsk; 1994. (in Russian)
6. Rovnaia OA, Il'in VN. Osobennosti adaptivnykh reakcij sistemy dykhaniia vysokvalificirovannykh sportsmenok sinkhronnogo plavaniia vo vremia interval'noj gipoksicheskoj trenirovki [Specific features of respiratory system's adaptation responses of elite synchronous swimmers during interval hypoxic training]. *Pedagogics, psychology, medical-biological problems of physical training and sports*, 2010;1:71-75. (in Ukrainian)
7. Rovnij AS, Rovnyj VA. Upravlenie sistemoj podgotovki iunykh begunov na 400 m s bar'erami [Management of junior 400 meters' hurdles-runners' training]. *Slobozhans'kij naukovo-sportivnij visnik*, 2009;1:72-75. (in Russian)
8. Kharitonova LG. Fiziologicheskie i biokhimicheskie aspekty adaptacii k intensivnym nagruzkam organizma begunov na 400 m s bar'erami [Physiological and bio-chemical aspects of adaptation to organism's intensive loads of 400 meters' hurdles-runners]. *Teoriia i praktika fizicheskoj kul'tury*, 1991;1:9-12. (in Russian)

9. Shi Dulin. Skorostno-silovaia podgotovka iunykh begunov na 400 m s bar'erami [Speed-power training of junior 400 meters' hurdles-runners]. *Slobozhans'kij naukovo-sportivnij visnik*, 2004. 1: 40-43. (in Russian)
10. Shi Dulin. Razvitie koordinacionnykh sposobnostej kak osnova sovershenstvovaniia tekhniki bega na 400 m s bar'erami [raining of coordination as the basis of perfection of 400 meters' hurdles technique]. *Slobozhans'kij naukovo-sportivnij visnik*, 2005;1:125-129. (in Russian)
11. Bailey DM, Davies B, Baker J. Training in hypoxia: modulation of metabolic and cardiovascular risk factors in man. *Med.Sci.Sports Exerc,* 2000;32(6):1058-1063.
12. Bennet S. *Training for 400 m*. Human Kinetics Pub; 1999.
13. Chick TW, Stark DM, Murata GH. Hyperoxic training increases work capacity after maximal training at moderate altitude. *Chest*; 1993;104:1759-1762.
14. Cheng Ping, Wang gig Yu. Technical training of 400 m Hurdle Race and the Rhythm among Hurdleg. *Journal of Shandong Sports Science & Technology*. 2002;3:12-14.
15. Hochachka PW, Rupert JI, Monge C. Adaptation and conservation of physiological system in the evolution of human hypoxia tolerance. *Comp. Biochem. Physiol*; 1999;124:1-8.
16. Levine BD. Intermittent hypoxic training: fact and fancy. *High Alt. Med. Biol.,* 2002;3(2):177-182.
17. Pearse WJ. Mechanisms of hypoxic cerebral vasodilatation. *Pharmac. Tner.,* 1995;65:75-78.
18. Tian zhong Yan. A research on the contest Rhythm of World mans 400 m Hurdles. *Journal of Shandong institute of Physical Education,* 2003;2:103-105.
19. Yang Hui. Analysis on Chinese Excellent Athlete Luli Xiana Score of 110 m Men Hurdle. *Journal of Beijing Sport University,* 2003;11:1579-1581.
20. Zhao Jia Gni. On the Training of teen-agers 400-meters Hurdle Race. *Journal of Anhui Polytechnic University Social Science*, 2001;1:143-144.

6

EFFECTS OF HIGH DOSE COFFEE INTAKE ON AEROBIC POWER IN DRAGON FEMALE ATHLETES

Ramin Shabani, Roya Rahmatian, Fatemeh Izaddoust
Department of Exercise Physiology, Rasht Branch, Islamic Azad University, Rasht, Iran

Abstract. *Background*: There are few studies that consider the effect of high doses of caffeine on aerobic power (VO2max). Also, to date, no study examined the effect of coffee intake on dragon boat paddler specifically on women. The purpose of this study was to investigate the effect of espresso coffee on improvement of aerobic power of dragon boat paddler. *Material*: Twenty women athletes of Guilan dragon bout team members of Malavan club of port city of Anzali (mean ±SD age, 23.60± 3.49 years; BMI,23.77±1.88kg/m^2; body fat, 30.32±4.65%) were recruited to this study, after they completed a primary test without consuming any coffee, they consumed 6mg/kg of coffee (espresso or decaffeinated) and following that they completed two experimental trials. A randomized, double-blind, repeated-measures, design was employed whereby paddlers complete a 2000m paddling dragon boat ergo-meter. *Results*: Coffee could improve VO2max (Without coffee =74.40±4.99, Espresso coffee =90.10±6.19, Decaffeinated coffee =91.00±5.67, $P \leq 0.05$). VO2max amount after exercise were significantly higher for both espresso coffee and decaffeinated coffee, when compared with without coffee condition. No significant differences were observed between espresso coffee and decaffeinated coffee ($P \leq 0.05$). *Conclusion*: The present study shows that both high doses of caffeine (espresso coffee) and decaffeinated coffee can enhance VO2max during aerobic exercise including 2000m dragon boat paddling. It seems that some compounds except caffeine in decaffeinated coffee can act improve VO2max. Further studies needed for considering the effect of high doses of coffee on endurance exercises. Also in other age ranges of women athletes and other sport athletes.
Keywords: caffeine, exercise, athletes, boating, VO2max.

Introduction

Dragon boat, a team paddling water sport, has developed in nearly 60 countries worldwide. Also annually over 50 million people in Asia are participant in dragon boat competitions. Dragon boat races are from 200 to 2000 meters and above. Cardiovascular endurance(In terms of VO2max) is one of the important skills for dragon boat paddlers [1] and a dragon boat paddler should ideally be able to maintain VO2max throughout the whole game [2].

Coffee contains mineral ingredients such as Ca, K, Fe, P, Ni, Mg, and Cr [3], polyphenols, melanoidin and caffeine [4]. Numerous studies have shown that caffeine can act as an ergo-genic aid, in long-term exercise [5-9]. Caffeine's primary ergo-genic mode of action is on the CNS [10]. Also it can be energetic with an increase in fat oxidation and a decrease in glycogen use [11]. Caffeine switches the substrate preference from glycogen to fat by increasing hormone sensitive lipase (HSL) activity and inhibition of glycogen phosphorylase activity [12].

Most research, have investigated the effect of low or moderate doses of caffeine consumption on performance, perceptual responses and Neuromuscular factors prior to endurance exercise [7-9,13, 14]. Nevertheless, there are a few studies that considered the effect of high doses of caffeine on endurance exercise [15, 16]. This may seem surprising as reports have shown that coffee is the most concentrated dietary source of caffeine as well as being one of the largest sources of caffeine used by athletes prior to competition [17]. However, according to our information to date, no study examined the effect of coffee ingestion on dragon boat paddler specifically on females.

In addition, a few studies indicated the effect of pre exercise coffee on endurance exercises [7, 8, 16, 18-20] and they demonstrated difference results. Hodgson et al. (2013) utilized coffee and caffeine in their Research and shown that both of caffeine and coffee (5mg/kg) consumption one hour prior to exercise can improve endurance exercise performance [8]. In contrast, Graham et al. (1998) Resulted that caffeine capsule could increase endurance compare to placebo but coffee don't have any effect on endurance [19]. In another study by Graham et al. (1995) they showed endurance enhanced with both 3 and 6 mg/kg of caffeine, whereas there was no significant effect with 9 mg/kg of caffeine [16]. Moreover, to our knowledge, there is the first study that considered the ergogenic effect of espresso coffee on aerobic performance compared to decaffeinated coffee or placebo.

Therefore, the purpose of this study was to determine the effects of high dose coffee (espresso coffee) on 2000m dragon boat women paddler compared to decaffeinated coffee or placebo.

Materials and Methods

Subjects

Participants.

Twenty women athletes of Guilan dragon bout team members of Malavan club of port city of Anzali (mean ±SD age, 23.60± 3.49 years; BMI, 23.77±1.88kg/m^2; body fat, 30.32±4.65%) with at least third time per week engaged in training and had competitive paddling experience were recruited for the study. The experiments were performed within the period of training phase. All participants didn't have any injuries and they were non-smokers. For inclusion in the study, volunteers should not use other nutritional supplements. All athletes were fully informed of the experimental trials and all risks and discomforts associated before providing written informed consent to participate in the study.

Ethical approval was obtained from the Islamic Azad University Rasht Branch Ethics Committee.

Research Design.

Method: The study utilized a double-blind, repeated-measures, design to identify the effects of espresso coffee and decaffeinated coffee on VO2max changes (2000m paddling). Research Subjects were asked to attend three laboratory sessions for doing two trails with coffee ingestion and one trail without coffee. All they took part in first session and two other sessions conducted 2 week apart and being performed at the same time in the morning to reduce the potential for circadian variability. In the first session participants pre-test measurements were assessed. Then they were performed the test without coffee and Subjects were given a questionnaire that measured feeling of perceived fatigue [21]. During the following two other visits, the subjects intake either the espresso coffee or a decaffeinated coffee and then remained seated for 60 minutes before the test. Athletes initially warmed up on a Dragon Boat Ergo-meter (D1-M) with the desired intensity and speed for 10 min. Then rested for 2 minute before the starting the tests. Then they performed 2000 meters paddling on a dragon boat ergo-meter that was calibrated prior each test by the athlete weight. Two second and third trails were separated by 24 h and the VO2max was recorded at the end of each test (showed by ergo-meter monitor). A Dragon Boat trainer that was Knows how worked a Dragon Ergo-meter and also was blind to the study protocol, supervised all sessions. Subjects were asked to maintain their habitual dietary intake and to abstain from coffee or vigorous physical activity for 24 h prior to each test. Also, all participants had previous experience with a dragon boat ergo-meter.

Pre-test assessment: Height and body weight (lightly dressed and barefooted) were measured to the nearest 0.1 cm nearest 0.01 kg, respectively, using a stadiometer and scale (Seca - Germany). Skinfold thicknesses were obtained at 3 sites (Triceps, Suprailiac, Thigh) according to the Standardization Reference Manual [22] using a Saehan caliper (SH5020, Korea), and body fat percentage were estimated using Jackson and Pollock nomogram. Body mass index were assessed using weight/height^2 (Quetelet, 1869).

Perceived fatigue: The perception of fatigue was performed using a Borg scale. The subjects indicated their own perception of fatigue immediately after the protocol on a scale of 0 to 10. Zero indicated least fatigue, and the ten indicated most fatigue.

Aerobic power assessment: Kayakers performed their 2000m test on ergo-meter task specificity trial on an air braked, drag adjustable Multistroke Dragon Boat Ergo-meter (D1-M). The ergo-meter consisted of a flywheel connected to a carbon shaft via a retractable cord attached at either end. Distance from seat to foot-bar was adjusted to match each individual's seat position in the kayak; hand position on the carbon shaft was also adjusted to match on-water paddling position. Paddler's weight in Kg was inputted in board console then accelerated the fan to a speed of 700 or over. Once the acceleration / speed is above 700, Was allowed the flywheel run freely until the fan had come to an unimpeded or un-accelerated stop, then the Drag Factor was automatically set. This calibration was performed prior to each test for all athletes according to manufacturer's recommendations. Subjects were performed 2000m paddling (determined by the covered distance was showed on monitor) in each session and one of the author's was supervised all sessions which was blind. VO2max were calculated at the end of each trail using the Dragon Boat ergo-meter, showed on ergo-meter monitor [23].

Coffee: three exercise trials were performed under three conditions, one with espresso coffee, the other one with decaffeinated coffee and third performed without any coffee. Subject ingested 6 mg caffeine/kg of espresso coffee, a range of 500-575 mg/kg, (based on a content of 145 mg caffeine/100 g coffee, Nestlé- NESCAFE) or 6 mg caffeine/kg of decaffeinated coffee (caffeine amount was negligible, Nestlé-NESCAFE) 60 minutes before the test [24]. Amount of Coffee needed was measured using electronic weighing machine (Sartorius GMBH by Gottingen Germany). Both espresso coffee and decaffeinated coffee were dissolved in 200 ml hot water and Not added any sweetener.

Statistical Analysis

Values are expressed as means ± SD. The normality of each data set was evaluated using the Kolmogorov–Smirnov test, which confirmed a normal distribution. Results were analysed using the general linear model with repeated measures. Where significant main effects were observed, Bonferroni post hoc tests were used to determine the differences. All data were analyzed using IBM SPSS Statistics version 21 for Windows (SPSS Inc., Chicago, IL, USA). A P value of less than 0.05 was considered to be statistically significant.

Results

Participants' (n = 20) descriptive statistics include age, weight, height, BMI, body fat percent and Borg perceived fatigue are listed (Table 1).

Table1. Participant characteristics (n=20).

Parameter	mean±SD
Age (year)	23.60±3.49
Weigh (kg)	61.70±4.32
Height (m)	162.90±6.20
BMI (kg/m^2)	23.77±1.88
Body fat percent	30.32±4.65
Borg perceived fatigue (0-10)	7.9±0.6

BMI=body mass index; BF%= Body fat percent

Repeated-measures ANOVA analysis used for assessment (espresso Caffeine= 90.10±6.19, Decaffeinated coffee= 91.00±5.67, Without Caffeine consumption =74.40±4.99, F=48.04, p=0.00). Information on espresso coffee, decaffeinated coffee and without coffee effects on 2000m dragon boat are conditions presented in Table 2.

Table2. Coffee effect on aerobic power in 2000m dragon boat paddling (N=20).

	Mauchly's W	Mean±SD	F	Df	Sig
Mauchly's Test	0.13			2	0.00*
Without coffee		74.40±4.99			
Espresso coffee		90.10±6.19	48.04	1.07	0.00*
Decaffeinated coffee		91.00±5.67			

Without coffee=pre-test; P≤0.05

Bonferroni post hock test was used for between group interaction and results indicated significant differences in espresso coffee vs. without coffee group and decaffeinated coffee vs. without coffee group. Although there was no significant difference between espresso coffee compare decaffeinated coffee group (Table3).

Table3. Bonferroni post hoc tests (N=20).

Group		Mean difference	Sig
without coffee	Espresso coffee	-15.70	0.00*
without coffee	Decaffeinated coffee	-16.60	0.00*
Espresso coffee	Decaffeinated coffee	-0.90	0.51

P≤0.05

Discussion

The current study determined the effects of high dose coffee (espresso coffee) on 2000m dragon boat women paddler compared to decaffeinated coffee or placebo. Numerous studies had been shown the effectiveness of caffeine on improve endurance exercise [6-9, 17]. Interestingly, current study showed that using coffee espresso (high dos coffee) on hour prior the exercise could significantly improve the VO2max compared with without coffee condition.

In support, most studies have shown this effect on aerobic endurance. Graham et al. (1995), examined the exercise responses of well-trained endurance athletes to various doses of caffeine (3, 6 and 9 mg/kg) one hour before ran at 85% of maximal O2 consumption to voluntary exhaustion and showed that endurance was enhanced with both 3 and 6 mg/kg of caffeine, whereas there was no significant effect with 9 mg/kg of caffeine. In contrast plasma epinephrine was increased in 6 and 9mg/kg. Similarly only the highest dos of caffeine resulted in increases in glycerol and free fatty acids. Thus, the highest dose had the greatest effect on epinephrine and blood-borne metabolites yet had the least effect on performance [16]. Caffeine acts as phosphodiesterase (PDE) inhibitor that causes an increase in cyclic adenosine monophosphate (cAMP) in the brain and leads to stimulation of catecholamines (i.e., epinephrine) [25, 26]. This elevation in epinephrine levels [27] would, in turn, improve performance by delaying carbohydrate utilization and preserving muscle glycogen content and it Cause a greater stimulation of lipolysis during exercise and a greater release of circulating FFAs into the blood stream [28]. Also this potential performance-enhancing mechanism may be particularly relevant for liver (Bischof et al. 2001) glycogen stores [29]. Spriet et al. (1992) found that ingestion of a high dose of caffeine (9mg/kg) before cycled to exhaustion at approximately 80% maximal oxygen uptake (VO2max) reduced muscle glycogenolysis in the initial 15 min of exercise by increasing free fatty acid (FFA) levels which inhibits glycolysis and spares glycogen for later use [11]. Also Costill and colleagues (1978) observed with their pioneering work on coffee consumption with caffeine (330 mg) in elite male and female cyclists. During exercise, this greater reliance on fat metabolism with caffeine intake spares muscle glycogen utilization, which likely limits fatigue during prolonged aerobic activities (30). Specifically, Essig et al. (1980) and Erickson et al. (1987) both reported 42% reductions in muscle glycogen use during cycling at 70% of maximal oxygen uptake following caffeine ingestion compared with a control–placebo [31].

Lamina et al. (2009) in a study on twenty non-athletes and non-regular users of caffeine African yang male in Different doses (5, 10 & 15 mg/kg) of caffeine, indicated no ergogenic effect of caffeine on VO2max in short maximum endurance performance [15]. Graham et al. (1991) showed that a high caffeine dose of caffeine (9mg/kg) or placebo one hour pre-exercise at approximately 85% VO2max; two trials running to exhaustion and two trials cycling to exhaustion had no effect on epinephrine concentration was with caffeine before running and cycling. Plasma glycerol was elevated only at exhaustion during cycling and Urinary increased after the running and cycling trials [32]. It seems that, difference result from different performance tests. Lamina et al used short maximum endurance, Graham et al. used a two trials running or cycling to exhaustion (85% VO2max) and we used 2000m paddling.

Also, this study demonstrated the effectiveness of decaffeinated coffee on improve VO2max compare with without coffee condition. Hodgson et al (2013) illustrated performance times during the time trail were significantly faster for both caffeine and coffee when compared to placebo and decaffeinated coffee performance, they were similar for both caffeine and coffee and no significant differences were observed between placebo and decaffeinated coffee during the time trail in eight trained male cyclists/triathlon athletes following 30 min of steady-state cycling at approximately 55% VO2max and consumption drinks consisting 5mg/kg of caffeine, instant coffee, instant decaffeinated coffee or placebo [8]. In a study by Graham et al. (1998), nine healthy, fit, young adults performed five trials after ingesting placebo (dextrose) capsules with water, caffeine capsules with water, regular coffee, decaffeinated coffee, or decaffeinated coffee plus caffeine. In all three Caffeine trials, the Caffeine dose was 4.45 mg/kg. After one hour of rest, the subject ran at 85% of maximal O2 consumption until voluntary exhaustion. The results showed plasma Caffeine and epinephrine was increased in the three Caffeine trials. But the plasma epinephrine increase was greater with Caffeine capsules than with Coffee and they suggested that there must be a component (s) of Coffee that moderates the actions of Caffeine [19].

In conclusion, caffeine can improve performance during aerobic exercise with low or moderate doses of caffeine. Furthermore, coffee can be effectiveness for enhance performance. The present study shows that high doses of caffeine can enhance VO2max during aerobic exercise including 2000m dragon boat paddling. Decaffeinated coffee could also have this effect. It seems that some compounds except caffeine in decaffeinated coffee can act improve aerobic power. A limitation of this study was the low number of volunteers obtained because of the total number of Club members was low. Also, subject habit in coffee consumption was not assessed. Further studies needed for considering the effect of high doses of coffee on endurance exercises. In addition more study needed for other age ranges of women athletes and other sport athletes.

Acknowledgements

This project was supported by Islamic Azad university of Rasht, Iran.

Conflict of interests

The authors declare that there is no conflict of interests.

References

1. Davies RC, Eston RG, Poole DC, Rowlands AV, DiMenna F, Wilkerson DP, et al. Effect of eccentric exercise-induced muscle damage on the dynamics of muscle oxygenation and pulmonary oxygen uptake. *J Appl Physiol,* 2008; 105 (5):1413-1421.
2. Singh R, Singh HJ, Sirisinghe RG. Physical and physiological profiles of Malaysian dragon boat rowers. *Br J Sports Med.,* 1995;29 (1):13-15.
3. Grembecka M, Malinowska E, Szefer P. Differentiation of market coffee and its infusions in view of their mineral composition. *Science of The Total Environment*, 2007;383 (1–3):59-69.
4. Vignoli JA, Bassoli DG, Benassi MT. Antioxidant activity, polyphenols, caffeine and melanoidins in soluble coffee: The influence of processing conditions and raw material. *Food Chemistry*, 2011;124 (3):863-868.
5. Doherty M, Smith PM. Effects of caffeine ingestion on exercise testing: a meta-analysis. *Int J Sport Nutr Exerc Metab.* 2004;14 (6):626-646.
6. Ganio MS, Klau JF, Casa DJ, Armstrong LE, Maresh CM. Effect of Caffeine on Sport-Specific Endurance Performance: A Systematic Review. *The Journal of Strength & Conditioning Research*, 2009;23 (1):315-324.
7. Skinner TL, Jenkins DG, Coombes JS, Taaffe DR, Leveritt MD. Dose response of caffeine on 2000-m rowing performance. *Medicine and science in sports and exercise*, 2010;42 (3):571-576.
8. Hodgson AB, Randell RK, Jeukendrup AE. The metabolic and performance effects of caffeine compared to coffee during endurance exercise. *PLoS One,* 2013;8 (4):555-561.
9. Ali A, O'Donnell J, Von Hurst P, Foskett A, Holland S, Starck C, et al. Caffeine ingestion enhances perceptual responses during intermittent exercise in female team-game players. *Journal of Sports Sciences,* 2015;1:1-12.
10. Fredholm BB, Battig K, Holmen J, Nehlig A, Zvartau EE. Actions of caffeine in the brain with special reference to factors that contribute to its widespread use. *Pharmacological reviews,* 1999;51 (1):83-133.
11. Spriet LL, MacLean DA, Dyck DJ, Hultman E, Cederblad G, Graham TE. Caffeine ingestion and muscle metabolism during prolonged exercise in humans. *The American journal of physiology*, 1992;262 (6):891-898.
12. Rush JWE, Spriet LL. Skeletal muscle glycogen phosphorylase akinetics: effects of adenine nucleotides and caffeine. *Journal of Applied Physiology,* 2001;91 (5):2071-2078.
13. Black CD, Waddell DE, Gonglach AR. Caffeine's Ergogenic Effects on Cycling: Neuromuscular and Perceptual Factors. *Medicine and science in sports and exercise*, 2015;47 (6):1145-1158.
14. Bortolotti H, Altimari LR, Vitor-Costa M, Cyrino ES. Performance during a 20-km cycling time-trial after caffeine ingestion. *J Int Soc Sports Nutr.* 2014;11:45-50.
15. Lamina S, Musa DI. Ergogenic effect of varied doses of coffee-caffeine on maximal aerobic power of young African subjects. *African Health Sciences*. 2009;9 (4):270-274.
16. Graham TE, Spriet LL. Metabolic, catecholamine, and exercise performance responses to various doses of caffeine. *Journal of applied physiology*, 1995;78 (3):867-874.
17. Desbrow B, Leveritt M. Awareness and use of caffeine by athletes competing at the 2005 Ironman Triathlon World Championships. *Int J Sport Nutr Exerc Metab*. 2006;16 (5):545-558.
18. McLellan TM, Bell DG. The impact of prior coffee consumption on the subsequent ergogenic effect of anhydrous caffeine. Int J Sport Nutr Exerc Metab. 2004 Dec;14 (6):698-708.
19. Graham TE, Hibbert E, Sathasivam P. Metabolic and exercise endurance effects of coffee and caffeine ingestion. *J Appl Physiol,* 1998; 85 (3):883-889.
20. Plaskett CJ, Cafarelli E. Caffeine increases endurance and attenuates force sensation during submaximal isometric contractions. *J Appl Physiol,* 2001; 91 (4):1535-1544.
21. Borg GA. Psychophysical bases of perceived exertion. *Med sci sports exerc.* 1982;14 (5):377-381.
22. Lohman TG, Roche AF, Martorell R. *Anthropometric standardization reference manual.* Champaign, IL: Human Kinetics Books; 1988.
23. *Welcome to KayakPro Europe Direct*. Available at: http://www.kayakpro.com/ (accessed 23.07.2016).
24. Graham TE. Caffeine and exercise: metabolism, endurance and performance. *Sports Med.* 2001;31 (11):785-807.
25. Graham TE, Battram DS, Dela F, El-Sohemy A, Thong FSL. Does caffeine alter muscle carbohydrate and fat metabolism during exercise? *Applied Physiology, Nutrition, and Metabolism*, 2008;33 (6):1311-1318.
26. Fredholm BB. On the mechanism of action of theophylline and caffeine. *Acta medica Scandinavica.* 1985;217 (2):149-153.
27. Greer F, Friars D, Graham TE. Comparison of caffeine and theophylline ingestion: exercise metabolism and endurance. *J Appl Physiol,* 2000;89 (5):1837-1844.

28. Ryu S, Choi S-K, Joung S-S, Suh H, Cha Y-S, Lee S, et al. Caffeine as a Lipolytic Food Component Increases Endurance Performance in Rats and Athletes. *Journal of Nutritional Science and Vitaminology,* 2001;47 (2):139-146.
29. Bischof MG, Krssak M, Krebs M, Bernroider E, Stingl H, Waldhäusl W, et al. Effects of short-term improvement of insulin treatment and glycemia on hepatic glycogen metabolism in type 1 diabetes. *Diabetes,* 2001;50 (2):392-398.
30. Costill DL, Dalsky GP, Fink WJ. Effects of caffeine ingestion on metabolism and exercise performance. *Med Sci Sports.* 1978;10 (3):155-158.
31. Essig D, Costill D, Van Handel P. Effects of caffeine ingestion on utilization of muscle glycogen and lipid during leg ergometer cycling. *Int J Sports Med,* 1980;01 (2): 86-90. doi:10.1055/s-2008-1034637
32. Graham TE, Spriet LL. Performance and metabolic responses to a high caffeine dose during prolonged exercise. *Journal of applied physiology,* 1991;71 (6):2292-2298.

7

ROLE OF STUDENTS' YOUTH IN STRATEGIC PLANNING OF EXTERNAL COMMUNICATIONS OF POPULATION PHYSICAL HEALTH "SPORTS FOR ALL" CENTERS

Kravchenko O.V.
National University of Physical Education and Sport of Ukraine

Abstract. _Purpose:_ to work out strategy of external communications system's improvement of population physical health and determine students' role in optimization of this system. _Material:_ we questioned 136 centers' functionaries and 338 representatives of groups of influence. SWOT-analysis was used. With the help of SWOT-analysis method we simulated 16 the most probable situations and strategic actions in case of their occurrence. For determination of experts' opinions concordance, we used concordance coefficient in SWOT-analysis. _Results:_ we found strong and weak sides of external communication centers' system, favorable opportunities and threats of this system. Strategies of centers' behavior in the most probable situations were worked out and students' youth role in them analyzed. It was determined that in every simulated situation participation of students-volunteers of physical culture-sports profile was very important. We also noted demand in increase of personnel's competence level, in attraction of specialists from other organization. _Conclusions:_ in conditions of limited resources and breadth of functioning the centers shall actively use students' assistance in organization and realization of different measures; attract them as consumers of the centers' services.
Key words: stakeholders, communications, interaction, SWOT-analysis, volunteers,

Introduction

Functioning of any physical culture-sports organization is connected with external communications, which ensure linking processes [12, 19, and 23]. They interact with interested physical and legal subjects, or groups of subjects (stakeholders). Centers "Sports for all" shall to involve wide population strata in motor functioning in time free of work or study [1-3]. Their functioning is oriented exclusively on health improvement of population and does not imply any profit. Financing is realized only by government or sponsors. Deficit of finances stimulates centers to receive free assistance from volunteers [4-6, 10]. For effective interaction it is necessary to use already created strategies of external communication [14, 22].

The most acceptable direction of the mentioned problems' solution can be application of SWOT-analysis. Effectiveness of such approach is sown in some researches.

As far as "Sports for all" movement and centers appeared in Ukraine not long ago their communication system has not been studied sufficiently yet and is imperfect. But their functioning is important for formation of population's demand in healthy life style, youth's socialization and students' adaptation at new place of study [7, 9, and 21]. That is why there is a demand in more detail analysis of functioning of population's physical health centers and students' role in optimization of this system.

Purpose, tasks of the work, material and methods

The purpose of the work is to develop strategy of external communications system's improvement of population physical health and determine students' role in optimization of this system.

For receiving of comprehensive information we questioned 136 centers' functionaries and 338 representatives of external groups of influence (stakeholders).

Statistical analysis

In our work we used SWOT-analysis. This method of strategic planning implies determination of factors of organization's internal and external medium and dividing them into four categories: strengths, weaknesses, opportunities and threats. For determination of experts' opinions concordance, we used concordance coefficient in SWOT-analysis. With the help of SWOT-analysis method we simulated 16 the most probable situations and strategic actions in case of their occurrence. The relevance of such approach is confirmed by other researches [12, 13, 15-18]. It permits to find strengths and weaknesses, opportunities and threats, which require the highest attention and efforts from organization [8]. Opportunities and threats can influence on system of centers' external communications but do not depend on "Sports for all" centers themselves. Strengths and weaknesses of this system depend on internal peculiarities of "Sports for all" centers.

Results of the research

Questioning and observations, conducted by us, resulted in determination of "Sports for all" centers' strengths and weaknesses as well as potential opportunities and threats (see table 1). In every group of factors we chose two main. Comparing them, we worked out 16 models of centers' behavior in different situations. Besides, we found ways of students' assistance in realization of "Sports for all" centers' strategic tasks. Some situations will facilitate development of the centers; other will require urgent measures for neutralization of negative factors.

Table 1. SWOT-analysis of system of centers' external communications центров

		Opportunities (O)		**Threats (T)**	
		1. increase of stakeholders' sponsoring of the centers	2. Increase of motor functioning popularity	1. Stoppage / weakening of voluntary stakeholders' interaction with centers	2. Reduction of governmental financing of centers' development and popularization
Strengths (S)	1.Many years' experience	Increase of projects' quantity and their participants	Expansion of centers' network and increase of consumers' quantity	Working out of programs for involvement of new participants and retention of old ones	Addressing to executive authorities, seeking of new investors
	2. Centers' realization of measures on attraction of stakeholders and intensification of communication with them	Increase of participants' quantity. Rising of efficiency of external communications	Increase of "ports for all" participants' quantity, covering of all Ukrainian territory	Involvement of new participants and retention of old ones with the help of new projects and programs	Attraction of new investors. Working out of programs of targeted governmental support
Weaknesses (W)	1. Weak material base	Increase of stakeholders' interest in communication with the help of already available channels for prevention from weakening or stoppage of interaction	Optimization and adaptation of available channels for communication with interested physical or legal subjects	Prevention from blocking of projects on stakeholders' interest intensification. Constructive working out of programs with usage of available communication means	Seeking of new investments and reasonable minimization of expenses
	2. Absence of specialists and department of external communications	Creation of position of profile specialist for maximizing of potential benefits	Creation of position of profile specialist for increase of movement's participants and intensification of communication with them	Attraction of qualified specialists from other organizations; seeking of volunteers-specialists in external communications	Attraction of qualified specialists for working out of programs with minimal governmental participation and minimal investments. Seeking of other sponsors Attraction of qualified specialists

In case S1-O1 (see table 1) favorable circumstances appear. In such case it would be purposeful to increase quantity of projects of "Sports for all" centers, in which more quantity of stakeholders (physical and legal subjects, influencing of centers' functioning) will participate as well as consumers. Higher quantity of participants will be required. Students of profile specialties already have required basic knowledge. They can help in organization and realization of measures and will receive necessary practical skills.

In case S1-O2 expansion of centers' activity is possible. It will permit to open new centers, i.e. to expand the network. Increase of motor functioning popularity implies strengthening of society's interest to it. In such situation assistance of students as volunteers is also required. Besides, formation of sports circles on the base of higher educational establishments is possible; realization of measures on popularization of healthy life style and centers' activity among students, as far as youth is the most important group of consumers.

In case S1-T1 it is necessary to minimize impact of negative factor and maximize influence of positive one. In such case experienced specialists of centers shall implement programs and take required measures for involvement of new interested subjects (sponsors, partners, consumers and etc.) as well as for prevention from stoppage of interaction with already available stakeholders. Direct realization of programs and projects will also require assistance of students, especially those, who master management. Besides practical experience it will help the students to quicker socialize in society.

In case S1-T2 seeking of voluntary stakeholders (sponsors, physical culture-sports organizations; mass media means and so on) becomes urgent. Besides, the strategy of interaction with governmental and local authorities, whom the centers subordinate, is required. The centers shall address to such boards. For this purpose the centers shall have visual materials, illustrating usefulness of their functioning. For collection of the materials the centers will require volunteers' assistance, which, mainly, can be rendered by students. In this case analysis of positive influence on youth and higher quantity of "Sports for all" young participants will add to reports and presentations' weight.

Combination of factors in case S2-O1 is a platform for increase of stakeholders groups' participants. In certain cases it is a platform for increase of the groups themselves and intensification of communication with them. Students will be regarded and actual and potential consumers; as mediators and supporters in interconnection with other stakeholders' groups. Other stakeholders (for example sponsors) can interact with youth for achievement their own targets.

Combination of factors S2-O2 permits to attract great number of new participants of movement "Sports for all", who will represent most of Ukrainian regions. For the centers it is important to support popularity of motor functioning and attract attention to themselves as to optimal place for practicing of physical culture exercises and sports. For example, for philanthropists and volunteers (including students), it important to demonstrate social usefulness of centers and other participants of "Sports for all" functioning. Interacting with the centers, students can familiarize with kinds of sports, presented by sports federations and associations, to understand use of motor functioning.

Combination of factors S2-T1 forces the centers to apply efforts to gain attention of volunteers. It is necessary to support interaction and watch its intensity. In case of resources' deficit it is necessary to use channels and means of communication with minimal financial expenses. Students shall be actively stimulated for cooperation as financially not motivated participants. It is very important in conditions of cost cutting. For this purpose it is necessary to stress on significance of their help, to cooperate with higher educational establishments, to encourage students with different bonuses.

In case S2-T2 the centers shall direct higher efforts to seeking of non governmental sources of financing, to more actively use the base of physical culture-sports organizations and use volunteers' assistance oftener. Besides, it is necessary to consider the cost of communicative channels and means. With it, cheap and high speed channels of communications can be used (mobile phones, e-mail).

Discussion

It should be noted that movement "Sports for all" appeared in Ukraine not long ago [1, 2, 6] and it is studied insufficiently. Previous model situations are more typical for physical-culture sports organizations and are not the topic of scientists' discussions [14, 23]. In this aspect model situations are more problematic and discussable. For example in situation W1-O1 weak material base can reduce success of increasing centers' support by stakeholders (it hinders effective communication). Therefore it is necessary to interest stakeholders by communication with the help of available communication channels and consideration of peculiar feature of every stakeholders group. In situation W1-O2 weak base can also hinder popularization of centers' activity in favorable conditions. Wide population strata will not be informed to full extent about peculiarities of motor functioning and centers' role in creation of conditions for such functioning.

With absence of required technical means for wide collection and transmitting of information it is purposeful to use students' assistance. Information about interests and potentials of stakeholders' groups, collected by them, can be used, when working out projects of the centers. Students can also help in propagating of information about motor functioning usefulness and about centers' "Sports for all" role in its popularization.

Dutchak M. [3, 4] wrote about importance of centers' "Sports for all" interaction with population. The author regarded "sports for all" as social phenomenon and underlined the role of state in its development. Results of our research point that state does not facilitate development of the centers properly. It is confirmed by other researches as well [11]. In our work deficit of programs on personal's vocational training is stressed on. It is especially important in situation W1-T1. With stoppage of interaction with voluntary stakeholders, weak material base will prevent the centers from creation of effective programs for struggle with such negative impact. It is necessary to increase interaction level with remaining stakeholders' groups and reasonably use available limited communication means. For this purpose it is necessary to perfect functionaries' skills. In case W1-T2 there happens ignoring of communication means' obsolescence in "Sports for all" centers by governmental and local authorities. Except active search of new material sources, it is necessary to attract attention of state, accentuating centers' significance in involvement of wide population strata in motor functioning; to underline importance of the centers in this process. One of the best methods is demonstration of great quantity of students. It facilitates their socialization [10, 7, and 9]. Other authors point at educational aspect of the centers' influence on students [7, 9, and 10]. These authors studied volunteers' movement in the whole, without accent on students [10].

Combination of factors W2-O1 restrains development of interconnections between centers and stakeholders. Due to deficit of specialists efficiency of communication with certain stakeholders' groups can weaken. Therefore, it is necessary to form a department or position of specialist, responsible for communication with external medium and be capable to watch groups' interests and activity and kept permanent links. However deficit of such specialists is rather acute. That is why it would be purposeful to attract students of appropriate specialties, who would cope with such important working aspect. Importance of volunteers of different specialties in centers' activity and competence of strategic planning were proved in other researches [10, 14, and 22].

In case of factors W2-O2 deficit of qualified specialists reduces role of centers in supporting prestige of motor functioning and healthy life style. In this case specialists of other profile are lack of time, knowledge and skills for effective external communication. Besides involvement of voluntary stakeholders it would be correct to create initiative programs. Such programs can be directed to governmental and local authorities. For this purpose specialists' assistance is required. In this case students of different related specialties can help. Other researches point at interconnection between support of local authorities and progress of "Sports for all" movement in Ukrainian regions as well as role of volunteers [1]. In general, authors, in their works, stressed on students' involvement as consumers [1, 4].

Combination of factors W2-T1 results in non effective communication and development of programs. It is required to raise the level of personnel's communication competence, to attract experienced specialists from other organizations or from volunteers; to work out projects on involvement of new participants. In W2-T2 conditions there appears a threat of increasing of centers' quantity and their programs. Projects can be closed by authorities or independently by centers due to lack of required resources. In such case more sponsors' or philanthropists' assistance is required. So specialists in work with stakeholders and in studying of their interests are wanted. It is purposeful to attract students of this profile on volunteer principles.

Conclusions

For profound analysis of the received in our research data we used SWOT-analysis of external communications system of centers of population physical health "Sports for all". Besides, it is a pattern for future independent analyzing works of the centers.

As far as weak material base is a key weakness of centers' external interaction, volunteers' assistance is required. We proved necessity of volunteer's assistance rendered by students of different specialties (especially in sphere of physical culture and sports management). Besides, students are important group of consumers, whose interests shall also be considered.

Conflict of interests

The author declares that there is no conflict of interests.

References

1. Varenik OM. *Organizacijna vzaiemodiia mizh sub'iektami sportu dlia vsikh na miscevomu rivni. Cand. Diss.* [Organizational interaction between subjects of sports at local level. Cand. Diss.], Kiev; 2014 (in Ukrainian)
2. Dutchak MV. *Sport dlia vsikh v Ukraini* [Sports for all in Ukraine], Kiev: Olympic Literature; 2009 (in Ukrainian)
3. Dutchak MV. *Teoretiko-metodologichni zasadi formuvannia sistemi sportu dlia vsikh v Ukraini. Dokt. Diss.* [Theoretical-methodological principles of formation of sports for all system in Ukraine. Doct. Diss.], Kiev; 2009 (in Ukrainian)
4. Dutchak M. Ekonomicheskie aspekty sporta dlia vsekh [Economic aspects of sports for all]. *Nauka v olimpijskom sporte,* 2010; 01-02: 101-112 (in Russian)
5. Kravchenko O. Stejkkholderi iak agenti zovnishnikh komunikacij v organizaciiakh sferi masovogo sportu ta sportu dlia vsikh [Stakeholders as agents of external communications in organization of mass sports and sports for all]. *Moloda sportivna nauka Ukraini,* 2014; 18: 47-52 (in Ukrainian)
6. Kravchenko OV. Rol' stejkkholderiv u stvorenni efektivnoi sistemi zovnishnikh komunikacij organizacij sferi masovogo sportu ta sportu dlia vsikh [Role of stakeholders in creation of effective external communications system in mass sports and sports for all]. *Teoriia i metodika fizichnogo vikhovannia i sportu*, 2014; 4: 107-110 (in Ukrainian)
7. Mal'ona S, Kindrachuk V. Pedagogichna sistema upravlinnia rozvitkom sportu dlia vsikh [Pedagogic system of management of sports for all development]. *Sportivnij visnik Pridniprov'ia*, 2013; 2: 222-226 (in Ukrainian)
8. Lipchuk VV. *Marketingovij analiz* [Marketing analysis], Kyiv: Akademvidav; 2008 (in Ukrainian)
9. Pozhar IIu. Rabota centrov «Sport dlia vsekh» sredi studencheskoj molodezhi v Ukraine [Works of "Sports for all" centers among students in Ukraine]. *XV Nauchnyj kongress «Olimpijskij sport i sport dlia vsekh», 12-15 sentiabria 2011, Kishinev* [15th scientific congress "Olympic sports and sports for all", September 12-15 2011, Chisinau], Kishinev; 2011. p. 135-137. (in Russian)
10. Prijmak M. Perspektivi rozvitku volonterstva u sporti dlia vsikh v Ukraini [Prospects of volunteers' movement in sports for all development in Ukraine]. *Aktual'ni problemi fizichnoi kul'turi i sportu*, 2014; 31 (3): 36-42 (in Ukrainian)
11. Prijmak M. Ocinka suchasnogo stanu pidvishchennia kvalifikacii fakhivciv sportu dlia vsikh v Ukraini [Assessment of modern state of sports for all specialists' advanced training in Ukraine]. *Aktual'ni problemi fizichnoi kul'turi i sportu*, 2014; 30 (2): 71-77 (in Ukrainian)
12. Beloborodko A. SWOT Analysis Approach for Advancement of Waste-to-energy Cluster in Latvia. *Energy Procedia.* 2015;72:163–169.
13. Can C. SWOT Analysis and Countermeasures of Ecological Agricultural Development of Jianshan Farm. *Journal of Northeast Agricultural University (English Edition).* 2015;22(1):12–21.
14. Daft RL. *Management.* Boston: Cengage Learning; 2014.
15. Driukov O.V., Conceptual principles of fencing development in children's sports schools in Ukraine. *Pedagogics, psychology, medical-biological problems of physical training and sports*, 2015;12:35-40. http://dx.doi.org/10.15561/18189172.2015.1206
16. Ghinolfi D. A model for southern mediterranean research institute self-assessment: A SWOT analysis-based approach to promote capacity building at Theodor Bilharz Research Institute in Cairo (Egypt). *Arab Journal of Gastroenterology.* 2014;15(3–4):92–97.
17. Glass JR, Kruse GH, Miller SA. Socioeconomic considerations of the commercial weathervane scallop fishery off Alaska using SWOT analysis. *Ocean & Coastal Management.* 2015;105:154–165.
18. Jaber JO. Employment of renewable energy in Jordan: Current status, SWOT and problem analysis. *Renewable and Sustainable Energy Reviews*. 2015;49:490–499.
19. Jones GR, George MJ. *Contemporary management.* 9th ed. New York: McGraw-Hill Education; 2015.
20. Krotee ML, Bucher CA. *Management of physical education and sport.* Boston: McGraw-Hill Higher Education; 2007.

8

FACTORIAL STRUCTURE OF PHYSICAL REHABILITATION GROUP STUDENTS' COMPLEX FITNESS

Sobko I. N., Ulaeva L.A., Yakovenko Y.A.
Simon Kuznets Kharkov National Economic University

Abstract. *Purpose:* differentiation of physical education process on the base of morphological-functional state and physical fitness indicators, psycho-physiological potentials of physical rehabilitation group's students. *Material:* 50 1st year students of 17-18 years' age participated in the research. Tests for assessment of students' morphological-functional state were used. Psycho-physiological testing was carried out with the help of computer program. *Results:* we marked out 5 factors, which characterize main components of students' physical condition. It was determined that low level of students' physical and functional potentials weakens functioning of organism's most important functions. It was found that the most important factors in complex fitness of physical rehabilitation group's students are power and functional potentials. *Conclusions:* it is necessary to purposefully work on formation of students' comprehensive motor potential. Results of the research permit to rationally distribute physical education means and methods in practical trainings of physical rehabilitation group.
Key words: physical rehabilitation, students, complex fitness, factorial analysis.

Introduction

Improvement of national higher educational system conditions optimization and upgrading of physical education. To day there is demand in development of effective means and methods, oriented on increase of students' education quality, considering age and personality aspects [1, 7, and 17]. It will create necessary pre-conditions for development of students' steady interest in independent motor functioning, formation of rational choice and usage of physical education means in their life activity skills [1, 3, 23, and 26]. This problem is rather urgent for physical education of boys [17] and girls [10].

Assessment of main group students' different kinds of sports sportsmen's morphological-functional state, physical fitness and psycho-physiological potentials was realized in many works [5, 6, and 8]. For determination of students' complex fitness characteristics scientists apply factorial and cluster analysis [6, 12, and 17]. There are data about application of special technologies in physical education of hard hearing girls [9, 11].

In physical education theory, there is intensive search of modern means, which would increase students' educational effectiveness (meaning students, trained in physical rehabilitation groups) [2, 3, 17, 18, 21, and 25]. Scientists regard questions of methodic and organization of special health groups and therapeutic physical culture groups students' physical education [4, 15]. They show positive influence of physical exercises and sports games elements on development of these groups' students' motor qualities and coordination [13, 18].

The program of discipline "Physical education" does not completely open content and orientation of education process for physical rehabilitation groups' students [16]. Recommendations on organization and technology of such trainings' construction have general character. It results in discrepancies and ambiguity in approaches to organization and building of practical classes with such contingent [22, 27, and 28]. Different character of students' diseases made to search adequate approaches to trainings. The more completely demand o such groups' students will be known the more significantly the methods of physical exercises' practicing will differ [2, 18, 28].

Thus, for effective work with physical rehabilitation group students, teachers shall have information about morphological-functional and physical fitness indicators, about students' psycho-physiological potentials. In its turn it will help to determine appropriate means and methods of physical education for this contingent.

Purpose, tasks of the work, material and methods

The purpose of the work is differentiation of physical education process with usage of adequate means and methods on the base of morphological-functional state and physical fitness indicators, psycho-physiological potentials of physical rehabilitation group's students.

The methods of the research: we used tests for assessment of morphological-functional state (body length, body mass, blood pressure, heart beats rate in rest), physical fitness (dynamometry of right and left hands; ball's passing in pairs for 30 sec. from 3 meters' distance; keeping legs under angle of 45°; bending and unbending arms in elbows with load of 1 kg for 30 sec.; throwing of tennis ball to target from 6 meters' distance), Romberg's test. Psycho-physiological testing was carried out with computer program "Psycho-diagnostic" [1]: we registered time of simple visual motor reaction and time of visual motor reaction of choice; tapping test.

50 1st year students of 17-18 years' age, who were trained in physical rehabilitation group, participated in the research.

Results of the research

For determination of complex fitness structure of physical rehabilitation group's students we applied factorial analysis by principle component method (see table 1).

Table 1. Matrix of components in factorial analysis of complex testing indicators of physical rehabilitation group's students

Description of factor	Indicators	Factors 1	2	3	4	5
Power potentials	Body length, cm	0.776				
	Body mass, kg	0.644				
	Dynamometry of right hand, kg	0.861				
	Dynamometry of left hand, kg	0.867				
	Ball passes in pars for 30 sec.	0.659				
	Arms' bending-unbending in elbows with 1 kg load for 30 sec., times	0.530				
Functional potentials	Systolic blood pressure, mm.merc.col.		0.668			
	Diastolic blood pressure, mm.merc.col.		0.860			
	Keeping legs under angle of 45º, sec.		-0.516			
Frequency of movements	Tapping test, times			0.772		
	Throwing of tennis ball to target, times			0.701		
Quickness of reaction	Time of simple visual motor reaction, m.sec.				0.821	
	Time of visual motor reaction of choice, m.sec.				0.597	0.563
Coordination potentials	Heart beats rate in rest, b.p.m.					0.851
	Romberg's test, sec.					0.634
Variance, %		25.23	12.54	9.84	9.15	8.06

First factor (power potentials) included the following indicators: "body length" (r = 0.776), "body mass" (r = 0.644), "dynamometry of right hand" (r = 0.861), "dynamometry of left hand" (r = 0.867) and "ball's passes in pairs for 30 sec." (r = 0.659). Indicators of body length, body mass and hands' strength are interconnected: hands' strength increases with increasing of body mass. For increasing of relative strength, considering excess body weight, it is necessary to use exercises for removal of excess fat.

Second by significance factor (functional potentials) contained the following indicators: "systolic b.p." (r = 0.668), "diastolic b.p." (r = 0.860), "keeping legs under angle of 45°" (r = - 0.516). These indicators are interconnected. The higher systolic and diastolic blood pressures are the less load of abdomen muscles can the tested endure. Low motor functioning of this contingent's students weakens functioning of most important muscular systems. It is the factor of reduction of cardio-vascular and respiratory systems' functional potentials.

Third factor (frequency of movements) included the following indicators: "tapping test" (r = 0.772), "throwing of tennis ball to target" (r = 0.701). It is not less significant: "fine motor skills" of hand indirectly is connected with operative thinking.

Forth factor (quickness of reaction) includes: "time of simple visual motor reaction" (r = 0.821) and "Time of visual motor reaction of choice" (r = 0.563-0.597).

Fifth factor (coordination abilities) includes indicators of heart beats rate in rest (r = 0.851) and Romberg's test (r = 0.634).

Factorial analysis resulted in determination that the tested group is heterogeneous. One part of students has low fitness level, other – average. It can be explained by the fact that 1st year students did not attend physical culture lessons, being pupils of school. Some pupils of special health group did not receive proper physical load, which was required for correction of their functional state, depending on disease.

Basing on the received data we produced the following recommendations on physical education of special health group's students. At first stage of educational process it is necessary to ensure as quick as possible recreation of functions, distorted by disease. For this purpose it is necessary to increase potentials of students' organism for practicing physical exercises though usual forms of motor functioning. At next stage it is required to start special trainings, considering disease of every student. It will ensure recreation of organism's general workability. At final stages of educational process it is necessary to train important motor qualities of this category's students.

In order to ensure complete compensation of available in physical rehabilitation group students' disorders, it is necessary to use basic variants of general physical and breathing exercises. Besides, purposeful work on formation of comprehensive motor potential with the help of aerobic loads, physical exercises of local and regional character is required. These recommendations facilitate increase of mental and physical workability through mastering of new physical exercises and motor skills [3, 14].

Discussion

Recent decades the quantity of special health groups' students has increased owing to reduction of health level [14, 21, 24, and 27]. Researchers [4, 15] confirm the data that students of this category can not master typical physical education program. The authors work out methodic and programs, which help students to strengthen their health and to raise physical fitness in process of physical education. Consideration of physical and psycho-physiological potentials of physical rehabilitation group's students is an important factor for increasing of educational process quality. The main task of physical rehabilitation group's students is achievement of maximal health improvement effect and removal of residuals of their diseases. That is why in trainings it is necessary to use strictly differentiated means and methods, depending on students' diseases.

As a result of our research we supplemented the data of other authors [6, 8, and 17] about usage of factorial analysis for determination of structure of students' complex fitness. The authors found that factorial structure of main group girls' fitness differs by great complexity, comparing with boys. In our research we found specific features of factorial structure of physical rehabilitation group's students. It permits for teacher to correctly select physical load.

Conclusions:

The fulfilled factorial analysis permits to determine rational correlation of means and methods for increasing of physical fitness and health strengthening of physical rehabilitation group's students. It was found that the most significant factors in complex fitness of physical rehabilitation group's students were power and functional qualities. In this connection it was offered to correct the program of discipline "Physical education" and content of practical trainings at every stage of educational process.

The prospects of further researches imply working out of physical education program for physical rehabilitation group's students and determination of its effectiveness.

Conflict of interests

The authors declare that there is o conflict of interests.

References:

1. Barybina LN, Kozina ZhL. Description of psychophysiological indexes of students of different sporting specializations. *Physical Education of Students*, 2010;4: 6-11.
2. Bismak OV. *Likuval'na fizichna kul'tura u special'nikh medichnikh grupakh* [Therapeutic physical culture in special health groups], Kharkiv, Brovin RH; 2010. (in Ukrainian)
3. Bodnar I. *Teoriia, metodika i organizaciia fizichnogo vikhovannia studentiv special'noi medichnoi grupi* [Theory, methodic and organization of special health group's students' physical education]. Lviv, Ukrainian technologies; 2005. (in Ukrainian)

4. Golod NR.,Principles of developing a well-rounded program of physical rehabilitation for female students in the special medical group with consideration of physical activity impairment. *Pedagogics, psychology, medical-biological problems of physical training and sports*, 2015;5:9-15. http://dx.doi.org/10.15561/18189172.2015.0502
5. Gurieieva AM, Klopov RV. Factor structure of physical state of female students of higher education institution. *Pedagogics, psychology, medical-biological problems of physical training and sports*, 2014;7:7-11. doi:10.6084/m9.figshare.1015378
6. Ivashchenko OV, Yermakova TS. Assessment of functional, coordination and power fitness of 7-8 form boys. *Pedagogics, psychology, medical-biological problems of physical training and sports*, 2015;9:20-25. http://dx.doi.org/10.15561/18189172.2015.0903
7. Kozina ZL, Iermakov SS. Analysis of students' nervous system's typological properties, in aspect of response to extreme situation, with the help of multi-dimensional analysis. *Physical Education of Students*, 2015;3:10-19. http://dx.doi.org/10.15561/20755279.2015.0302
8. Kozina ZhL, Sobko IN, Kolomiec NA, Jagiełło Władysław, Jagiełło Marina. Allocation algorithm for athletes group to form tactical tasks in game team sports using the methods of multivariate analysis (illustrated women Ukrainian team basketball with hearing impairments). *Pedagogics, psychology, medical-biological problems of physical training and sports,* 2014;12: 40-48. doi:10.15561/18189172.2014.1208
9. Kozina ZhL, Sobko IN, Prokopenko AI, Guba AV, Iermakov SS, Prusik Krzysztof, Cieślicka Mirosława. Methods of technical and tactical training basketball players with hearing impairments using innovative technologies. *Physical Education of Students*, 2014;3:30-39. doi:10.6084/m9.figshare.978699
10. Kozina Zh.L. Osnovnye polozheniia avtorskogo kursa podgotovki beremennykh k estestvennym zdorovym rodam "Raskrytie cvetka" [Main principles of author's training course for preparation of pregnant women to natural healthy childbirth "Opening of flower"]. *Pedagogics, psychology, medical-biological problems of physical training and sports,* 2008;3:81–92.
11. Kozina ZhL, Sobko IN, Klimenko AI, Sak NN. Comparative characteristics of psychophysiological features skilled basketball players-women with hearing and skilled basketball players healthy. *Pedagogics, psychology, medical-biological problems of physical training and sports*, 2013;7:28-33. doi:10.6084/m9.figshare.735962
12. Kozina Zh.L. Faktorni modeli fizichnoi pidgotovlenosti volejbolistok visokogo klasu riznogo igrovogo amplua [Factorial models of physical fitness of different game roles' elite female volleyball players]. *Pedagogics, psychology, medical-biological problems of physical training and sports,* 2007;9:80–85.
13. Kudelko VE, Ulaieva LO, Shevchenko OO. Pozitivnij vpliv vprav dlia rozvitku koordinacii u studentiv, iaki zajmaiut'sia fizichnim vikhovanniam u grupi LFK [Positive influence exercises for coordination on students, who train in TPC]. *Pedagogics, psychology, medical-biological problems of physical training and sports,* 2011;7:49–54.
14. Kudelko VE, Ulaieva LO, Sobko IM. *Metodichni rekomendacii z navchal'noi disciplini «Fizichne vikhovannia» dlia studentiv special'nikh navchal'nikh grup usikh napriamiv pidgotovki* [Methodic recommendations on discipline "Physical education" for students of special health groups of all directions of training], Kharkov: KhNUE; 2012. (in Ukrainian)
15. Kuzmin VA, Kopylov YuA, Kudryavtsev MD, Galimov GY, Iermakov SS. Substantiation of effectiveness of trainings on health related methodic for students with weakened motor fitness. *Physical Education of Students*, 2015;6:43-49. http://dx.doi.org/10.15561/20755279.2015.0606
16. Marakushin AI, Piddubnij OG, Cimbaliuk ZhO, Sobko IM, Cherednichenko AV. *Robocha programa navchal'noi disciplini «Fizichne vikhovannia» za obranim vidom organizovanoi rukhovoi aktivnosti dlia studentiv usikh napriamiv pidgotovki dennoi formi navchannia* [Working program of discipline "Physical education" by chosen kind of organized motor functioning for full time students for all directions of training], Kharkov: KhNUE; 2014. (in Ukrainian)
17. Prusik Krzysztof, Prusik Katarzyna, Kozina ZhL, Iermakov SS. Features of physical development, physical preparedness and functional state of boys and girls - students of Polish higher educational establishments. *Physical Education of Students*, 2013;1:54-61. doi:10.6084/m9.figshare.96415

18. Sobko IN, Ulaeva LA. Razvitie vynoslivosti na zaniatiiakh po fizicheskomu vospitaniiu v gruppe LFK [Training of endurance at physical education classes in TPC groups]. *XI Mezhdunarodnaia nauchnaia konferenciia "Fizicheskoe vospitanie i sport v vysshikh uchebnykh zavedeniiakh", 23 –24 aprelia, 2015, Khar'kov* [9th International scientific conference "Physical education and sports in higher educational establishments", April, 23 –24, 2015. Kharkov], Kharkov; 2015. (in Russian)
19. Becker CM, Glascoff MA, Felts WM, Kent C. Adapting and using quality management methods to improve health promotion explore. *The Journal of Science and Healing*. 2015;11:222–228.
20. Cameron MH, Monroe L. *Physical rehabilitation: evidence-based examination, evaluation, and intervention*. St. Louis: Elsevier Health Sciences; 2007.
21. Goforth M, Almquist J, Matney M, Abdenour TE, Kyle J, Leaman J, Montgomery S.Understanding organization structures of the college, university, high school, clinical, and professional. *Clinics in Sports Medicine,* 2007;26:201–226.
22. Hong Xia M. Effects of different sports events on the physical self of deaf college students. *Journal of Physical Education*, 2010; 17: 55–59.
23. McLeod JD, Uemura R, Rohrman S. Adolescent mental health, behavior problems, and academic achievement. *Journal of Health and Social Behavior,* 2012;53:482–497.
24. Norma GC, Barton M, Bowles E, Scott BM. Multilevel analysis of student and school-level variables on students' health-related fitness. *Medicine & Science in Sports & Exercise,* 2015;47:47– 52.
25. O'Sullivan SB, Schmitz TJ. *Physical Rehabilitation*. Philadelphia: F.A. Davis Company; 2006.
26. Symons AB, Morley CP, McGuigan D, Elie A. A curriculum on care for people with disabilities: effects on medical student self-reported attitudes and comfort level. *Disability and Health Journal,* 2013;7:88–95.
27. Varela-Mato V, Clemes S, Cancela-Carral J. Physical activity and sitting time measured in Spanish university students. *Journal of Science and Medicine in Sport,* 2012;15:20–25.
28. Young Hui-Ju, Erickson ML, Johnson KB, Johnson MA, McCully KK. A wellness program for individuals with disabilities. *Disability and Health Journal,* 2013;8:345–352.

9

GENERAL LAWS OF COMPETITION DUEL AND UNIVERSAL REQUIREMENTS TO TECHNICAL-TACTIC FITNESS OF ELITE WRESTLERS

Korobeynikov G.V.[1], Latyshev S. V.[2], Latyshev N.V.[3], Korobeynikova L.G.[1], Goraschenko A.U.[4]
[1]National University of Physical Education and Sport of Ukraine
[2]Rostov State University of Civil Engineering
[3]Donetsk National University
[4]State University of Physical Education and Sport the Republic of Moldova

Abstract. *Purpose:* to determine and formulate general technical-tactic laws (rules) of competition duel in modern free style wrestling. *Material:* competition functioning of free style wrestlers at Olympic Games has been analyzed. Results of authors' own pedagogic observations and advanced experience of free style wrestling specialists have been generalized. *Results:* it was found that victory in duel can be resulted only from attacking tactic of duel. It was determined that wrestlers' activity (quantity of actual attacks in unit of time) varies from 1 to 2.2 attacks per minute. Reliability of attack (ratio of quantity of assessed attacks to quantity of actually fulfilled attacks) is within 0.33-0.63. Reliability of defense (ratio of quantity of successfully repelled opponent's attacks to general quantity of his actual attacks) is from 0.55-0.78. Efficiency of fighting in stance is within 0.6-1.3 points per minute. Efficiency of ground fighting is 1.3-2.3 points per minute. *Conclusions:* coach shall bring the formulated laws in compliance with specificity of his functioning and consider them, when planning training process of junior wrestlers.
Key words: wrestling, competition, laws, technique, tactic.

Introduction

In modern sports, only talented sportsman can achieve high international results. His talents, abilities and characteristics shall adequately correspond to requirements of modern competition functioning in the chosen kind of sports [7 - 10, 14, 15].

This statement is true for all kinds of sports. For martial arts, its interpretation and practical realization have significant specificity. It is connected with the fact that genotype predisposition to martial arts is conditioned by sportsman's bents and systemic interconnection of practically all qualities (characteristics): anthropometrical, physical, psychic, social-psychological [7 - 9, 12, 13

With it, compensatory factor is rather substantial in sport wrestling, when some qualities can be compensated by other [7 - 9, 12, 15]. For example, deficit of strength can be compensated by high endurance or coordination and flexibility. It forms its individual style of combat, its peculiar technique. With it, level of separate motor qualities can substantially differ in wrestlers of close sportsmanship but different combat styles [7, 12, and 13].

Combat style is determined by dominantly expressed development of one or several motor qualities in combination with relevant features of sportsman's body composition and psyche. Every elite wrestler conducts successful duels strictly as per his own (individual) combat style (which is, as a rule, typical). It is the basis of his successful competition functioning [5 - 7]. Every typical combat style has its own features of competition technique and combat tactic [6 - 8].

Generalization of coaches' experience and results of competition functioning show that it is possible to outline the most general laws (rules) of competition duel's conduct. They are intrinsic to all elite wrestlers, independent on weight category or combat style in free style wrestling. These laws condition certain universal (for all elite wrestlers) requirements to technical-tactic fitness.

To large extent, coaches rely on their experience and do not consider universal requirements of technical-tactic training. Coaches often make mistakes in sequence of mastering and in accentuation of attention in process of technical-tactic training. In the whole, it is connected with coach's not systemic choice of trainings' content at stage of basic training. It often results in great losses in wrestler's sports functioning.

For optimization of trainings, coach shall clearly and definitely understand general laws, consequences of which determine methodic and practical aspects of technical-tactic training. They shall be considered by coach when making working programs and correcting of junior wrestlers' training. These facts condition the importance of our work.

Purpose, tasks of the work, material and methods

The purpose of the work is to determine general technical-tactic laws (rules) of competition duel in modern free style wrestling as well as to formulate universal requirements to wrestler's technical-tactic fitness.

Materials and methods of the research: generalization of results of analysis of scientific-methodic literature, pedagogic observations, video-analysis of competition duels and specialists' advanced experience.

Results of the research

We have analyzed competition functioning of free style wrestlers at Olympic Games [2 - 4, 11]. Besides, we generalized results of own pedagogic observations and advanced experience of free style wrestling specialists [1, 7 - 9, 12, 13]. It permitted to outline general laws of competition duel's conduct and present some universal principles of elite wrestlers' technical – tactic fitness. Below we give these laws and principles (requirements).

1.Wrestling stance

Stance is main position in initial period of contact with opponent, when wrestler touches mat only by feet. Adequacy (correctness) of wrestling stance is initial condition of combat effectiveness and of duel in general. Elite wrestler conduct duels in reliable for defense and convenient for attack wrestling stance. Such stance can be called "correct" and adequate to combat conditions.

"Correct" wrestling stance implies steady wrestler's position under external impacts imposed by opponent. It shall permit easy maneuvering and quick transition to attack, defense or counter-attack. It is achieved at the account of wrestler's body weight uniform distribution on all foot and proper position of legs and torso.

Usually wrestler's feet are located at one and half shoulder width. With it one foot (by half of its length) is in front of the other. It ensures required (reliable) stability when opponent tries to imbalance wrestler forward-backward or to the right-to the left. Legs shall be compulsory bent a little in knees (with angle between ankle and hip of about 150-165°) and relaxed for timely attacks and defenses.

Torso shall be bent in respect to the line of horizon. It ensures defense of legs against opponent's attacks and prevents from headlock or capture of arm by opponent. Angle of torso bent shall be kept during all duel period in spite of increasing fatigue. The value of angle is chosen, considering wrestler's anthropometric characteristics.

Arms shall be bent in elbows (approximately by 90°) and their projection on mat shall be approximately by length of hand in front of shoes' toes.

Specific features of wrestling stance and other technical and tactic actions on next stages of training are conditioned by choice of own individual combat style.

2. Distance

Distance of combat is chosen depending on combat style and for increasing convenience of duel conduct.

3. Moving on mat

Moving on mat is directed at seeking favorable moment for attack or advantageous position in respect to opponent. Elite wrestler usually moves forward, to the right or to the left in competition duel He tries to "press" opponent constantly with speed-power actions, with false attacks. With it, the main thing is to keep "correct" stance. Backing shall be excluded.

The mentioned law is realized in combat on the base of several requirements (conditions). When backing, it is practically impossible to fulfill efficient attack with face directed forward. Backing is punished by referees. If wrestler makes his opponent to back, he deprives him of possibility to attack. Active moving and onset ensure also psychological confidence in success of combat and initiative. It is especially important when equal by sportsmanship wrestlers are fighting.

4. Grasp

Grasp implies strong connection with body part of opponent or parts of own body for fulfillment of technique action or blocking of opponent's action. Fight for "own" grasp and its hold are important components of duel. They can serve as parameters of competition functioning simulation. In such case time of being in own grasp is proportional to probability of actual attack and saving advantages. Since the first seconds of combat successful wrestler tries to fulfill (to impose) own grasp. Grasp can be attacking (as a rule) and blocking. In such grasp opponent can not fulfill attack. He must impose his own grasp. It requires additional efforts.

In general case (60% of time sportsman is in his own grasp and 40% - in opponent's grasp) wrestler has 1.5 times more opportunities to execute attack and not to admit opponent' attack.

5. Attacking actions

Attacking actions are the basis of attacking strategy. It is a determining one in building of modern duel in free style wrestling. Attack consists of various preparatory actions and attacking technique (resulting part). Means of technical tactic preparation for technique's fulfillment are rather various. With it, techniques have rather stable space time and power structure. Preparation for technique's fulfillment is directed to distraction of opponent's attention from actual attack. Elite wrestler shall have in his arsenal minimum 2-3 (better 3-4) main technical-tactic actions (TTA) for fighting in stance. With it, these TTA shall be selected so that wrestler should be able to attack opponent from the right and from the left. This condition is compulsory, when selecting attacking TTA for their perfection. Junior wrestler will never become elite sportsman, if he can fulfill attacks only from one side. For elite wrestler it is very easy to defend reliably one side.

It is desirable for wrestler to have in arsenal of main techniques minimum one throw. It can be applied at the beginning of combat, when opponent is not too sweaty and grasp can be fulfilled reliably. Thus, it is possible to receive significant advantage. Throw also can be applied at the end of fight, when fight result can not be saved by one or two points and it is necessary to risk and fulfill throw.

For ground fighting sportsman shall be able to fulfill minimum one (better two-three) main techniques, connected with each other. There are some elite sportsmen (Olympic champions), who do not fulfill any TTA in ground fighting. But it is an exclusion from the rules.

Elite wrestler shall be able to fulfill main techniques in fight with any opponent of his weight category minimum 1-2 times.

6. Defense actions

Defense actions are the main confusing factor, hindering opponent's TTA. With active usage of own body parts, in defense wrestler destroys opponent's attack and tries to quickly create convenient situation for counter attack.

Characteristic (distinctive) feature of elite wrestlers is psycho-physiological ability to fight to the end. Analysis of competition functioning and accumulated experience shows that even in completely losing positions elite wrestlers do not lose points and even can win. It is explained by the fact that in fight for points sportsmen are in state of maximal physical and psychic-emotional tension. Sportsmen spend forces very quickly. That is why, in such conditions opponent can simply feel lack of forces for efficient completion of TTA or he can make mistake, caused by fatigue.

In ground fighting reliability of elite wrestlers' defense is ensured practically by 100%. Losing of points by elite wrestler in ground fighting is connected with occasional factors. Such high reliability of defense is conditioned by the fact that defense requires much less efforts. That is why it is much easier not to lose points (i.e. neutralize opponent's efforts) than to win points (i.e. to create favorable conditions for attack and fulfill it).

7. Counter attacking actions

Counter attacking actions are responding TTA after organization of defensive actions or for anticipation of opponent's attack. Success of counter attacking actions is ensured by high quickness and coordination.

Elite wrestler shall have carefully trained technique of responsive attack in response to opponent's attack by legs. Responsive attacks (as system of counter attacking actions) can be conventionally divided into three groups, depending on how quickly the attacked wrestler responds to attack; in which phase of attack he meets the opponent.

First group - the attacked wrestler responds practically immediately. He fulfills counter movement, followed by overturn by twisting. Second group – the attacked wrestler responds a little later and, having met the opponent, he fulfills attack to legs (to the nearest leg of opponent). Third group – the attacked wrestler responds too late and responsive attack implies positioning behind the opponent.

8. Fighting in "standard" positions

In every fight wrestlers get in some, rather definite positions, for several times. These typical positions are called "standard". In such standard positions wrestler shall be able to fight as per perfectly trained patterns. Let us regard two standard positions, which are met very often.

The first position appears, when wrestler grasped leg and did not manage to finish technique (because of opponent's timely defense). In 80% elite wrestler brings fulfillment of this TTA to referee's assessment. The second position is grasping of head and shoulder. It appears, when wrestler tries to attack opponent's legs, but the opponent timely responds (does not permit for attacking wrestler to grasp legs). In this position attacking wrestler shall be able to realize reliable (practically in 100% of cases) defense. Wrestling in the mentioned positions shall be paid special attention to, when planning training of junior wrestlers.

9. Stance-ground fighting

Fight is started in stance. Since the first seconds fight is directed to move opponent into ground fighting.

With moving opponent into ground fighting, attacking wrestler always strives to fulfill technique in ground fighting, when opponent is not ready for defense.

Elite wrestler shall compulsory have this skill. We give two the most effective transitions from stance fighting to ground fighting as examples: 1 – attack of legs with head being outside, then transition to overturn; 2 – attack of legs with head being inside, then transition to overturn by twisting with cross grasp of shins.

Discussion

As analysis of competition functioning shows [2 - 4, 11] as well as experience of advanced specialists in sport wrestling [1, 7 - 9, 12, 13] only attacking tactic can result in victory. Defensive fighting is not intrinsic to elite wrestlers. It is acceptable only for preservation of score. In most cases in fighting, wrestler combines different kinds of tactic, depending on certain tasks, which he solves in definite moment of time. With it elite wrestler keeps mainly attacking tactic in competition duel.

For realization of attacking tactic wrestler shall meet the mentioned above 9 requirements. These results confirm and supplement the researches of other authors. For example, authors [12, 14] pay special attention to formation of "correct" stance. It is the basis of effective competition functioning.

In works [13, 15] authors accentuate attention on variability of preparatory actions and rather rigid structure of main technique of elite wrestler. It is confirmed by item 5 of our results.

Results, received in items 6, 7, 8, 9 supplement researches of authors [1, 8, 9, 12, 13, 15]. These data characterize distinctive features of elite wrestlers: ability to fight to the end (for points); having perfect responsive attacking techniques; ability to fight in standard positions; ability to realize transition from stance to ground fighting without pauses.

Training of elite wrestlers requires strict individualization [5, 6, 10, and 11]. Depending on style of combat, wrestler chooses the following: attacking and blocking grasps; distance of duel conduct; directions of moving on mat. With it, in choice there are general patterns, intrinsic to all elite wrestlers. They are presented in items 2, 3, 4 of our results.

Attacking style of duel conduct is intrinsic to all elite wrestlers. However, quantitative characteristics of competition functioning substantially depend on combat style. Analysis [2 - 4, 11] of wrestlers' competition functioning at Olympic Games shows that activity (quantity of actual attacks per unit of time) of wrestlers (who won 1-5 places) varies from 1 to 2.2 attacks per minute. Reliability of attack (ratio of assessed attacks to quantity of actually fulfilled attacks) is within 0.33-0.63. Reliability of defense (ratio of quantity of successfully repelled attacks to total quantity of actual attacks) is within 0.55-0.78. Efficiency of fighting in stance is within 0.6-1.3 points per minute. Efficiency of ground fighting is 1.3-2.3 points per minute.

Generalizing these data we can affirm that in stance fighting elite wrestler shall fulfill in average 4-5 actual attempts to fulfill technique. In this case every second-third attempt shall result in good points. Ground fighting is approximately two times more efficient than fight in stance. The formulated above regularities shall be complied by coach with specificity of his functioning and considered when planning training process of junior wrestlers.

Conclusions

On the base of analysis of competition functioning and generalization of experience of advanced specialists in sport wrestling we found and formulated general laws of competition duel conduct in modern free style wrestling. On this ground we presented universal peculiarities and requirements to technical-tactic fitness of elite wrestlers.

The prospects of further researches: the received results can be regarded as the basis for further profound analysis of competition functioning as well as for further specification and correction of working training programs at stages of basic training. It is anticipated development of definite training tasks on technical tactic and on special physical fitness.

Conflict of interests

The authors declare that there is no conflict of interests.

References:

1. Korobeynikov GV, Radchenko UA. Osoblivosti tekhnichnoi pidgotovlenosti borciv greko-rims'kogo stiliu visokoi kvalifikacii [Specific features of technical fitness of Greco-Roman elite wrestlers]. *Pedagogics, psychology, medical-biological problems of physical training and sports*, 2009;7:81–85. (in Russian)
2. Latishev NV, Latishev SV, Gavrilin VA. Analiz sorevnovatel'noj deiatel'nosti finalistov igr XXIX Olimpiady v Pekine po vol'noj bor'be [Analysis of competition functioning of free style wrestlers-finalists of 29th Olympic Games]. *Teoriia i metodika fizichnogo vikhovannia*, 2008;1:173–180. (in Russian)
3. Latishev SV. Analiz taktiko-tekhnichnikh dij borciv vil'nogo stiliu na Igrakh XXVI Olimpiadi v Atlanti [Analysis of technical-tactic actions of free style wrestlers at 26th Olympic Games in Atlanta]. *Teoriia i metodika fizichnogo vikhovannia i sportu,* 2000;2–3:20–23. (in Ukrainian)
4. Latishev SV, Gromakov AU, Chocharay ZU. Sravnitel'nyj analiz kharakteristik sorevnovatel'noj deiatel'nosti borcov vol'nogo stilia na Olimpijskikh igrakh v Atlante i Sidnee [Comparative analysis of competition functioning characteristics of free style wrestlers at Olympic Games in Atlanta and Sydney]. *Pedagogics, psychology, medical-biological problems of physical training and sports*, 2001;2:45–52. (in Russian)
5. Latishev SV. Stili protivoborstva v sovremennoj vol'noj bor'be [Combat styles in modern free style wrestling]. *Fizichne vikhovannia, sport i kul'tura zdorov'ia u suchasnomu suspil'stvi*, 2011;1:69–73. (in Russian)
6. Latyshev S, Korobeynikov G, Korobeinikova L. Individualization of training in wrestlers. *International Journal of Wrestling Science*, 2014;4(2):28-33.
7. Latyshev SV. Kolichestvennaia ocenka kharakteristik uspeshnosti vedeniia poedinka dlia sportsmenov s razlichnymi stiliami protivoborstva v vol'noj bor'be [Quantitative assessment of characteristics of duel's success for different combat styles' wrestlers in free style wrestling], *Moloda sportivna nauka Ukraini,* 2011;15(1):168–174. (in Ukrainian)
8. Novikov AA. *Osnovy sportivnogo masterstva* [Principles of sportsmanship], Moscow: Soviet sport; 2012. (in Russian)
9. Piloyan RM. *Uzlovye voprosy mnogoletnej podgotovki borcov* [Key issues of many years' training of wrestlers], Moscow: MOGIFK; 1988. (in Russian)
10. Platonov VN. *Sistema podgotovki sportsmenov v olimpijskom sporte* [The system of preparation of sportsmen in Olympic sport], Kiev: Olympic Literature; 2004. (in Russian)
11. Podlivaev BA, Korzhenevsky A. Variation of the performance in qualified wrestlers in Greco-Roman wrestling by their level of functional skills. *International Journal of Wrestling Science*, 2013;3(2):14 - 21.
12. Tumanian GS. *Strategiia podgotovki chempionov* [Strategy of champions' training], Moscow: Soviet sport; 2006. (in Russian)
13. Shahmuradov UA. *Vol'naia bor'ba* [Free style wrestling], Moscow: High school; 1997. (in Russian)
14. Emma Sandberg, Natha T. Bell. *Coaching Youth Wrestling*. Illinois: Human Kinetics; 2007.
15. Ryan T, Sampson J. *Elite Wrestling*. New York: McGraw–Hill; 2006.
16. Korobeynikov G, Mazmanian K, Korobeynikova L, & Jagiełło W. Psychophysiological states and motivation in elite judokas. *Archives of Budo,* 2010;6(3):129-136.

17. Korobeynikov GV, Radchenko YA. Demonstration of intuitive thinking in conditions of competitive activity depending on athletes' psychophysiological state. *Pedagogics, psychology, medical-biological problems of physical training and sports,* 2012;6:87-91.
18. Korobeynikova LG. Determinant of psychophysiological state of sportsmen of high qualification with different emotional characteristics. *Pedagogics, psychology, medical-biological problems of physical training and sports,* 2011;4:94-97.
19. Latyshev SV, Korobeynikov GV. Approach of the systems to problem of individualization of training of fighters. *Physical Education of Students*, 2013;5:65-68. http://dx.doi.org/10.6084/m9.figshare.771109
20. Zapovitriana EB, Korobeynikov GV, Korobeinikova LG. Peculiarities of vegetative regulation of heart rate in wrestlers of different age groups. *Pedagogics, psychology, medical-biological problems of physical training and sports,* 2015;4:22-26. http://dx.doi.org/10.15561/18189172.2015.0404

10

PSYCHOLOGICAL MEANS OF RECREATION SPORTSMEN'S PSYCHIC WORKABILITY

Gant H.Y., Orlenko O.M.
Kharkov State Academy of Physical Culture

Abstract. *Purpose:* to study recreation of sportsmen's psychic workability under influence of psychological methods. *Material:* Students-sportsmen, practicing boxing and kickboxing (n=45, age17-23 years) participated in he research. Express assessment methodic for "Self-feeling, activity and mood", "Correcting tests" was used. *Results:* sportsmen's subjective assessment of own state depends on the stage of competition functioning. This assessment is rather favorable in pre-competition and competition periods. In pre-competition period unconscious weakening of psychic workability happens. Psychic workability weakening in competition period is of functional character and can be reduced in post-competition period. *Conclusions:* application of art-therapeutic methodic results in sportsmen's more recreated, relaxed and hardy. Singing and drawing can be used as the method of stabilization of sportsmen's activity, mood and self-feeling.
Key words: art therapy, psychology, sportsmen, boxing, psychic workability.

Introduction

Recent time the problem of human psychic activity regulation has been attracting attention of many researchers. Importance of this problem is determined by its significance for solution of many tasks of fundamental and applied psychology. Indeed, human ability to control own functioning for solution of the chosen tasks is of key importance for its adaptation in different life activity and sports spheres [24, 29, 31]. Solution of this problem is of special importance in physical education of youth [6].

In modern society high requirements are set to sportsman on development of his regulatory processes, which would permit for him to be a genuine subject of own behavior and to independently determine own prospects [4, 5, 7]. Formation of sportsmen's abilities of psychic self-regulation is important for maximal realization of their potentials in extreme conditions of sports functioning. Among factors of self regulation mechanisms' formation central place belongs to psychic workability, which determines direction and level of subject's functioning [17, 22]. Such functioning is a component of martial arts sportsmen's training [1, 26]. In this case it is necessary to objectively assess sportsmen's potentials for quick recreation of his physical and psychic workability. Recreation of psychic workability takes more time than recreation of physical workability. That is why one of promising directions of the research is study of psychic functioning arbitrary regulation in stress conditions. It was found that absence of ability for arbitrary regulation of psychic functioning under stress factors' influence is one of reasons of sportsmen's affective and behavioral dysfunctions [20, 22, 28].

Analysis shows that ability of psychic workability recreation is the basic component of sportsmen's successful psychological training. It ensures holistic training and competition processes in martial arts [15, 20, 26]. Alongside with it, at present there are no systemized ideas about laws of psychic workability's effective recreation mechanisms' formation in martial arts in training and competition periods. The question of training and competition extreme conditions' influence on sportsmen's functional state has been remaining practically not studied. It emphasizes on the urgency of this research. Need in scientific working out of tools for complex assessment of sportsmen's psychic workability is evident. Its important component is development of programs for recreation of sportsmen's psychic workability at different stages of sports functioning. For solution of this, rather difficult, circle of problems special complex psycho-diagnostic study, oriented on analysis of the whole spectrum of sportsmen's psychic workability mechanisms, is required. It is of great significance for working out the program of sportsmen's psychic workability recreation and for predicting their professional functioning successfulness.

The purpose of the work is to study recreation of sportsmen's psychic workability under influence of psychological means.

Material and methods

Participants: students-sportsmen, practicing boxing and kickboxing (n=45, age17-23 years) participated in he research. Among them there were 19 elite sportsmen. Randomly the sportsmen were divided into 2 groups: control and experimental.

Organization of the research: the research was carried out in several stages. For studying psychic workability (concentration of attention, stability of attention, re-switching of attention) in control and experimental groups we used methodic (Correction tests). Testing was conducted: before training, just after training and 40 minutes after training. We used special forms with lines of randomly located letters. Sportsmen looked through the form line by line and crossed out the pointed in instruction letters. With it (after every 60 seconds) by command they marked the looked through quantity of letters by vertical line [23]. The methodic of express assessment of self-feeling, activity and mood (SAM) was used for assessment of sportsmen's actual state. The sportsmen were offered to describe their state in the given moment with the help of table, consisting of 30 pairs of polar qualities. In every pair it was necessary to choose the quality, which describes sportsman's state the most accurately and mark the number, which corresponds to degree of this characteristic's expressiveness [17].

The next stage of the research was study of art-therapeutic techniques for recreation of sportsmen's psychic workability. Experimental group sportsmen were offered to sing in chorus: just after training; during changing cloth and hygienic procedures. After singing sportsmen assessed their mood, state and activity by SAM scale [17] and fulfilled methodic "Correcting tests" [23].

Besides, as art-therapeutic methodic for sportsmen's psychic workability recreation we used technique "Intuitive drawing". This technique implies topic-free drawing. Experimental group sportsmen were offered to draw picture just after training. Drawing shall be fulfilled alternatively by right and left hands wit open and closed eyes. Topics and materials were chosen by sportsmen independently. Time for picture drawing was unlimited. After drawing sportsmen assessed their mood, state and activity by SAM scale [17] and passed "Correcting tests" [23].

Statistical analysis: for every studied indicator we calculated mean values and mean square deviation. Confidence of differences between mean values was determined by Student's t-criterion at 1% and 5% of significance levels [11].

Results of the research

Before training process we found in sportsmen the following: mean values of "self-feeling" indicators (good self-feeling) (5.93±1.07); feeling own strength (5.93±0.73); feeling workability (5.71±1.44); feeling power (5.50±1.29); cheerfulness (5.14±1.10); feeling hardy (5.29±1.68); feeling healthy (6.07±1.00). These indicators were at satisfactory level. After training sportsmen felt certain fatigue (3.07±1.73); exhausted (3.79±1.19); very tired (3.71±1.82) and more tensed (4.00±1.11). After singing experimental group sportsmen note that they are more fresh (5.33±1.44) and hardier (5.58±1.16). By these maximal indicators differences were not confident ($p<0.05$). Besides, they not that they are rested (5.33±1.44) and more relaxed (5.58±1.16) (differences are confident at $p<0.05$). After drawing pictures control group sportsmen noted wish to work (4.71±1.89) and increased attention (5.71±0.87). In pre-training period mean values of this criterion stabilized up to initial level (differences are not confident, $p>0.05$).

In pre-training period the following mean values of indicators are at rather satisfactory level: "activity" (feeling of activity-passivity, 5.43±1.16); mobility (5.57±1.28); quickness (5.14±1.17); wish to function (5.50±1.09); feeling of indifference-enthusiasm (5.46±0.93); indifference – excitement (4.79±1.19); drowsiness – excitement (4.00±1.62); distraction –attention (5.07±1.21). Just after training mean values of indicators "activity" differ from mean values of "activity" before training: sportsmen feel themselves less quick (4.86±1.03); more distracted (4.93±1.21); having wish to rest (3.57±1.91). With it this differences are not confident. Confident differences were in indicator: feel more excited (5.29±1.68), than before training.

40-60 minutes after singing technique sportsmen note growth of wish to work (4.58±1.78). Mean values by this criterion are stabilized up to initial level in pre-training period (differences are not confident, $p>0.05$). Besides, there is confident reduction by indicators "drowsiness-excitement" (3.33±1.83). 40-60 minutes after drawing pictures' technique experimental group sportsmen not increased wish to work (4.71±1.89). Mean indicators by this criterion stabilize up to initial level in pre-training period (difference are not confident, $p>0,05$).

In pre-training period rather at satisfactory level are indicators "mood": feeling joyful-sad (5.50±1.70); happy-unhappy (5.89 ±1.18); cheerful-cheerless (5.57±1.34); satisfied (5.86±1.03); full of hopes (5.57±1.70). By results of after training testing we registered rising of mood (6.14±1.10), enthusiasm (5.29±1.07), feeling of satisfaction (6.29±1.07) but weakening of optimism (5.57 ±1.28) and state of relaxation (4.79±1.42). The differences are not confident (p>0,05).

After "Song" technique, before training sportsmen's indicators are higher than initial training: "happy" (6.42±0.51); "cheerful" (6.33±0.89); "joyful" (6.08±0.90). Indicators "calm" (5.42±1.24), "optimistic" (6.08±0.90) stabilized up to initial level. With it difference were confident at (p>0.05). After drawing, before training indicators by criteria "happy", "cheerful", "joyful" also increased higher than initial level and indicators be criteria "calm" and "optimistic" stabilized up to initial level with not confident differences at (p>0.05).

After application art-therapeutic techniques indicators of concentration of attention in control (58.3±5.9) and experimental (69.8±13.8) groups had statistically not confident differences at p>0.05. The same was with indicator of attention stability. Indicators of attention re-switching in control group were insignificantly lower than in experimental group (p>0,05).

Discussion

We received new data, permitting to timely correct content of sportsmen's psychological recreation program of in conditions of training process with the help of art-therapy. We found peculiar features of sportsmen's psychological workability, self-feeling, activity and mood on different stages of training process.

In opinion of S. Skeify indicators for art-therapy in sportsmen are: difficulties of emotional development, actual stress, depression, weakening of emotional tonus, emotional deprivation, lability, impulsivity of emotional reactions, feeling of emotional rejection, feeling of isolation, conflicts in interpersonal relations, non satisfaction in family, jealousy, increased anxiety, fears, phobias, low self-assessment, and low degree of self-perception [19]. In our study we used art-therapeutic techniques for recreation sportsmen's psychic workability.

Correcting potentials of art-therapy are connected with providing a client with practically unlimited opportunities for self-expression and self-realization in art [2, 8, 12, 16]. We found that after free singing and intuitive drawing pictures sportsmen's actual state improves. Free singing and intuitive drawing positively influenced on recreation of sportsmen's psychic workability. So we can say that art-therapeutic techniques can be used for recreation of sportsmen's psychic workability. It will permit to stabilize sportsmen's activity, mood and self-feeling.

General principles of art-therapy correction potentials are presented in works by A.I. Kopytin [12, 13]. When drawing pictures, client shall have opportunity to tell about the picture; to describe definite forms, objects, characters. Sportsman shall have opportunity to focus attention on colors. In other research it is noted that focusing on colors helps to understand actual emotions and feelings [10]. In drawing pictures we recommended sportsmen to pay special attention to the absent parts of picture and empty space on sheet as well as to tell about own feeling in the process of drawing, before it and after it. In research [12] author notes that client shall have opportunity to work in convenient for him temp. The client shall comprehend future picture and reflect his state in it. In our research we gave sportsmen opportunity to feel that they control drawing process and its results by themselves.

In other work it is noted that free singing positively influences on human targeted functioning. Positive emotional feelings, when singing pleasant melodies, strengthen attention, activate emotional central nervous system and stimulate intellectual activity [21]. Results of our research prove that free singing confidently improves sportsmen's mood.

A.I. Kopytin thinks that free singing and drawing are good stress-releasing and emotional stability keeping means. In free thinking and drawing those emotions are felt and splashed out, which can not be released even with tears [12]. We found that after singing or drawing sportsmen felt themselves fresher, headier, relaxed.

With it G. Ruthann [18] notes that singing favorite melodies positively influences on human targeted functioning. Such approach facilitates such organism's rhythmic tuning, which results in more effective processes in organism. Positive emotional feelings, when singing pleasant melodies, strengthen attention, activate central nervous system and stimulate intellectual activity [3, 13, 18, and 27].

The main criterion for psychological methods' selection for sportsmen' psychic workability recreation shall be desire of sportsmen themselves to sing or to draw [8]. In our study we determined effectiveness of the offered exercises and techniques for recreation of psychic workability. It permits to recommend their application in trainings and out of trainings.

Coaches are recommended to control main indicators of sportsmen's psychic workability during all year. It will permit to select effective means and methods of influence on the studied characteristics, the level of which determines sportsmen's readiness for effective interaction and high sport efficiency. Analysis of correlation of some indicators of sportsmen's functional state showed that in pre-competition period there is unconscious weakening of psychic workability. In conditions of competition functioning such weakening is of functional character and can be reduced in post-competition period.

Conclusions

Sportsmen's subjective assessment of their state depends on the stage of competition functioning as well as on pre- and post- competition periods.

After singing or drawing, sportsmen notice increase of freshness and relaxation of their state (5-7 minutes after training). Such indicators are absent in case of usual after-training rest (during 30-40 minutes). After singing, wish to work appears in sportsmen. Besides, indicators by criteria "happy", "cheerful", "joyful" increase up to level above initial (before training). In pre-training period we observed stabilization of indicators up to initial level by criteria "calmness", "optimistic". Singing and drawing can be used as method of sportsmen's psychic workability recreation. It stabilizes their activity, mood and self-feeling.

Conflict of interests

The authors declare that there is no conflict of interests.

References

1. Belykh SI. Effektivnye metody podgotovki kikbokserov [Effective methods of kick-boxers' training*], Slobozhans'kij naukovo-sportivnij visnik,* 2009; 3: 332–335 (in Russian)
2. Bekker-Glosh V. *Art-terapiia v aleksianerovskoj psikhiatricheskoj bol'nice* [Art-therapy in alexianery psychiatric hospital], Sankt Petersburg; 2001. (in Russian)
3. Burno ME. *Klinicheskaia psikhoterapiia* [Clinical psycho-therapy], Moscow; 2000. (in Russian)
4. Belykh SI, Eremenko VV, Marabian AV. *Usovershenstvovanie trenirovochnogo processa v khode podgotovki kikbokserov* [Perfection of training process in kick-boxers' training], Slobozhans'kij naukovo-sportivnij visnik, 2007; 11: 9–122. (in Russian)
5. Bleer AN. Psikhologicheskie faktory obespecheniia ustojchivosti psikhomotornykh dejstvij v edinoborstvakh [Psychological factors of psycho-motor actions' stability in martial arts]. *Sportivnyj psikholog*, 2008; 2: 26-30. (in Russian)
6. Gant OIe. Vpliv profesijnogo stresu na osobistist' sportsmeniv [Influence of professional stress on sportsmen's personalities]. *I Mizhnarodna konferenciia Ievrazijs'kogo naukovogo rozvitku, Viden', Avstriia, kviten' 2014* [1st International conference of Euro-Asian scientific development, Vienna, Austria, April, 2014], 2014. P. 250-255. (in Ukrainian)
7. Gant OIe. Vpliv situacii ekstremal'noi sportivnoi diial'nosti na samoocinku sportsmeniv [Influence of extreme sport functioning on sportsmen's self-assessment]. *XVIII regional'naia nauchno-prakticheskaia konferenciia uchitelej "Obrazovanie kak faktor formirovaniia innovacionnogo chelovecheskogo potenciala", Khar'kov, 14 aprelia 2012 g.* [18th regional scientific-practical conference of teachers "Education as factor of formation of human innovative potential", Kharkov, April 14, 2012], 2012. P. 64-69. (in Ukrainian)
8. Gant OIe. *Metodi art-terapii u roboti sportivnogo psikhologa* [Art-therapy methods in work of sports psychologist], Kharkiv: KHFAFK; 2014. (in Ukrainian)
9. Gant OIe, Malik IaK. Sportivna diial'nist' iak osoblivij vid profesional'nogo funkcionuvannia liudini [Sport functioning as special kind of human professional functioning]. *Problemi ekstremal'noi ta krizovoi psikhologii*, 2014;17: 62-73. (in Ukrainian)
10. Inkmann L, Kunst Haus Kannen. *Art-terapiia* [Art-therapy], Sankt Petersburg; 2001. (in Russian)
11. Kobzar' AI. *Prikladnaia matematicheskaia statistika* [Applied mathematical statistic], Moscow; 2006. (in Russian)
12. Kopytin AI. *Sistemnaia art-terapiia [*Systemic art-therapy], Sankt Petersburg; 2001. (in Russian)

13. Kopytin AI. *Teoriia i praktika art-terapii* [Theory and practice of art-therapy], Sankt Petersburg; 2002. (in Russian)
14. Makarov VV. *Lekcii po psikhoterapii.* [Lectures on psycho-therapy], Moscow; 2000.(in Russian)
15. MakNiff Sh. Tvorchestvo za ramkami privychnogo: rasshirenie vozmozhnostej psikhologicheskikh issledovanij s pomoshch'iu iskusstva [Creative work out of usual: expansion of potentials with the help of art], *Isceliaiushchee iskusstvo*, 2002;5(3):8-25. (in Russian)
16. Peredel'skij AA. *Sport i illiuziia sporta* [Sports and illusion of sports], Moscow; 2011. (in Russian)
17. Rajgorodskij DIa. *Prakticheskaia psikhodiagnostika* [Practical psycho-diagnostic], Samara: Bahrah-M; 2001. (in Russian)
18. Rutan Dzh, Stoun U. *Psikhodinamicheskaia gruppovaia psikhoterapiia* [Psycho-dynamic group psycho-therapy], Sankt Petersburg; 2002. (in Russian)
19. Skejfi S. *Dialektika art-terapii* [Dialectic of art-therapy], Sankt Petersburg; 2001. (in Russian)
20. Sopov VF. *Psikhicheskie sostoianiia v napriazhennoj professional'noj deiatel'nosti* [Psychic states in tensed professional functioning], Moscow: Triksta; 2005. (in Russian)
21. Uajteker P. Dvizhenie, improvizaciia i telesnye oshchushcheniia v art-terapii [Movements, improvising and body feeling in art therapy], *Isceliaiushchee iskusstvo*, 2002;5(1): 37-39. (in Russian)
22. Chikova OM. *Psikhologicheskie osobennosti sportivnoj deiatel'nosti i lichnosti sportsmena* [Psychological peculiarities of sport functioning and sportsman's personality], Minsk; 1993. (in Russian)
23. *Enciklopediia psikhodiagnostiki. Psikhodiagnostika vzroslykh.* [Encyclopedia of psycho-diagnostic. Psycho-diagnostic of adults]. Samara; 2009. (in Russian)
24. Aghyppo A, Tkachov S, Orlenko O. Role of physical education on the formation of a healthy lifestyle outside of school hours. *Journal of Physical Education and Sport*, 2016;16(2):335 – 339.
25. Belcaro G. Pycnogenol® Improves cognitive function, attention, mental performance and specific professional skills in healthy professionals age 35–55. *J Neurosurg Sci*, 2014;58: 239-248.
26. Förstl H. Boxing-acute complications and late sequelae: from concussion to dementia. *Dtsch Arztebl Int*, 2010;107(47): 835-839.
27. Gavett BE, Stern RA, McKee AC. Chronic traumatic encephalopathy: a potential late effect of sport-related concussive and subconcussive head trauma. *Clinics in sports medicine*, 2011;30(1): 179-188.
28. Iermakov S, Podrigalo L, Romanenko V, Tropin Y, Boychenko N, Rovnaya O, Kamaev O. Psycho-physiological features of sportsmen in impact and throwing martial arts. *Journal of Physical Education and Sport*, 2016;16(2):433–441. doi:10.7752/jpes.2016.02067
29. Luzzi R. Pycnogenol® supplementation improves cognitive function, attention and mental performance in students. *Panminerva medica*, 2011;53(3):75-82.
30. Neselius S. CSF-biomarkers in Olympic boxing: diagnosis and effects of repetitive head trauma. *PloS one*, 2012;7(4): 533-606.
31. Slobodanka Gašić-Pavišić, Snežana Joksimović, Dragan Janjetović. General Self-Esteem And Locus Of Control Of Young Sportsmen. *Zbornik Instituta za pedagoshka istrazhivana*, 2006;38:385-400.

11

FORMATION OF SELF-REGULATION CULTURE OF PHYSICAL EDUCATION FACULTY

Kudin S.F.
Chernigov National Pedagogical University

Abstract. *Purpose:* to experimentally substantiate effectiveness of pedagogic conditions of self-regulation culture formation of future physical culture teachers. *Material:* in the research 110 3rd year students of physical education faculty participated. The students were questioned. The level of students' anxiety was assessed. *Results:* Implementation of the author's course in educational process facilitated formation of students' self-regulation skills and abilities; raises confidence and self estimation; influences positively on functional state. It was found that students acquire ability to consciously observe their own verbal constructs of negative thinking and create positive alternatives. *Conclusions:* preparing of future physical culture teachers stipulates his (her) ability to effectively fulfill professional functioning in the aspect of health preservation. The necessary conditions of self-regulation culture formation are formation of students' holistic value-meaningful attitude to individual health and health of surrounding people.
Key words: physical culture, professional training, self-regulation, self-regulation culture.

Introduction

Protection and strengthening of children and youth's health are one of main tasks of social program in many countries. At present stage of Ukrainian society's development protection of young generation's health is still an acute question. Indicators and tendencies still remain unsatisfactory [15]. Realization of state policy of health protection also can not be considered excellent. It is proved by many scientific researches [13, 14, 18, and 20]. School shall create all conditions for health protection of its disciples. At the same time school also is rather specific risk factor in aspect of pupils' morbidity [1, 12]. Constant physical, intellectual and emotional overloads, stress situations cause discomfort in pupils and teachers [9].

Health, by its essences, shall be the first demand of man. But satisfaction of this demand has complex, contradictory character. It results not always in desirable way that is conditioned by many circumstances. In particular, health culture, as system of health control yet has not taken important place in hierarchy of demands and values of pupils and students [2, 4, 6, 7, 13, 15, 17, 19, 21-24].

Analysis of literature sources and the author's many years' experience in system of higher pedagogic education permits to speak about urgency of this problem. This problem is conditioned by contradiction between society's demand in physical culture teachers and insufficient level of scientifically substantiated approaches to formation of pupils', students' and teachers' self-regulation culture [3, 5, 8, and 11].

Purpose, tasks of he work, material and methods

The purpose of the work is to test experimentally effectiveness of pedagogic conditions of self-regulation culture formation of physical education faculty students.

The task of work is to test the author's training-methodic complex for students. The complex includes: working program, methodic recommendations on study of special course: Psycho-valueology", tasks for independent training, automated testing system "Camomile Net" for final control of knowledge [9, 10]. The logic of building of training work implies students' gradual mastering of the following: theoretical principles of human health and self-regulation; methodic of individual health assessment; practical skills of self-regulation, which can be used by future physical culture teachers in their professional functioning and everyday life. Important component of this course is worked out by the author methodic of studying of self-regulation theoretical principles and practical means of its application [10]. In formation of self-regulation skills special accent was made on teaching students to conscious observation of own verbal constructs of negative thinking and on techniques of positive alternatives' construction.

In the research 3rd year 110 (82 boys and 28 girls) students of physical education faculty of Chernigov National Pedagogical University, named after T.G. Shevchenko, participated. In experiment we used observation methods, talks, questioning, and psycho-diagnostic testing of students' anxiety by methodic of anxiety's assessment of Spielberg Ch.D. and Khanin Yu.L.; experts' assessment and self assessment of emotional self-feeling by the worked out by the author scale

[9]; statistical methods. Confidentiality of results was assessed by Student's criterion.

Results of research

For determination of effectiveness of self-regulation culture formation's pedagogic conditions we questioned students of experimental group. Analysis of questioning results (see table 1) showed that students' awareness of modern self-regulation means is rather low (18.1%). However, significant part of students would like to acquire knowledge in this field for stabilization of individual psycho-emotional state (47.1%). Students consider it an important component of their professional qualities (40.6%).

Table 1. Questioning results, %

Questions	Answers		
	Yes	No	Difficult to answer
Do you know modern self-regulation means?	18.1	28.2	53.7
Is it necessary to study in the courses of principles of medical knowledge, valueology, psycho-valueology, psycho-physiology, principles of self-regulation?	48.5	23.4	28.1
Do you think that self-regulation could help you in your future profession?	40.6	22.9	36.5
Do you think that self-regulation techniques can help you to better regulate own psychic and physical condition in everyday life?	47.1	13.3	39.6

Effectiveness of our methodic is witnessed about by results of diagnostic of students' anxiety at control stage of research (see table 2). In experimental group we found no confident differences between anxiety indicators (2.76%, $p<0.05$); in control group anxiety indicator increased by 24.86%, with high degree of confidence ($p<0.001$).

Table 2. Indicators of students' anxiety

Group	Stating stage	Control stage	Differences		
	M±m		Absolute	%	p
Experimental group	33.49±0.76	34.48±0.574	-0.99	2.76	>0.05
Control group	33.52±0.653	42.29±1.217	-8.76	24.86	<0.001

Notes: M – mean arithmetic; m – mean error of mean arithmetic; p –coefficient of confidence of differences.

Reduction of anxiety indicators in experimental group we explain by students' ability to consciously use self-regulation means. In control group anxiety indicator was higher. It can be connected with the fact that finish of training process and start of examination session create situations of increased intellectual and emotional overloads for students. With it not skilled in self-regulation students can not always resist such overloads. On control stage of experiment we conducted diagnostic of self-feeling of experimental and control groups' students before and after special course "Psycho-valueology". Comparative results are given in table 3.

Table 2. Indicators of students' self-feeling

Group	Stages	Self-feeling (points) M±m Before experiment	After experiment	Differences Absolute	%	t	p
Experimental	Stating	3.28 ± 0.123	3.36 ± 0.114	0.08	2.4	0.47	>0.05
	Control	3.96 ± 0.108	4.68 ± 0.095	0.72	18.2	5.00	<0.001
Control	Stating	3.40 ± 0.115	3.68 ± 0.125	0.28	8.2	1.64	<0.05
	Control	3.76 ± 0.133	3.60 ± 0.115	0.16	44.3	.0.91	>0.05

Notes: M – mean arithmetic; m – mean error of mean arithmetic; p –coefficient of confidence of differences.

After special course, indicators of experimental group students showed positive dynamic at control stage: improved by 17.3% ($p<0.001$). Marks were in the range: "self-feeling is better than usually" and "good self-feeling". It confirms effectiveness of our methodic. In control group, self-feeling indicators improved only by 4.1%. It also witnesses about effectiveness of our methodic. Thus, acquiring of self-regulation skills facilitated improvement of students' emotional and general condition.

Indicators of self-regulation culture's formation are ability to control own psycho-emotional state and conscious readiness to apply required means for this purpose. We determined indicators by self-assessment of theoretical knowledge formation, by students' practical and professional skills. They also were determined by experts' assessment of theoretical knowledge, practical and professional skills in application of self-regulation means. Comparative analysis is given in table 4.

Table 4. Students' readiness to apply self-regulation means (points)

Kinds of readiness	Assessment of readiness	Stating stage M ± m	Control stage M ± m	Absolute	%	t	p
Theoretical	Self-assessment	1.30±0.093	2.25±0.093	-0.95	70.0	6.73	<0.001
	Experts' assessment	1.33±0.095	1.90±0.123	-0.57	40.8	3.50	<0.001
Practical	Self-assessment	1.45±0.09	1.90±0.123	-0.46	30.1	2.78	<0.001
	Experts' assessment	1.41±0.097	2.18±0.088	-0.77	52.1	5.39	<0.001
Professional	Self-assessment	1.30±0.09	2.13±0.100	-0.83	61.6	5.81	<0.001
	Experts' assessment	1.33±0.09	2.29±0.095	-0.95	68.0	6.73	<0.001

Notes: M – mean arithmetic; m – mean error of mean arithmetic; p –coefficient of confidence of differences.

By criterion of theoretical readiness students' self-assessment increased by70.0%, experts' assessment increased by 40.8%. By criterion of practical readiness (which characterizes students' ability to use self-regulation complex for stabilization of own psycho-emotional state) self assessment increased by 31.6%. Experts' assessment increased by 52.1% that was higher than students' self assessment.

Discussion

Professional training of future physical culture teachers in modern conditions implies training of specialist, capable to fulfillment certain social role and his (her) readiness to form the culture of control of individual health in their disciples. It is that we call culture of self-regulation. In this important activity good results are not possible at the account of one or several methods' application [3, 11, and 16]. In process of health's formation and strengthening it is important to remember about complex character of the approach [15].

We completely support scientific approaches of specialists, who search pedagogic ways of health related technologies' implementation in educational system. The authors regard this process in wide cultural aspect [4, 14]. Our approach means that with determination of pedagogic conditions of health related technologies' implementation, accent shall be put on formation of students' conscious, value-oriented attitude to own health and health of surrounding people [13, 14, and 15]. With such approach we create conditions for preservation and strengthening of rising generation's health as well as for possible solution of socially important problem – overcoming of crisis of culture – by future generations.

Conclusions:

1. Training of future physical culture teacher envisages his (her) readiness to effectively fulfill professional functioning in health-related aspect. That is why formation of self-regulation culture is an integral component element of his (her) professional competence.
2. Formation of students' value-meaningful attitude to individual health and health of surrounding people are the necessary conditions of self-regulation culture's formation.
3. The conducted by us experimental research showed that implementation of special course "Psycho-valueology" in practice of physical culture teachers' training gives positive health related effect.

Acknowledgements:

The research has been fulfilled as per topic of Chernigov National Pedagogical University, named after T.G. Shevchenko "Methodological principles of future physical culture teachers' professional training to culture of healthy life style formation in modern youth" (state registration №0110U000020 dt. January 29, 2010).

Conflict of interests

The author declares that there is no conflict of interests.

References:

1. Balakirieva OM, Bondar TV, Artiukh OR. *Stan ta chinniki zdorov'ia ukrains'kikh pidlitkiv* [Condition and factors of Ukrainian adolescents' health], Kiev: KIS; 2011. (in Ukrainian)
2. Bashavec' NA. *Teoretiko-metodichni zasadi formuvannia kul'turi zdorov'iazberezhennia iak svitogliadnoi oriientacii studentiv vishchikh ekonomichnikh navchal'nikh zakladiv. Dokt. Diss.* [Theoretical-methodic principles of formation of health protection culture as world vision orientation of higher economic educational establishments' students. Dokt. Diss.], Odessa; 2012. (in Ukrainian)
3. Golenkova IuV. *Samoreguliaciia iak faktor formuvannia majbutnikh vchiteliv fizichnoi kul'turi. Cand. Diss.* [Self-regulation as factor of formation of future physical culture teachers. Cand. Diss.], Kharkiv; 2011. (in Ukrainian)
4. Gorashchuk VP. *Teoretichni i metodologichni zasadi formuvannia kul'turi zdorov'ia shkoliariv. Dokt. Diss.* [Theoretical and methodological principles of formation of pupils' health culture. Dokt. Diss.], Kharkiv; 2004. (in Ukrainian)
5. Grin'ova MV. *Teoretichni osnovi doslidzhennia zmistu samoreguliacii diial'nosti liudini* [Theoretical principles of research of human self-regulation content]. Vitoki pedagogichnoi majsternosti, 2010;7:73–77. (in Ukrainian)
6. Dzhurins'kij PB. *Teoretichni i metodichni zasadi pidgotovki majbutnikh uchiteliv fizichnoi kul'turi do zdorov'iazberezhuval'noi profesijnoi diial'nosti. Dokt. Diss.* [Theoretical and methodic principles of future physical culture training to health protective professional functioning. Dokt. Diss.], Odessa; 2013. (in Ukrainian)
7. Iezhova OO. *Zdorov'iazberigaiucha diial'nist' v osvitnikh zakladakh* [Health related functioning in educational establishments]. Osvitni innovacii, 2007;1:61–66. (in Ukrainian)
8. Kudin SF, Savonova OV. Dosvid roboti z formuvannia valeologichnogo svitogliadu majbutnikh pedagogiv [Practical experience in formation of valuelogic world vision of future pedagogues]. *Visnik Chernigivs'kogo derzhavnogo pedagogichnogo universitetu*, 2005;28:15–19. (in Ukrainian)
9. Kudin SF. *Osnovi psikhovaleologii* [Principles of psycho-valueology], Chernihiv: CSPU Publ.; 2005. (in Ukrainian)
10. Kuz'omko LM, Kudin SF, Savonova OV. *Psikhovaleologiia* [Psycho-valueology], Chernihiv: CSPU Publ.; 2007. (in Ukrainian)

11. Lisenko-Gelemb'iuk KM. *Samoreguliaciia iak chinnik rozv'iazuvannia mizhosobistisnikh konfliktiv students'koi molodi. Cand. Diss*. [Self-regulation as factor of solution of students' inter-personal conflicts. Cand. Diss.], Kiev; 2011. (in Ukrainian)
12. Nosko MO, Bojko DO, Diatlov VO. *Vishcha pedagogichna osvita i nauka Ukraini* [Higher pedagogic education and science in Ukraine], Kiev: Knowledge of Ukraine; 2012. (in Ukrainian)
13. Nosko MO, Grishchenko SV, Nosko IuM. *Formuvannia zdorovogo sposobu zhittia* [Formation of healthy life style], Kiev: MP Lesya; 2013. (in Ukrainian)
14. Nosko MO, Iermakov SS, Garkusha SV. Teoretiko-metodichni aspekti zmicnennia fizichnogo zdorov'ia uchnivs'koi ta students'koi molodi [Theoretical-methodic aspects of strengthening of pupils' and students' physical health]. *Visnik Chernigivs'kogo nacional'nogo pedagogichnogo universitetu*, 2010;76:243–247. (in Ukrainian)
15. Nosko MO, Garkusha SV, Voiedilova OM. *Zdorov'iazberezhuval'ni tekhnologii u fizichnomu vikhovanni* [Health related technologies in physical education]. Kiev: SPD Savchinska N.V.; 2014. (in Ukrainian)
16. Titarenko EV. *Professional'naia podgotovka budushchikh specialistov fizicheskoj kul'tury na osnove kompleksa sredstv psikhoreguliacii. Cand. Diss*. [Professional training of future physical culture specialists on the base of complex of psycho-regulation means. Cand. Diss], Stavropol; 2006. (in Russian)
17. Iermakova TS. Education of children in Polish family in a context of forming health culture. *Pedagogics, psychology, medical-biological problems of physical training and sports,* 2014;11:17–22. http://dx.doi.org/10.15561/18189172.2014.1104
18. Iermakova TS. Development of the idea of forming health culture of a person in the world educational thought. *Pedagogics, psychology, medical-biological problems of physical training and sports*, 2014;4:8–12. http://dx.doi.org/10.6084/m9.figshare.950949
19. Iermakova TS. The peculiarities of work of the European network of health promoting schools (comparative analysis). *Pedagogics, psychology, medical-biological problems of physical training and sports*, 2013;10:93–96. doi:10.6084/m9.figshare.775339
20. Ivashchenko OV, Yermakova TS. Assessment of functional, coordination and power fitness of 7–8 form boys. *Pedagogics, psychology, medical-biological problems of physical training and sports*. 2015;9:20–25. http://dx.doi.org/10.15561/18189172.2015.0903
21. Ivashchenko OV, Yermakova TS, Cieslicka M, Muszkieta R. Discriminant analysis as method of pedagogic control of 9–11 forms girls' functional and motor fitness. *Journal of Physical Education and Sport,* 2015;15(3):576–581.
22. Ivashchenko OV, Yermakova TS. Structural model of in-group dynamic of 6–10 years old boys' motor fitness. *Pedagogics, psychology, medical-biological problems of physical training and sports,* 2015;10:24–32. http://dx.doi.org/10.15561/18189172.2015.1004
23. Yermakova TS. Individualization of forming health culture in schoolchildren of Polish schools. *Pedagogics, psychology, medical-biological problems of physical training and sports,* 2015;1:29–33. http://dx.doi.org/10.15561/18189172.2015.0106
24. Żukowska Hanna, Szark-Eckardt Mirosława, Muszkieta Radosław, Iermakova TS. Characteristics of body posture in the sagittal plane and fitness of first-form pupils from rural areas. *Pedagogics, psychology, medical-biological problems of physical training and sports*, 2014;7:50–60. http://dx.doi.org/10.6084/m9.figshare.1015583

12

MODERN METHODIC OF POWER CARDIO TRAINING IN STUDENTS' PHYSICAL EDUCATION

Osipov A.Yu. [1,2], Kudryavtsev M.D. [1,3,5], Kramida I.E. [3], Iermakov S.S. [4], Kuzmin V.A. [1], Sidorov L.K. [5]
[1] Siberian Federal University, Russia
[2] V.F. Voino-Yasenetsky Krasnoyarsk State Medical University, Russia
[3] Siberian State Aerospace University, Russia
[4] Kazimierz Wielki University, Poland
[5] Krasnoyarsk State Pedagogical University of V.P. Astafyev, Russia

Abstract. *Purpose:* significant increase of students' physical condition and health level at the account of application of modern power cardio training methodic. *Material:* 120 students (60 boys and 60 girls) participated in the research. The age of the tested was 19 years. The research took one year. We used methodic of power and functional impact on trainees' organism (HOT IRON). Such methodic is some systems of physical exercises with weights (mini-barbells), to be fulfilled under accompaniment of specially selected music. *Results:* we showed advantages of power-cardio and fitness trainings in students' health improvement and in elimination obesity. Control tests showed experimental group students achieved confidently higher physical indicators. Boys demonstrated increase of physical strength and general endurance indicators. Girls had confidently better indicators of physical strength, flexibility and general endurance. Increase of control group students' body mass can be explained by students' insufficient physical activity at trainings, conducted as per traditional program. *Conclusions:* students' trainings by power-cardio methodic with application HOT IRON exercises facilitate development the following physical qualities: strength and endurance in boys and strength, flexibility and endurance in girls. Besides, it was found that such systems of exercises facilitate normalization of boys' body mass and correction of girls' constitution.
Key words: health, physical condition, students, physical education, power-cardio training, HOT IRON.

Introduction

Recent years there has been observed negative tendency to noticeable worsening of modern young people: students' and pupils' physical condition and health [11, 30]. K. Hardman in his works expresses serious trouble about significant falling of students' physical health standards and growth of obesity in developed European countries and developing countries of Africa and Asia [12, 13]. It was found that young people's excessive involvement in internet activity and computer games was a serious threat to their physical and psychic health [22-24]. For correction of this negative situation scientists recommend to raise everyday level of young people's physical functioning. However, specialists note that physical functioning level of most of young people does not correspond to optimal parameters. As per the data of D. Basset most of USA youth do not realize the recommended 60 minutes a day of physical functioning [4]. It is also noted that youth of Russian Federation has insufficient level of motor functioning [30]. In this connection it is necessary to introduce substantial changes in acting to day physical education programs for youth in educational establishments. In opinion of M. Chin, attitude to pedagogic aspects of physical education teaching in modern schools and universities shall be significantly re-thought for liquidation of global threats to health of our planet population – excessive weight and deficit of every day motor functioning [9].

The studies, conducted in a number of Norwegian universities witness that in the process of students' physical education it is necessary to use methodic, which would motivate young people for active participation in working out training programs, choosing form of classes and selecting physical exercises [1]. P. Sabramaniam also says about importance of development of students' interest to physical culture practicing. In his opinion students' interest to trainings can be noticeably increased at the account of changes of some aspects of young people's educational medium [34]. In general demand in substantial increase of students' motivation for regularly and active physical culture and sports practicing is discussed by many specialists [5, 21, 32, 33]. Chinese scientists L. Song and J. Chen note the absence of any interest to physical exercises in national HEEs students. It is connected with deficit of management and absence of encourage from physical education teachers [364]. Negative attitude to existing academic physical culture programs is demonstrated also by many American students [10].

The key to this problem's solution can be changes in physical education programs for students. Besides, it is necessary to raise the quality of young people's training. Rather important are modern training methodic, permitting for teachers to use new effective forms and methods of physical education in educational process. Scientists throughout the world discuss new styles of teaching in higher educational establishments [2, 3, 14-16]. The authors note that new styles of teaching permit for a student to actively participate in educational process and achieve the set targets with high effectiveness.

Specialists also note the absence of students' right for choosing the most favorable training programs in many higher educational establishments [37]. General orientation of physical education programs in higher educational establishments of Russian Federation, built on strict regulation of academic material is very serious pedagogic problem. Such orientation of physical education means and forms seriously restricts development of students' personal physical culture. It does not facilitate formation of their active interest to regular practicing physical culture and sports.

The demand in creation effective system of students' involvement in regular physical activity and healthy life style is pointed at by many scientists: A. Bolotin [6], Yu. Kopylov [18], A. Osipov [30, 31], M. Kudryavtsev [25, 26], I. Kramida [23], S. Iermakov [19, 20, 22, 27] et al. Modern fitness-technologies [35] and programs, based on power-cardio training can facilitate achievement of this target. It was found that significant part of modern youth desires to practice physical functioning. Such functioning includes dances, fitness-aerobic, power training in gyms. M. Byra affirms that active fitness-methodic can be successfully applied by HEE teachers in different forma of students' training [7]. Success of fitness-programs' application in students' health improvement is proved by studies of W. Chen [8]. Success of power-cardio programs' application in students' health improvement is proved by L. Konovalova [17].

Hypothesis: it is assumed that for successful solution of students' physical condition, physical fitness and health worsening it is necessary to change the form and methodic of physical culture classes in HEEs. It is offered to use methodic of power and functional training, known as HOT IRON. This methodic is a system of training exercises with mini barbells, oriented on increase of students' power endurance. The main exercises are: lunges with barbell on shoulders; squats with barbell; bench press of barbell, fulfilled under accompaniment of specially selected music. Positive effect of HOT IRON trainings are: reliable correction of body figure, loosing weight, growth of muscular tissues. Many scientists note that improvement of appearance (athletic body constitution, harmonious muscles and physical attractiveness) is an important stimulus for young people's regular trainings. This fact permits to use HOT IRON methodic in mixed and separate groups. It is known HOT IRON trainings can be practiced only with instructor\, who was trained in special centers and received appropriate certificate. That is why most of HOT IRON trainings are practiced in private fitness-centers, but not in educational establishments [29]. Therefore, HOT IRON application in education establishments is a kind of scientific novelty.

The purpose of the research: is significant increase of students' physical condition and health level at the account of application of modern power cardio training methodic.

Material and methods

Participants: 120 students (60 boys and 60 girls) participated in the research. The age of the tested was 19 years. All students gave consent for their participation in experiment.

Organization of the research: the researches were conducted in 2014-2015. The researches lasted one year. In training of experimental groups the author used methodic of power-cardio training on the base of HOT IRON program. The trainings were conducted by qualified instructors, who were trained in specialized HOT IRON centers. This fact guaranteed high quality of students' trainings. At the beginning of the research all students passed medical examination in university polyclinic and were admitted for physical trainings without any limitations. After it the tested were divided into 2 control groups (1st boys group and 3rd – girls' group) and 2 experimental groups (2nd – boys group and 4th- girls' group).

Control groups were trained on the base of sport and outdoor games. They were trained in gym. Experimental groups were trained as per HOT IRON programs under accompaniment of special music (power exercises with weight). At the beginning and at the end of the researches all students passed a number of control tests for assessment their physical condition and physical fitness. Strength was estimated by quantity of chin ups on horizontal bar (for boys) and quantity of pressing ups in lying position (for girls). Endurance was assessed by Cooper's test – running the most possible distance for 12 minutes. Flexibility was assessed by forward bending from position standing on pedestal< on which there were marks for measurements. Students fulfilled forward bent with straightened legs, touching the pedestal by hands fingers. !00 meters' run was used for assessment quickness.

Statistical analysis: was fulfilled with the help of SPSS program. Difference between mean values was found with Student's t-criterion.

Results

At the beginning of the research test results did not show any confident differences between experimental and control groups' students. At the end of experiment boys of experimental group were confidently far ahead of his peers from control group in strength (P<0.01) and endurance (P<0.05). Besides, difference in body mass values was also found. Body mass of experimental groups' students practically did not change. Body weight of control groups' students confidently increased (P<0.05). Results of boys' control tests are given in table 1.

Table 1. Physical condition and physical fitness indicators of the tested boys

Physical qualities	Before experiment		After experiment	
	Control group	Experimental group	Control group	Experimental group
Strength (chin ups, q-ty of times)	9±3	8±4	10±3	15±2**
Flexibility (forward bents, cm)	4±2	5±2	5±2	6±2
Quickness (100 meters' run, sec.)	13±4	14±4	13±2	12±4
Endurance (Cooper's test, km)	2.3 ±0.4	2.2±0.3	2.2±0.2	2.5±0.4*
Body mass, kg	72±4	73±3	77±4*	72±4

Notes: * - P<0.05; ** - P<0.01.

At the end of experiment girls of experimental group were confidently far ahead of his peers from control group in strength (P<0.01), flexibility (P<0.01) and endurance (P<0.05). Body mass of experimental group's girls confidently reduced (P<0.05). In control group the girls' body weight increased (P<0.05). The girls' control tests results are given in table 2.

Table 2. Physical condition and physical fitness indicators of the tested girls

Physical qualities	Before experiment		After experiment	
	Control group	Experimental group	Control group	Experimental group
Strength (chin ups, q-ty of times)	12±2	11±2	14±2	24±3**
Flexibility (forward bents, cm)	9±3	10±2	10±3	15±4**
Quickness (100 meters' run, sec.)	16±2	17±3	15±3	14±2
Endurance (Cooper's test, km)	1.8±0.4	1.9±0.4	2.0±0.3	2.3 ±0.4*
Body mass, kg	55±3	56±2	58±3*	53±2*

Notes: * - P<0.05; ** - P<0.01.

Discussion

The received data are interesting because they permit to objectively assess different programs of students' physical education. The results of the experiment coincide with the data of other studies [18, 24, 35]. The trainings by HOT IRON methodic demonstrate significant increment of students' physical strength and endurance. Increment of these indicators took place both in girls and boys. It permits to recommend such methodic for mixed contingent of trainees. Trainings based on traditional physical education programs (general physical training, sport and mobile games) do not permit to achieve significant results in training of physical qualities.

We registered disturbing tendency of body mass increase in control groups' students. The increase was in average from 3 to 4 kg. This tendency permits for the authors to agree with specialists' conclusions about insufficient effectiveness of the existing standard physical education programs for students [4, 9, 12, 36]. At classes conducted by HOT IRON methodic demonstrate preservation of body mass at previous level or its reduction within body figure correction. It permits for the authors to agree with statements of other specialists about advantages of power-cardio and fitness training in students' health protection and obesity liquidation. Students' body mass increase in control groups can be explained by insufficient physical functioning of young people on physical culture trainings, conducted by traditional program.

Specialists note that students' technical fitness in sport games is insufficient. Teachers have to spend a lot of time for training of the simplest technical elements instead of sport perfection and increase of trainees' game experience [11, 24, 28]. That is why motor density of such trainings remains to be low and students' motor functioning – insufficient.

Conclusions

The research permits to make the following conclusions:

1. Analysis of scientific data witnesses about substantial decrease of physical condition, physical fitness and health of most of modern young people. The sharpest threat, as considered by specialists, is deficit of youth's everyday motor functioning. The reasons of low physical functioning are: deficit of youth's motivation for regular practicing of physical exercises and absence of interest to acting in HEEs physical education programs.
2. For substantial increase of students' motivation for regular physical culture trainings at HEEs specialists recommend to apply new, effective forms and methods of physical education. Such methods can include students' physical culture trainings, based on power-cardio training. Successfulness of different fitness programs' application in students' health improvement is proved by domestic and foreign specialists.
3. For solution the problem of students' bad physical condition and health the author recommends to use HOT IRON exercises system at physical culture lessons in HEEs.

Conflict of interests

The author declares that there is no conflict of interests.

References:

1. Abildsnes E, Stea TH, Berntsen S, Omfjord CS, Rohde G. Physical education Teachers' and public health Nurses' perception of Norwegian high school Students' participation in physical education – a focus group study. BMC Public Health [Internet]. 2015 Dec [cited 2016 Nov 9]; 15(1). Available from: http://www.biomedcentral.com/1471–2458/15/1295
2. Adyrkhaev SG. Modern technology of physical education of disabled students in conditions of inclusive education. *Pedagogics, psychology, medical-biological problems of physical training and sports,* 2016; 1: 4-12. doi:10.15561/18189172.2016.0101
3. Al-Haliq M, Oudat M, Al-Taieb M. The effect of using video on developing physical fitness of physical education students at the Hashemite University. *Asian Social Science,* 2014; 10(1): 21–27. doi:10.5539/ass.v10n1p21
4. Basset D, Fitzhugh E, Heaz G, Erwin P, Frederick G, Wolff D, et al. Estimated energy expenditures for school-based policies and active living. *American Journal of Preventive Medicine,* 2013; 44(2): 108–113. doi:10.1016/j.amepre.2012.10.017
5. Bliznevsky AA, Kudryavtsev MD, Iermakov SS, Jagiełło W. Formation of active-effective attitude of 12-13 years' judo athletes to sports functioning in competition period. *Archives of Budo,* 2016;12: 101-115.
6. Bolotin A, Bakayev V. Structure and content of the educational technology of managing students' healthy life-style. *Journal of Physical Education and Sport,* 2015; 15(3): 362–364. doi:10.7752/jpes.2015.03054
7. Byra M, Sanchez B, Wallhead T. Behaviors of students and teachers in the command, practice, and inclusion styles of teaching. *European Physical Education Review,* 2014; 20(1): 3–19. doi:10.1177/1356336X13495999
8. Chen W, Mason S, Hypnar A, Hammond-Bennett A. Association of quality physical education teaching with students' physical fitness. *Journal of Sports Science and Medicine,* 2016; 5: 335–343.
9. Chin M, Edginton K. *Physical Education and Health: Global Perspectives and Best Practice*. Sagamore Publishing LLG; 2014.
10. Davis S. *Factors Influence High School Students' Enrollment in Elective Physical Education: A Mixed Method Study.* [PhD thesis]. 2016 [cited 2016 Nov 24]. Available from: http://digitalcommons.odu.edu/hms_etds/7
11. Gaskov AV, Kuzmin VA, Kudryavtsev MD, Iermakov SS. Successfulness of general and special physical qualities' development on different stage of students-boxers' training. *Physical Education of Students,* 2016;20(1):4–11. doi:10.15561/20755279.2016.0101
12. Hardman K. Physical education in schools: a global perspective. *Kinesiology,* 2008; 40(1): 5–28.

13. Hardman K. The situation of physical education in schools: A European perspective. *Human Movement,* 2008; 9(1): 5–18. doi:10.2478/v10038-008-0001-z
14. Iermakov SS, Arziutov GN, Jagiełło W. Quick training of students to judo techniques. *Archives of Budo,* 2016;12: 15-24.
15. Iermakov SS, Podrigalo LV, Jagiełło W. Hand-grip strength as an indicator for predicting the success in martial arts athletes. *Archives of Budo,* 2016;12: 179-186.
16. Ilchenko SS. Motor and sport components in hierarchy of non physical culture profile pedagogic specialties students leisure. *Pedagogics, psychology, medical-biological problems of physical training and sports*, 2016; 5: 33-37. doi:10.15561/18189172.2016.0505
17. Konovalova L. Fitness technology in physical education of students. *Modern Research of Social Problems,* [Internet]. 2013 [cited 2016 Nov 9]; 2013;7(27):26. doi:10.12731/2218-7405-2013-7-26 Available from: http://cyberleninka.ru/article/n/fitness-technology-in-physical-education-of-students
18. Kopylov Yu, Jackowska L, Kudryavtsev M, Kuzmin V, Tolstopyatov I, Iermakov S. The concept of structure and content of health related trainings for higher educational establishments' students. *Physical education of students,* 2015; 5: 23–30. doi:10.15561/20755279.2015.0504
19. Kopeikina EN, Drogomeretsky VV, Kondakov VL, Kovaleva MV, Iermakov SS. Modification of Harvard step-test for assessment of students' with health problems functional potentials. *Physical Education of Students*, 2016;20(4):44-50. doi:10.15561/20755279.2016.0405
20. Kozina ZL, Iermakov SS, Kadutskaya LA, Sobyanin FI, Krzeminski M, Sobko IN, Ryepko OA. Comparative characteristic of correlation between pulse subjective indicators of girl students' and school girls' reaction to physical load. *Physical Education of Students*, 2016;20(4):24-34. doi:10.15561/20755279.2016.0403
21. Kretschmann Rolf. Comparison of 9th grade students' physical activity levels during recess and regular class periods using objective measurement. *Pedagogics, psychology, medical-biological problems of physical training and sports*, 2016;4:59-63. doi:10.15561/18189172.2016.0409
22. Kudryavtsev M, Kramida I, Kuzmin V, Iermakov S, Cieślicka Mirosława, Stankiewicz Błażej. Influence of study in HEE on ubiquity and strength of students' computer gambling. *Physical education of students,* 2016; 3: 13–22. doi:10.15561/20755279.2016.0302
23. Kudryavtsev M, Kramida I, Osipov A. Influence of monitor bad habits on healthy lifestyle of students. *Theory and Practice of Physical Culture,* 2016; 6: 24–26.
24. Kudryavtsev MD, Kopylov YuA, Kuzmin VA, Ionova OM, Yermakova TS. Personality oriented system of strengthening of students' physical, psychic and social-moral health. *Physical education of students,* 2016;3:43–52. doi:10.15561/20755279
25. Kudryavtsev MD, Kramida IE, Iermakov SS. Influence of studying in higher educational establishment on students' harmful computer habits. *Physical Education of Students*, 2016;5:17–23. doi:10.15561/20755279.2016.0503
26. Kudryavtsev MD, Kramida IE, Kuzmin VA, Iermakov SS, Cieslicka Miroslawa, Stankiewicz Blazej. Influence of study in hee on ubiquity and strength of students' computer gambling. *Physical education of students*, 2016;(3):13–22. doi:10.15561/20755279.2016.0302
27. Kuzmin VA, Kopylov YuA, Kudryavtsev MD, Galimov GY, Iermakov SS. Substantiation of effectiveness of trainings on health related methodic for students with weakened motor fitness. *Physical education of students,* 2015;6:43–49. doi:10.15561/20755279.2015.0606
28. Osipov A, Dankova M, Tarasenko A, Shnarkin S. Sport-oriented approach to physical education of student youth at higher educational institutions of the Krasnoyarsk territory (on the example of such sports specializations as volleyball and soccer). *Bulletin of Krasnoyarsk State Pedagogical University named after V.P. Astafiev,* 2014; 3(29): 88–91.
29. Osipov A, Gibaeva N, Kachaeva Yu, Pereus O. The method of HOT IRON as a means of increasing the level of physical development of students and formation of their motivation for regular physical exercise. *Bulletin of Krasnoyarsk State Pedagogical University named after V.P. Astafiev,* 2014; 4(30): 82-86.
30. Osipov A, Vonog V, Prokhorova O, Zhavner T. Student learning in physical education in Russia (problems and development perspectives). *Journal of Physical Education and Sport,* 2016;1:688–693. doi:10.7752/jpes.2016.s1111
31. Osipov A, Vonog V. Ensuring a possibility of high quality training of students as sports volunteers for competitions in terms of organizing and running Universiade – 2019. *Journal of Physical Education and Sport,* 2016; 2: 361 – 364. doi:10.7752/jpes.2016.02057
32. Perlman D, Piletic C. The influence of an adapted physical education course on preservice teacher instruction: Using a self-determination lens. *Australian Journal of Teacher Education,* 2012; 37(1): 1–17.

33. Podrigalo LV, Iermakov SS, Alekseev AF, Rovnaya OA. Studying of interconnections of morphological functional indicators of students, who practice martial arts. *Physical Education of Students*, 2016;1:64-70. doi:10.15561/20755279.2016.0109
34. Sabramaniam P. Motivational effects of interest on student engagement and learning in physical education: A review. [Internet]. [Cited 2016 Nov 2]. Available from: http://www.unco.edu/cebs/psychology/kevinpugh/motivation_project/resources/subramaniam.pdf
35. Skurikhina NV, Kudryavtsev MD, Kuzmin VA, Iermakov SS. Fitness yoga as modern technology of special health groups' girl students' psycho-physical condition and psycho-social health strengthening. *Physical education of students*, 2016;2:24–31. doi:10.15561/20755279.2016.0204
36. Song L, Chen J. University students' conceptions of an excellent physical education teacher in China. *European Physical Education Review,* 2012; 19(1): 110–126. doi:10.1177/1356336X12465512
37. Warner B. An exploration of engagement, motivation and student-centered learning in physical education. *Journal of Unschooling and Alternative Learning,* [Internet]. 2015 [cited 2016 Nov 09]; 2015;9(18). Available from: http://jual.nipissingu.ca/wp-content/uploads/sites/25/2015/03/v9181.pdf

13

ACMEOLOGICAL PRINCIPLES OF FORMATION DYNAMIC OF PHYSICAL EDUCATION SPECIALISTS' ACMEOLOGICAL COMPETENCE ACTIVITIES' COMPONENT

Dereka T.Hr.
Borys Grinchenko Kyiv University

Abstract. *Purpose:* to determine characteristics of archeological competence's activities component formation in physical education specialists and find correlation of its components. *Material:* in the research students of specialty "Physical education" (n=194) participated. Activities' component of acmeological competence was determined by results of fulfillment of individual scientific research task. The content of such tasks was enriched with acmeological component. *Results:* we analyzed correlation and intra-influence of parts of acmeological competence's activities component ion respect to its formation level. By results of factorial analysis we grouped, classified acmeological competence components and made them compactly visual. The most significant factors of acmeological competence components are marked out. *Conclusions:* we formed activities' component of acmeological competence in process of students' independent and scientific research work.
Key words: acmeology, competence, component, professional, physical education.

Introduction

In documents of European Council ability to study (without mentioning education level) is characterized as human ability to manifest consistency and persistence in studies, as well as ability to organize own studying individually and in groups, controlling information and time effectively [6, pg. 346]. Such competence implies awareness of educational process. It is determined by demands of an individual and his (her) abilities to overcome obstacles. It envisages acquiring, processing and mastering new knowledge and skills as well as search and usage of recommendations [15]. Ability to study implies usage of previously received knowledge and life experience. It is required for application of knowledge and skills in different contexts: at home, at work, in process of study, in vocational training.

In the frames of analytical research Bologna project TUNING they marked out (from 85) the most important components of work by specialty (in order of their significance) [7, pg. 32-33]: 1) ability for analysis and synthesis; 2) ability to study; 3) ability to realize knowledge in practice.

Thus, ability to study is one of key competences. It is a universal tool of modern continuous education system, without which human self-realization is impossible [8, pg. 33]. To master this ability it is necessary to use own positive experience of independent studies.

Multi-levels integral personality-activities' quality permits to set and to effectively solve the tasks and problems of different complexity. It is required for self-actualization, self-perfection, and self-realization in different aspects of personality's life. In first turn it related to professional functioning. Such functioning is characterized by acmeological competence [3, pg. 54]. Such competence characterizes specialist as a subject of professional self-development. It reflects his ability to plan own gradual development in different spheres of life activity with constant complicating of tasks and growth of achievements' level. In this process human psychological and acmeological resources realize to the fullest extent.

The problems of acmeological approach implementation in educational process were regarded the following contexts:

- Perfection of educational process when practicing different forms of physical education in comprehensive schools. The prospects of such approaches' realization were marked out [18];
- Physical culture teachers' readiness for implementation of new technologies. Setting of goals and the tasks, corresponding to them for students, considering "acme" as personal "top" of every student, were studied [19];
- Implementation of active teaching methods, which are connected with development of specialist's personality and formation of his (her) didactic thinking [22];

- Effectiveness of acmeological approach in the process of future physical culture teacher's professional training [12];
- Influence of stimuli for success, self-realization with training means; formation of individual style on quality of students' vocational training. Besides, technology for ensuring future teacher's readiness for professional-pedagogic self-realization are offered [14];
- Determination of ways for creative potential peaks' achievement in conditions of information-educational space. It was noted that in conditions of information intensification in education acmeological technologies facilitate optimization of teachers' professional formation [11];
- Creation of effective educational technologies, pointed at development of higher educational establishment students' professionally-oriented communication competence [10];
- Psycho-pedagogic conditions of education's realization, concentrated on acmeological orientation of graduate's personality [17];
- Understanding of creative-acmeological approach and its content in study of teacher's professional progress. It was noted that creative activity was conditioned by demand in success in professional sphere; achievement of professional competence and self-organization [16].

In our previous works we substantiated the structure and components of physical education specialists' acmeological competence. We offered conception and model of specialists' continuous professional training, based on acmeology. We also studied the principles of content formation, forma and methods of specialists' continuous professional training, based on acmeology [1, 2, and 3].

Thus, the task of professional training is formation of competent specialist, who would be able to constantly, systemically generalize world and domestic experience as well as innovative search of self-realization ways in conditions of modern society. Continuity of knowledge acquiring, professional competence, value attitude to own physical condition and national health in the whole become leading, essential characteristics of professional fitness.

The purpose of the research: to determine characteristics of ability to study formation in process of physical education specialists' continuous professional training based on acmeology.

Material and methods

Participants: in the research students of specialty "Physical education" (n=194) participated. For pedagogic experiment we formed control (n=98) and experimental (n=96) groups of students.

Procedure: the researches were conducted on the base of Kiev University, named after Boris Grinchenko. In period 2010-2015 in educational process of physical education specialists we used acmeologically enriched content of academic disciplines of professional and practical cycles. Activities' component of acmeological competence we determined by results of individual scientific-research works, fulfilled by students. The content of such tasks was enriched with acmeological component. Besides, activities' component included results of students' questioning about every day independent preparation for lectures (hours/day). Physical education specialists' acmeological component includes also integral indicator of activation's motivation. This indicator includes: inner motive, cognition motive, motive for failures avoiding, competition motive, motive for change of activity, self-respect, significance of results, complexity of task, will effort, assessment of achieved results, assessment of own potential, the planned mobilization of forces, expected results, regularity of results, initiative [1, pg. 442].

Statistical analysis: we determined mean values, Student's t-criterion; correlation analysis was fulfilled. In this work we used «Statistica» programs.

Results of the research

The author's conception of physical education specialists' continuous professional training, based on acmeology, shall be realized in educational process of higher educational establishments. Professional training if oriented on formation of acmeological competence on all levels of higher physical culture education. In formation of acmeological competence in specialists' continuous training accents are shifted from initial cycle of higher education to bachelor's and master's cycles.

Thus, in the future specialist with formed acmeological competence will be able to solve the problems of different difficulty. Graduate will constantly self-perfect and self-realize in professional functioning. At master's level of higher education professional training is accented on formation of specialist's activities' component. The formation process is realized in independent and scientific-research students' work.

Formation of activities' component takes place with the help of acmeologically oriented active means of teaching: lectures (information lectures, problem lectures, binary lectures, topical lectures, reviews, conferences, lecture-visualization and consultations) and seminars (inter-disciplinary seminars, seminars-conferences, discussions, seminar research, role game, "brain storm", and analytical seminar).

Now let us analyze interconnections and inter-influence of activities' component parts in respect to its formation level.

Integral indicator of activity's motivation consists of motivation structure's fifteen components. By the value of correlation coefficient and closeness of connection this indicator influences to the largest extent on level of acmeological competence activities' component formation (r = 0.82).

Students independent and scientific research work have significant correlation with level of activities' component formation (r = 0.61 and r = 0.54, accordingly). Students spend from one to three hours for independent preparation for classes every day. One hour a day for preparation for classes is pent by 18.57% of students. Two hours a day – by 58.57% of students. Three hours – by 22.86%.

Ability to study shall be formed in the process of studying at higher educational establishment. It is necessary to encourage acquiring professional scientific, learning and methodic literature. Questioning results showed that only 58.6% of students buy literature periodically. 41.4% of students do not buy such literature at all.

Thus, it is important to form activities' component, teach students to work regularly and independently. It is also necessary to facilitate formation of internal demand in independent learning. The formed specialists' competence will ensure ability and acme-motivation of personality for constant learning, self-perfection, and self-development during all life. The formation of the component facilitates steady positive attitude to independent study; forms and fixes personality-significant sense of learning actions.

Correlation analysis showed interconnection of activity-motivation indicators and activities' component. High correlation with the level of component's formation had motive of self-respect (r = 0.85) and cognitive motive (r = 0.83). Self respect motive is expressed in object's strive for more and more difficult goals in one-type activity. Cognitive motive characterizes subject's interest to results of his (her) activity. Cognitive motive is a criterion of society. This motive can conceal rather wide circle of more personal motives, which require satisfaction by studying.

The next group of activity's motivation indicators has significant correlation with the level of the component's formation. Assessment of results in respect to potentials in certain kind of human activity was r = 0.7. Assessment of own potential was r = 0.69. Motive for avoiding was r = 0.68. It should be noted that negative, exciting value of result is intrinsic to motive for avoiding or, to be more exact, fear to show low result and after effects of it.

The next group of activity's motivation indicators has also significant correlation with the level of the component's formation. It characterizes correlation of pre-set level of motivation for efforts, required for achievement of results (r = 0.64) and expected level of activity's results (r = 0. 4). For determination of holistic structure of competence cognitive criterion, subject's understanding of reason factors' educational process is very important. They include subject's understanding of result's dependence on correlation of chance and personal potentials (r = 0.66) as well as understanding of to what extent setting of tasks is initiative of directive (r = 0.54). Competition motive (r = 0.54) is a specific in group of motives, connected with result. The content of this motive is determined by to what extent increase of its level is important for the subject.

Moderate correlation with formation level of the component has internal motive (r = 0.47). It is directly connected with the process of activity. This motive is a generalized and demonstrates enthusiasm with fulfillment of task, with educational process. .

Assessment of complexity of the fulfilled task (r = 0.39) and assessment of will effort in the process of the task solution (r = 0.38) have also moderate correlation with component's formation level. It shall be considered, when filling academic disciplines with acmeological component; when planning lectures and practical classes.

Motive for change of activity (r = - 0.1) has weak correlation with the component. It opens subject's feelings and tendency to stop the work. Personal significance of activity's results (r = - 0.3) also has weak feedback with the component. That is why in the process of specialists' professional training influence of teacher and educational medium of educational establishment are rather important. They facilitate formation and manifestation of personality's activity in the process of professional formation and constant perfection of specialist.

Thus, level of component's formation in experimental group is 68.54%. In control group this indicator is 55.6%.

Analysis of pedagogic experiment results shows that in experimental group we registered statistically significant distinctions in competence level and in level of its components' formation ($p < 0.05$). I control group we observed certain dynamic but there were no statistically significant distinctions in competence formation level and in the studied components ($p > 0.05$) (see fig.1).

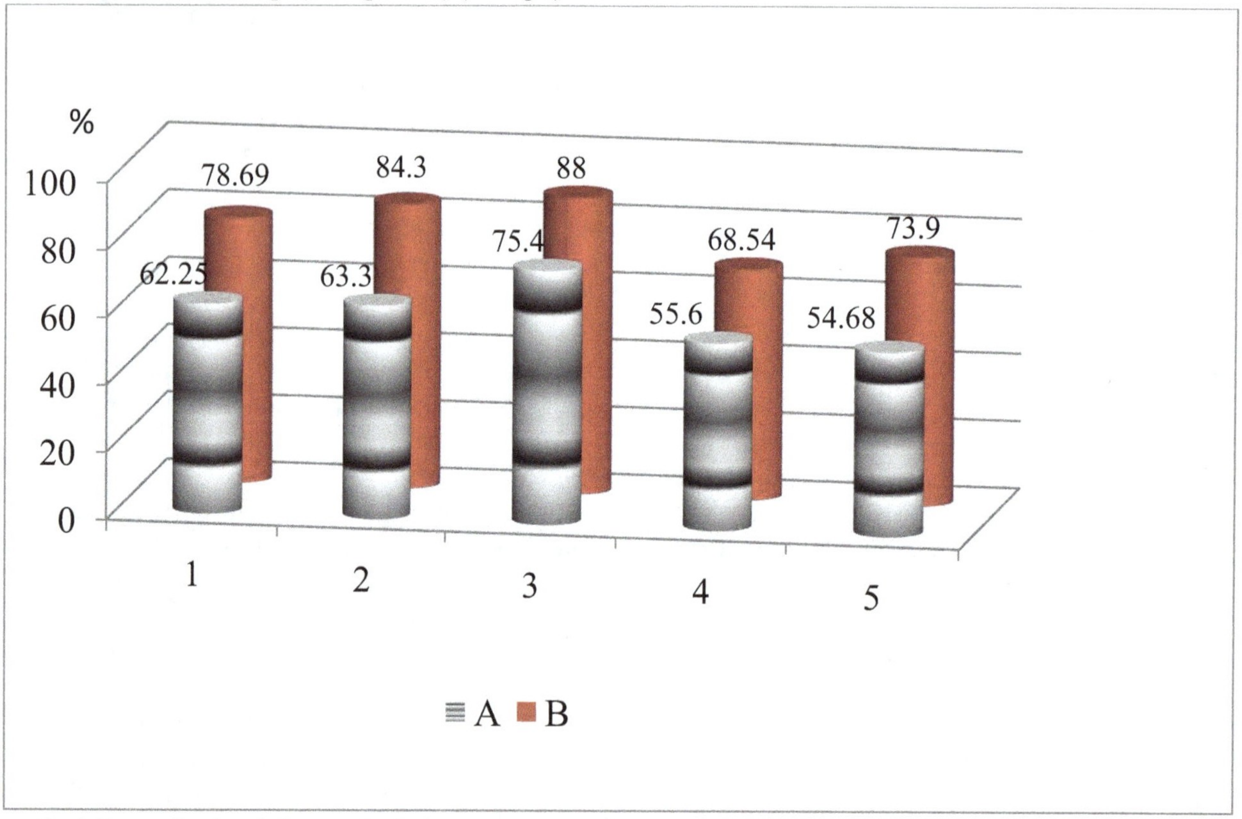

Fig.1. Formation level of acmeological competence and its components in process of continuous professional training of physical education specialists: A – control group of students; B – experimental group of students; 1 – acmeological competence; 2 –acme-motivation; 3 – cognitive component; 4 – activities' component; 5 – personality's component.

Discussion

The conducted study permitted to substantiate demand in students' involvement in fulfillment individual and group scientific-research tasks as well as fulfillment of scientific topic of department, writing scientific-research students' works, participation in scientific-research seminars, conferences and international grants.

The received results witness that students' scientific functioning is oriented on formation of future scientists and on increase of professional duties' fulfillment. For modern physical education specialist it is characteristic to constantly study and generalize new material, questions of allied sciences [13, 21]. In professional functioning of modern physical culture teacher (coach of any kind of sports) there are elements of scientific-research character. That is why experience of scientific work in students' years helps to solve them effectively [1, pg. 388].

The results of this research substantially supplement theoretical ideas about formation of motivation for achievement. By the data of foreign scientific works the main motive of highly productive scientist's activity is "motive for achievement" [5]. Motive for scientific search is cognitive demand, which creates scientist's readiness to manifest intellectual activity in emerging problem situation [4]. There is also other point of view. Formation of "motive for achievement" to large extent depends on education of child in family, starting from early childhood (day regime, child's orientation on independence) [5]. Scientists also introduced term "motivation of effectiveness" [20]. A person is active, when he (she) feels demand in effect of his (her) actions. Satisfaction of this demand results in feeling of competence accompanied by gladness and pleasure. It is evident that this kind of motivation is close to motivation of achievement [4]. Researchers note that insistence is also connected with "motive of achievement".

Our studies supplemented theoretical principles, devoted to realization of independent functioning. Independent work is main mean of students' mastering learning material [9]. Results of our research point at the fact, that such kind of teaching is necessary for mastering academic disciplines and for general skills of work in professional, scientific and teaching spheres formation. They also facilitate formation of ability to take responsibility and to solve any problem independently as well as to find effective solutions, way out from crisis situations [2].

Thus, independent functioning facilitates formation of adequate self-assessment, active life position. It also expands creative experience of physical education specialist [1, pg. 390]. In the base of students' independent work there is conception of independence. In our opinion students' independent activity is possible only is steady motivation is present. The strongest motivating factor is preparation for future professional functioning.

Conclusions

1. In process of future physical education specialists' training it is necessary to use acmeologically oriented forms and methods. Acmeological enrichment of academic disciplines' content forms specialists' acmeological competence.
2. It was found that parts of activities' component influence on its formation level.

Acknowledgements

The research has been fulfilled in compliance with combined plan of scientific-research works of Kiev University, named after Boris Grinchenko "Philosophical, educational and methodic principles of competence personality-professional multi-profile university education" (PK № 0110u006274) for 2011-2015.

Conflict of interests

The author declares that there is no conflict of interests.

References:

1. Dereka TG. *Neperervna profesijna pidgotovka fakhivciv fizichnogo vikhovannia* [Continuous professional training of physical education specialists], Kyiv: Edelweiss; 2016. (in Ukrainian)
2. Dereka TG. Formuvannia diial'nisnogo komponenta akmeologichnoi kompetentnosti fakhivciv fizichnogo vikhovannia [Formation of activities' component of physical education specialists' acmeological competence]. *East European Scientific Journal*, 2016;3(7):26-29. (in Ukrainian)
3. Derkach AA, Sajko EV. *Samorealizaciia – osnovanie akmeologicheskogo razvitiia* [Self-realization – the basis of acmeological development], Moscow: MPSI; 2010. (in Russian)
4. Illin IeP. *Motivi i motivaciia* [Motives and motivation], Ternopol: Teaching book – Bogdan; 2013. (in Ukrainian)
5. MakKleland D. *Motivaciia cheloveka*. [Motivation of man]. Sankt Petersburg: Peter; 2007. (in Russian)
6. Andrushchenko VP, Ziaziun IA, Kremen' VG, Maksimenko SD, Nichkalo NG, Sisoieva SO, Cekhmister IaV, Chalij OV. *Neperervna profesijna osvita* [Continuous professional education], Kiev: Scientific thought; 2003. (in Ukrainian)
7. Rashkevich IuM. *Bolons'kij proces ta nova paradigma vishchoi osviti* [Bologna process and new paradigm of higher education], Lviv: Lviv polytehnyka; 2014. (in Ukrainian)
8. Savchenko OIa. *Uminnia vchitisia – kliuchova kompetentnist' molodshogo shkoliara* [Ability to study – key competence of junior schoolchild], Kiev: Pedagogical thought; 2014. (in Ukrainian)
9. Ficula MM. *Vstup do pedagogichnoi profesii* [Introduction to pedagogic profession], Ternopol: Teaching book – Bogdan; 2005. (in Ukrainian)
10. Atamanova IV, Bogomaz SA, Kozlova NV, Kashirina VI. An Educational Technology for Developing Professionally-Oriented EFL Communicative Competence: Its Acmeological Potential. XXVI annual

international academic conference, language and culture. *Procedia Social and Behavioral Sciences*, 2015;200:236-242. doi:10.1016/j.sbspro.2015.08.058

11. Dragnev YV. Acmeology aspect of professional becoming of the future teacher of physical training in conditions of information of education. *Pedagogics, psychology, medical-biological problems of physical training and sports,* 2010;10:43-46.
12. Dragnev YV. Informative and educational spaces in higher educational establishment and their influence on professional development of future teacher of physical culture. *Pedagogics, psychology, medical-biological problems of physical training and sports,* 2011;3:46-49.
13. Quennerstedt M, Larsson H. Learning movement cultures in physical education practice. *Sport, Education and Society,* 2015;20(5):565–572. doi:10.1080/13573322.2014.994490
14. Rybalko LS. The method of preparation and realization of professional and pedagogical self-actualization experiment on the acme base. *Pedagogics, psychology, medical-biological problems of physical training and sports,* 2009;11:90-94.
15. Rychen DC. *Key Competencies for Successful Life and Well-Functioning Society*. OECD: Hogrefe and Huber; 2003.
16. Segeda NA. The Content of the Creative-Acmeological Approach to the Teacher's Professional Development. *Pedagogics, psychology, medical-biological problems of physical training and sports,* 2009;4:106-110.
17. Turgunbayeva B, Bekzhanova B, Uaidullakyzy E, Arkhabayeva DA. Akmeological approach in professional training of the undergraduates in terms of postgraduate education. 2nd Cyprus international conference on educational research (CY-ICER 2013). *Procedia Social and Behavioral Sciences*, 2013;89:544-548. doi:10.1016/j.sbspro.2013.08.891
18. Vaskov UV. Innovative approaches are in organization of educational process of pupils general schools. *Physical education of students*, 2012;1:24-29.
19. Vas'kov YV. Acmeological approach to physical education of students of secondary schools in the aspect of personality-oriented training. *Pedagogics, psychology, medical-biological problems of physical training and sports*, 2015;3:3-9. doi:10.15561/18189172.2015.0301
20. White RW. Personality psychologist. *Harvard Gazette,* 2001;1:1-2.
21. Wuest DA, Bucher ChA. *Foundations of Physical Education, Exercise Science and Sport*. St. Louis: Mosby: YearBook Inc.; 2003.
22. Yarmoschuk OO. Didactic games in the system of specialist's preparation of physical culture and sport. *Pedagogics, psychology, medical-biological problems of physical training and sports,* 2011;12:139-142.

14

APPLICATION OF REAL-METHODIC FOR MASTERING ARM WRESTLING TECHNIQUES

Bezkorovainyi D.A.
Kharkiv National University of Municipal Economy

Abstract. *Purpose:* to substantiate application of REAL-methodic for training of students-sportsmen at initial stage of arm wrestling. *Material:* in the research 25 1st and 2nd year students participated. The students attended 3 trainings every week. Each training session lasted 2 hours. REAL-methodic was used at initial stage of training at the beginning of the first semester and after one month of trainings. The research took two months (September – October 2015). At each training session REAL-methodic used three times: in first part (warming up); in second (main) – in rest pauses for understanding of discipline; in third part (final) for recreation and relaxation. *Results:* 23 from 25 students-sportsmen accurately fulfilled two main arm wrestling techniques: attack over top and attack in hook; two sportsmen made little mistakes in attacking techniques. It was found that effectiveness of this methodic application to large extent depends on students' motivation, on comfort condition of their nervous system; on presence of mutual trust and positive micro-climate in students' group. *Conclusions:* application of REAL-methodic at initial stage of students-sportsmen's training accelerated perception of training technologies and arm wrestling techniques, shortened period of techniques' mastering, permitted to quicker pass to preparatory period of sport training basic stage.
Key words: arm wrestling, sport training, REAL-methodic, schema, pattern.

Introduction

Arm wrestling is a traumatic kind of sports due to its power orientation and technical complexity. That is why it is extremely dangerous to admit students-sportsmen to competition functioning without their clear understanding of arm wrestling techniques. When mastering techniques at initial training stage there appears some difficulties. The main difficulty for young sportsmen is perception, systemizing, processing and reproduction of verbal and motor (non verbal) information, rendered by coach. This difficulty can be solved with the help of REAL-methodic, offered by N.M. Maslova and her followers [5, 9–13].

Health related component of REAL-methodic completely justifies itself if it is used in physical culture – sport sphere. It protects, corrects and improves health due to starting of self regulation mechanism [15]. General approaches to determination of purpose, tasks and content of environmental pedagogic, including physical education means, are elucidated in monograph of Prof. L.N. Necheporenko [16]. In work by N.A. Oleynik et al. [17] content of discipline "Physical culture" was analyzed from environmental position and correspondence to conception of noosphere education. The authors present all groups of means and methods of psycho-physical self-regulation, which are used in students' physical education. The authors note that specificity of most of kinds of sports implies usage of right-side and left side movements. That is why specialists in physical culture and sports shall understand it by themselves, feel it and promote it among supporters of noosphere education. In work by N.N. Zavidivska [6] noosphere pedagogic paradigm was substantiated as conceptual basis of students' health-related physical culture education. The author reveals noosphere essence of physical education and health related education of students as well as generalizes main aspects of noosphere pedagogic paradigm oriented on fundamentalization of health related physical culture education. In this work the following necessities are noted: cultivation of holistic, sound thinking; provisioning of person with tools for independent practicing of healthy life style. Besides, ability to set aims, to choose physical culture means and foresee after effects of own actions in health are marked out.

In the works by V.M. Klochko and D.O. Bezkorovayniy [8], V.M. Klochko and T.V. Bondarenko [11] it is noted that application of REAL-methodic at initial stage of students-sportsmen's training in arm wrestling gives positive result, accelerates perception of training technologies and arm wrestling techniques, shortens period of techniques' mastering as well as speeds up transition to preparatory basic stage of sport training [8, 11]. Alongside with it there is a demand in continuation of such researches for prevention from traumatism in arm wrestling.

Purpose, tasks of the work, material and methods

The purpose of the work is to substantiate application of REAL-methodic for training of students-sportsmen at initial stage of arm wrestling during their studying in HEE of engineering specialties.

The tasks of the work: 1) to study literature on the researched problem; 2) to work out schema-pattern – of sportsman's skillfulness; 3) to substantiate purposefulness of application of the worked out schema-pattern in the process of training session.

Material and methods of the research: in the research 1st and 2nd year students of KhNUME participated (n = 25). Students attended trainings three times every week. Each training session lasted 2 hours. REAL-methodic was used at initial stage of training at the beginning of the first semester and after one month of trainings. From that moment student received initial idea about this kind of sports, about elements of sportsmanship, familiarized with principles of techniques and tactic of duel.

The research took two months (September – October 2015). At each training session REAL-methodic used three times: in first part (warming up); in second (main) – in rest pauses for understanding of discipline; in third part (final) for recreation and relaxation.

At the end of the research sportsmen's fulfillment of techniques was assessed by experts. It was noted that 23 from 25 students-sportsmen accurately fulfilled two main arm wrestling techniques: attack over top and attack in hook; two sportsmen made little mistakes in attacking techniques.

Results of the researches

Arm wrestling is a power kind of sports, in which important role is played by technical tactic fitness of sportsmen. By the latter arm wrestling is very close to wrestling. Arm wrestling is full fledged and attractive kind of sports with well developed system of trainings and competitions. Initial stage is of special importance for a sportsman. In arm wrestling one must not start main training loads and direct duels without proper technical training. Traumas are quite possible and it would result in disappearing of motivation.

Arm wrestling technique develops on the base of analysis of content of sportsmen's competition functioning [3, 4, 8]. It implies registration and evolution of basic requirements and rational variants of techniques, considering limbs' positions in space, their trajectories, distribution of opponent's forces. Arm wrestling techniques are rather conservative because they are restricted by rules of competitions and small space of sportsmen's interaction. Increase of general and special fitness, training of sportsmen's individual abilities – all these influence on technique and its elements. With it main mechanism of movements preserves. Formation and development of every sportsman's technique is realized with consideration of his weight-height indicators and strength of main muscular groups. Correct assessment of movements' technique permits for sportsman to use main and auxiliary training exercises in more correct way. Perfection of sportsmen's technical actions shall be continuous and constant (cyclic-evolutional) with increasing of his fitness level [6, 8, 9].

For quicker mastering of arm wrestling techniques we offered to use holistic systemic bio-adequate methodic, which was developed under guidance of academician N.V. Maslova [3, 5, 9, 11]. This methodic is a combination of coach's and sportsman's coordinated actions targeted at motivation and activation of holistic and dynamic thought-forms of sport orientation and skills of work with them. Organization of work was built on integral synthesis of evolving physiological, mental, psychic and moral functions of trainees.

Specific features of REAL-methodic:

– Relaxation stages alternated with active stages;

– Against relaxation background there takes place accumulation of information (work of right semi-sphere). With activation left semi-sphere's functions are trained (logic, analysis, structuralizing of information);

– Calm atmosphere of training results in improvement of psycho-physical parameters of students-sportsmen's self feeling.

Compulsory condition of bio-adequate training is involvement of sensor motor and symbol stage of work with information. Effectiveness of this methodic application to large extent depends on students' motivation, on comfort condition of their nervous system; on presence of mutual trust and positive micro-climate in students' group.

In every training active and relaxation stages of information perceiving and mastering go turn by turn. Active stage implies the following kinds of work [1, 2, 7, 8, 13]:

– Discussion of studied problems;

– Personal experience exchange with perceiving of meaning space of the studied questions;

– Oral questioning of students on the studied material.

In relaxation stage the following work shall be done:

– Listening to the studied material and its visualization;

– Listening to musical compositions for creation of positive psycho-emotional background; these compositions shall differ from compositions of active stage;

– Projecting of virtual models of the studied information by switching brain's projective function in work;

– Construction of thought scheme (pattern) of virtual model of the studied information;

– Creation of comfort zone of training process participants' thinking: "coach-students' group", "coach-student", "student-student".

Table 1. Stages of work with information as per *REAL-methodic* (by N.V. Antonenko et al.)

Stages of work at training session №	Description of stage and its orientation	Student's psycho-physiological condition	Student's tasks and actions	Task of impact
1	Sensor motor	relaxation	Listen to information and visualize it	Introduction of new material considering student's personal experience and choice
2	Symbol	activity	Draw symbol, pattern, information; discussion of information	Involve brain's different centers in work
3	Logical	relaxation	Listening to text (task)	Understanding of information through logical thinking
4	Linguistic	activity	Reading the text (task). Analysis, translation and etc.	Mastering of material

Pattern is reference thought form, filled with complete structuralized information in algorithmic order. On of its important tasks is to switch in operation all channels of perception, basing on personal experience of a trainee or archetypes (stable pictures of unconscious). Image is result and ideal form of reflection of material or ideal object in human mind. It appears on the base and in form of symbols in conditions of practice and cognition.

In work with 1st and 2nd year students we tested REAL-methodic we received positive result. As the basis we took pattern of professional workmanship of T.V. Bondarenko [5], which was used by the author in training of KhNUME students to discipline "Management of professional workability" (fig.1).

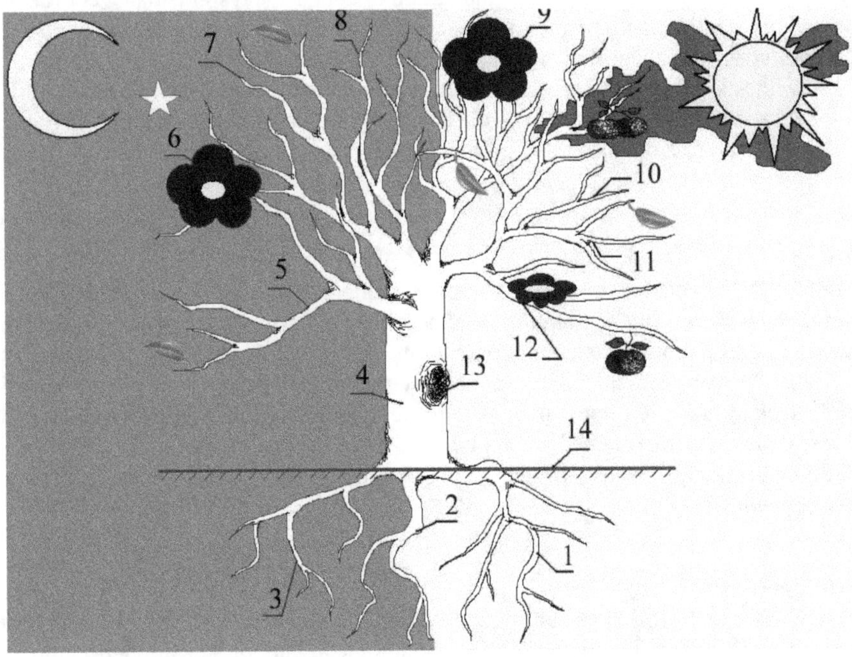

Fig.1. Schema-pattern "Professional functioning of specialist" (by T.V. Bondarenko)
1 – psychic state. 2 – physical health, 3 – social health, 4 – professional workability, 5 – qualification, 6 – labor productivity, 7 – professional fitness, 8 – quality of production, 9 – creative potential, 10 – labor activity, 11 – professional ethic, 12 – physiological cost of work, 13 – harmful habits, 14 – professional health.

In our case tree in the schema is sportsman's personality. The tree's foundation (success in realization of sportsmanship) is single root system (sportsman's health), represented by three branches (physical, psychic and social health). Status of root system (health) conditions vital capacity of tree (sportsman) and depends on ground, on which he lives as well as on many endogenous and exogenous factors, including natural ones (cloud), daily and other biological rhythms (sun-moon). For feeding and strengthening of tree fertile soil is required (sport health). The state and composition of soil influence on growth of the whole tree (height, volume of crown), on its ability to blossom and give fruits (flowers, apples).

The trunk of tree (thought form of sport workability) is the main indicator of progress (sport achievements). Damages of trunk (harmful habits) significantly limit harmony of growth and influence on tree's (sportsman) vital capacity in the whole. Sportsmanship is tree's crown, which can have different volume. As it is known there is close connection between crown (sportsmanship) and root system (health): on surface of ground their area is approximately equal. Crown consists of combination of branches) components of sportsmanship: qualification, efficiency, activity, sport ethic and so on), on which (as indicator of sport functioning's quality) beautiful flowers (realization of sport functioning, creative potential) bloom or not bloom. If technology of wood care (sport regiment) violates physiological laws, the flowers can be flawed (invested funds do not justify result) and fruits (results in money or other form) will be wormy or not appear at all.

Discussion

Organization of training process in arm wrestling requires consideration of many factors, which characterize personality of sportsman and his coach [18–24]. Prevention of sportsmen from traumatism is especially important. All these taken together determine success of sportsmen's and coach's actions.

The results, received by us, confirm the opinion of many other authors [5, 6, 8–11, 17] about effectiveness of REAL-methodic application in education and physical culture-sport activity. The researches by N.V. Maslova et al. [15] confirm urgency and effectiveness of this methodic usage for economy of human thinking and improvement of health. The authors think that structuralizing of academic information as per principle of gold proportions is a preventive measure in solution of pedagogic task of health protection.

The offered by us methodic is based on combination of coach's and sportsman's coordinated actions. The main direction of such interaction is motivation and activation of holistic thought forms of sport orientation and skills of technological work with them. In training process important role is played by integral preparation, the basis of which is synthesis of physiological, mental, psychic and moral functions of sportsmen. Especial importance has thought pattern of sport workability. This thought pattern is the main indicator of sport achievements. Such approach to construction of training process permits to more effectively control sportsmen's actions.

Conclusions:

Application of REAL-methodic at initial stage of students-sportsmen's training in arm wrestling gave positive result, accelerated perceiving of trainings' technologies and arm wrestling techniques, shortened period of techniques' mastering and permitted to quicker pass to preparatory basic stage of sport training.

It is noted that 23 from 25 students-sportsmen accurately fulfilled two main arm wrestling techniques: attack over top and attack in hook; two sportsmen made little mistakes in attacking techniques.

Further researches will be oriented on application of REAL-methodic on stages of basic training and direct, pre-competitions' training. For assessment of this methodic it is planned to use special tool methods of students' health assessment.

Acknowledgement

The research has been fulfilled as per combined plan of scientific-research works in sphere of physical culture and sports for 2011–2015 by topic 3.7 "Methodological and organizational-methodic principles of determination of human physical condition's individual norm" (state registration number 0111U000192).

Conflict of interests

The author declares that here is no conflict of interests.

References:

1. Antonenko NV, Ul'ianova MV. *Pedagogika noosfernogo razvitiia* [Pedagogic of noosphere development]. Moscow: Ekon-Inform; 2007. (in Russian)
2. Astaf'ev BA. *Osnovy Mirozdaniia* [The foundations of the Universe]. Moscow: White Alva; 2002. (in Russian)
3. Bezkorovajnij DO. *Navchannia tekhnici borot'bi na rukakh* [Training of arm wrestling technique]. Kharkiv: HNAMG; 2009. (in Ukrainian)
4. Bezkorovajnij DO. Bazova sistema trenuvannia ta sistema bezposeredn'oi pidgotovki do zmagan' v armsporti [Basic system of training and system of directpre-competitions' training in arm wrestling]. *Pedagogics, psychology, medical-biological problems of physical training and sports,* 2010;1:13–16 (in Ukrainian)
5. Bondarenko TV, Zazdravnov AP, Panina EL. *Noosfernoe myshlenie* [Noosphere thinking]. Kharkov: SPD District Brovin; 2012. (in Russian)
6. Zavidivs'ka NN. Noosferna pedagogichna paradigma iak konceptual'na osnova fundamentalizacii fizkul'turno-ozdorovchoi osviti studentiv [Noosphere pedagogic paradigm as conceptual basic of fundamentalization of students' health related physical culture education]. *Pedagogics, psychology, medical-biological problems of physical training and sports,* 2012;1:68–71. (in Ukrainian)
7. Zviaginceva IM. *Silova ta fizichna pidgotovka* [Power and physical training], Kharkiv: HNAMG; 2009. (in Ukrainian)
8. Klochko VM, Bezkorovajnij DO. *Sportivni iedinoborstva* [Sport martial arts], Kharkiv: HNAMG; 2005. (in Ukrainian)
9. Klochko VM. *Innovacijni pedagogichni tekhnologii formuvannia psikhofizichnikh i shvidkisno-silovikh iakostej iedinoborciv* [Innovative pedagogic technologies of formation of martial arts sportsmen's psycho-physical and speed-power qualities], Kharkiv: HNAMG; 2012. (in Ukrainian)
10. Klochko VM. *Ocenka zdorov'ia studentov* [Assessment of students' health], Kharkiv: HNAMG; 2012. (in Russian)
11. Klochko VM, Bondarenko TV. Primenenie bioadekvatnykh metodik fizicheskogo vospitaniia pri formirovanii noosfernogo myshleniia studentov [Application of bio-adequate physical education methodic with formation of students' noosphere thinking]. *Noosfernoe obrazovanie v Ukraine*, 2008;2:119–125. (in Russian)
12. Maslova VN. *Noosfernoe obrazovanie* [Noorsphere education], Moscow: Institute Holodinamiki; 2002. (in Russian)
13. Maslova NV. Noosfernoe obrazovanie [Noorsphere education], *XXI Mezhdunarodnaia nauchnaia prakticheskaia konferenciia "Noosfernoe obrazovanie – fundament ustojchivogo razvitiia obshchestva", Sevastopol'* [21st International scientific practical conference "Noosphere education – as foundation of society's stable development', Sevastopol], 2007. P.30–50. (in Russian)
14. Maslova NV. *Periodicheskaia sistema obshchikh zakonov poznaniia i postizheniia* [Periodic system of general laws of cognition and comprehension], Moscow: Institute Holodinamiki; 2007. (in Russian)
15. Maslova NV, Antonenko NV, Ul'ianova MV, Kulikova NG, Mazurina LV, Klyshko ZhM, Vancian IE. *Bioadekvatnaia metodika prepodavaniia* [Bio-adequate methodic of teaching], Moscow: Center of Natural Sciences "Planet Seven-I."; 2008. (in Russian)
16. Necheporenko LS. *Ontopedagogika ta invajromental'na pedagogika* [Onto-pedagogic and environmental pedagogic], Kharkiv; 2001.(in Ukrainian)
17. Olejnik NA, Bondarenko TV, Zajcev VP, Kramskoj SI. Invajromental'naia napravlennost' fizicheskogo vospitaniia i ego mesto v sisteme noosfernogo obrazovaniia [Environmental orientation of physical education and its place in system of noosphere education]. *Physical education of students of creative specialties,* 2008;3:83–93. (in Russian)
18. Dragnev YV. General not specialized subject armsport in conditions of profile training within the framework of base general not specialized subject physical culture. *Pedagogics, psychology, medical-biological problems of physical training and sports*. 2009;10:51 – 53.
19. Kamaev OI, Bezkorovainyi DO. Influence of the experimental program of trainings in armsport on the power indexes of basic muscle groups of 16–17–years-old armwrestlers. *Pedagogics, psychology, medical-biological problems of physical training and sports,* 2013;1:34–39. http://doi.org/10.6084/m9.figshare.106936
20. Podrigalo LV, Galashko MN, Galashko NI. Study and evaluation of indicators of relationships motor analyzer sportsmen of armsport. *Physical Education of Students,* 2013;3:46–49. http://doi.org/10.6084/m9.figshare.669671
21. Podrigalo LV, Galashko MN, Galashko NI, Prusik Krzysztof, Cieślicka Mirosława. Research of hands' strength and endurance indications of arm sport athletes having different levels of skills. *Physical education of students,* 2014;2:37–40. http://doi.org/10.6084/m9.figshare.907140

22. Podrigalo LV, Galashko NI, Galashko MN. Goniometric researches of armwrestling sportsmen. *Physical Education of Students,* 2013;1:45–49. http://doi.org/10.6084/m9.figshare.156357
23. Podrigalo LV, Galashko NI, Galashko MN. Using ergonomic approaches for increasing effect of preparation at arm sport. *Physical Education of Students,* 2012;1:87–90.
24. Podrigalo LV, Iermakov SS, Nosko MO, Galashko MN, Galashko NI. Study and analysis of armwrestlers' forearm muscles' strength. *Journal of Physical Education and Sport*, 2015;15(3):531–537.

15

EFFECT OF HIGH-INTENSITY INTERVAL TRAINING ON BODY COMPOSITION AND BIOENERGETIC INDICES IN BOYS-FUTSAL PLAYERS

Fatemeh Balbasi, Ramin Shabani, Marzieh Nazari
Department of exercise physiology, Rasht Branch, Islamic Azad University, Rasht, Iran

Abstract. *Background:* High-intensity interval trainings (HIIT) can result in the best improvement of body fitness among athletes in the shortest possible time. The impact of HIIT on bioenergetic factors of futsal players has not been studied extensively. The objective of the present study was to investigate the effect of 3-week HIIT on body composition indices, maximum aerobic power, and maximum anaerobic power, anaerobic power among boys - futsal players. *Material:* 30 boys - futsal players (mean± SD age, 13.49±1.03 years; BMI, 20.95±1.78 kg/m^2) participated in the study voluntarily. They were randomly assigned to experimental (n=15) and control (n=15) groups. HIIT lasted for three weeks, three sessions a week for 12-36 minutes on treadmill. Weight, body mass index (BMI), waist to hip ratio (WHR), thickness of body fat, maximal aerobic power, and maximum anaerobic power were recorded before intervention and 48 hours after the final training session. Aerobic power was measured with 20-m shuttle run, and maximum anaerobic power was measured with RAST test. Paired sample t-test was used to determine pretest-posttest differences, and independent t-test was used to determine between-group differences. The significance level was set to $P < 0.05$. *Results*: Significant differences were found in weight, BMI, thickness of body fat, maximum aerobic power and maximum anaerobic power in experimental group ($P = 0.001$) before and after training intervention, but the change in WHR was not significant ($P < 0.05$). No significant differences were observed in selected body composition between experimental and control groups, but they exhibited significant differences in maximum aerobic power and maximum anaerobic power ($P = 0.001$). *Conclusion*: According to the results, HIIT can be an effective training program for improving the performance of bioenergetic indices of futsal players. Also, it is recommended to study the effect of similar trainings with longer durations on other indices in other sports in future studies.
Keywords: HIIT, VO_{2max}, Maximum anaerobic power.

Introduction

Most sports need performance of short-time, quick activities with the maximum power efficiency. So, coaches and sport specialists have been always seeking new trainings to improve athletes' aerobic and anaerobic power in the shortest possible time [1]. High-intensity interval trainings (HIIT) are new interval methods interested by athletes, coaches, and researchers in recent years. Though there is no comprehensive definition of HIIT, it generally refers to repetitions of short-time interval exercises with full intensity or intensities close to what results in maximal oxygen uptake. Depending on training intensity, an HIIT effort may last for several seconds to several minutes in which the intervals are separated with a cool-down period of a few minutes or low-intensity activity [2].

Futsal is a high-intensity athletic activity. The fact that professional futsal players should perform repeated, rapid activities in smaller field with shorter rest than soccer players shows that aerobic and anaerobic power are necessary in futsal [3].

Maximum aerobic power (VO_{2max}) is a common way to measure aerobic performance. It shows the maximum possible oxygen that human body can intake in one minute, and it is closely related to body endurance and aerobic activity and depends on the performance of skeleton, muscular, and cardiovascular systems [4]. In addition, maximum anaerobic power (p_{max}) is the ability of all muscles to produce more force with high speed in sprint activities for a very short time [5]. Given the strong correlation of health with fat level, the evaluation of body composition (especially body fat percent) is an important component of physical fitness [6].

Doğramacı et al. (2006) estimated that futsal players reached 75% of maximum heart rate and 90% of maximum oxygen intake in high-intensity, competitive games [7]. Many studies have specified HIIT advantages as improving athletic capacity and the factors related to endurance performance including muscle oxidative capacity and VO_{2max} [8, 9, 10, 11]. In addition to improving aerobic power due to the rest periods between activities, these trainings increase speed or the ability of maintaining speed in long-time intervals [12]. Also, post-HIIT adaptations show that these adaptations improve skeleton muscle glycogen at rest and maximize glycolytic and oxidative enzymes, and also, it is reported that maximum oxygen intake does not change after HIIT programs [13].

There are disagreements about the impact of HIIT training on body composition and bioenergy level, so that whilst some studies report the reduction of body composition such as weight, BMI, fat percent, and waist circumference [14, 15], others report no significant improvement [11, 16]. On the other hand, significant improvements are reported in aerobic and anaerobic power by some studies [9, 10, 11], whereas others did not observe any influences [16, 17]. High-quality, low-volume trainings are, in essence, used to find a training program with the appropriate intensity, duration, and repetition which can result in rapid and concurrent improvement of aerobic and anaerobic power. Therefore, since few studies have been reported on the effect of HIIT training on the improvement of aerobic and anaerobic performance among futsal players [18, 19] and yet they have yielded inconsistent results, and given the possible usefulness of HIIT training and the importance of bioenergetic indices in futsal, the present study was aimed at examining the effect of HIIT training on body composition and bioenergetic indices.

Material and Methods

Participants

Thirty boys - futsal players (mean± SD age, 13.49±1.03 years; BMI, 20.95±1.78 kg/m^2) playing in futsal club of Roodbar city in Guilan Province, Iran volunteered to participate in this study. They were randomly assigned to experimental (n = 15) and control (n = 15) groups. The conditions for participation were player's consent, no illness record, and training experience of at least six months to two years, and the conditions for the exclusion of subjects included injury so severe that he could not keep training, and absence for two consecutive or three non-consecutive sessions.

The research was approved by Human Studies Review Committee at Islamic Azad University, Rasht Research Design.

One week before the fulfillment of the protocol, the volunteers were briefed to get familiarized with high-intensity interval training. The day after getting their consent, their height, weight, thickness of body fat, BMI, WHR, VO_{2max}, and P_{max} were measured. The tests were administered one week before and 48 hours after the last training session. The height was measured with a ruler with the precision of 1 mm. The subjects were weighed with a scale (made by Beurer Co., Germany) with the precision of 0.1 kg, in which they were asked to go on scale without shoes and with the least clothes. The height was recorded in centimeter and the weight in kilogram. The waist circumference was measured at the point midway between the lowest rib and the iliac crest in standing position. To measure thickness of body fat, the thickness of subcutaneous fat layer was measured with a caliper (SAEHAN, South Korea) on abdomen, chest and thigh [20]. Then, the recordings were used to estimate Total thickness of body fat by Jackson and Pollock's formula. Body mass index (BMI) was measured in kg m^{-2} by

$$BMI = weight\ (kg) / height\ (m)^2$$

To ensure the reliability and validity of the measurements, they were all carried out in a single day. Aerobic power was measured with 20-m shuttle run test and anaerobic power was measured with RAST test. In shuttle run test, the subjects were asked to run a 20-m course periodically with uniform increase in pace. The test was designed in 21 levels (each level with its own number of shuttles). The subjects departed from the start line covering the course between two consecutive obstacles to reach the next pace [21]. In RAST test, a 30-m course was selected with plenty of empty space in either side. The subjects were asked to warm up for at least seven minutes. At the outset, they were weighed. Then, they started running. They should rest for 10 seconds at the end of the course. Immediately afterwards, they should run back. The subjects should run the course six times with their highest speed [22].

Trainings protocol

The trainings lasted for 10 sessions, three sessions a week. The subjects were completely trained one week before the research, and they run on a treadmill for one session as a test. The training sessions included warm-up (15 minutes), main training phase, and cool-down for experimental group. HIIT group warmed up in general and specific manner (including jogging, stretching, sit-up with medicine-ball, skipping rope, push-up, and workout with ball), and cool-down phase included jogging, resting, and stretching for recovery. In the main phase of the training, the subjects run on treadmill on the basis of VO2peak. Rest time was 1:3 and training duration was 12-18 minutes in the first week, 25 minutes in the second week, and 36 minutes in the third week. The trend of the trainings is presented in Table 1.

Table1. High intensity interval training program

session	Rest Time Second	Activity Time	Replete	Speed Treadmill	Total Time

		Second					
1	90	30	2	8	7.5	7	12
2	90	30	3	8	7.5	7	18
3	90	30	3	8	7.5	7	18
4	135	45	3	9	8.5	8	25
5	135	45	3	9	8.5	8	25
6	135	45	3	9	8.5	8	25
7	135	45	3	10	9.5	9	25
8	135	45	3	10	9.5	9	25
9	135	45	4	10	9.5	9	36
10	135	45	4	10	9.5	9	36

Statistical analysis

Data were descriptively analyzed by mean, standard deviation. After Kolmogorov-Smirnov Test and given the normal distribution of data, paired sample t-test was used to determine pretest-posttest differences, and independent t-test was used to estimate between-group differences. All statistical analyses were carried out with SPSS (Ver. 22) Software Package. The significance level was set to less than 0.05.

Results

Table 2 presents some anthropometric descriptive of the subjects including age, height, weight, total thickness of body fat, BMI, and WHR (Table 2).

Table2. Baseline characteristics of study participants (mean± SD)

variable	Control mean± SD	Experimental mean± SD
Age (year)	13.53±1.06	13.46±1.18
Height(m)	149.00±4.97	159.27±3.61
Weight(kg)	45.86±3.06	47.87±4.04
Thickness of body fat(mm)	17.17±1.00	15.15±1.51
BMI(kg/m^2	20.66±1.15	21.24±2.14
WHR	0.85±0.02	0.86±0.01

BMI: body mass index; WHR: waist to hip ratio

As is evident in Table 3, HIIT significantly affected weight, BMI, and thickness of body fat of subjects in experimental group ($P < 0.05$). However, no effect was observed on WHR ($P > 0.05$). Control group showed significant change just in thickness of body fat between pre-test and post-test ($P < 0.05$) and other variables did not change significantly ($P > 0.05$). On the other hand, HIIT resulted in significant change in VO_{2max} and P_{max} of experimental group between pre-test and post-test ($P < 0.05$, Table 3).

Table 3. Effects of HIIT training according paired t-tests (n=30)

	Group	Before	After	t	p
Weight(kg)	Control	45.86±3.06	45.72±2.87	1.16	0.2
	Experimental	47.87±4.4	47.56±3.96	3.2	0.005*
BMI(kg/m^2)	Control	20.66±1.15	20.60±1.11	1.1	0.2
	Experimental	21.24±2.14	21.11±2.13	3.31	0.005*
WHR	Control	0.85±0.02	0.86±0.01	0.1	0.89
	Experimental	0.86±0.0	0.86±0.00	0.1	0.8
Thickness of body fat(mm)	Control	17.17±1.0	16.62±0.8	5.9	0.000*
	Experimental	15.15±1.51	14.62±1.38	7.4	0.000*
Vo2max	Control	41.01±5.09	41.17±5.10	0.7	0.4
	Experimental	42.30±4.84	47.94±5.33	10.18	0.000*
P_{max}	Control	42.58±40.72	41.88±36.97	3.1	0.007*
	Experimental	47.15±47.87	54.91±55.01	14.13	0.000*

$p \leq 0.05$

According to Table 4, there was no significant difference in BMI between control and experimental groups ($P > 0.05$). But, there was significant difference in VO_{2max} and P_{max} between control and experimental groups ($P < 0.05$). In other words, HIIT improved VO_{2max} and P_{max} in experimental group as compared to control group.

Table 4. In depended t-test between groups (n=30)

	Group	Mean± Difference	t	DF	p
Weight(kg)	Control	0.14±0.48	-0.9	28	0.3
	Experimental	0.29±0.34			
BMI(kg/m²)	Control	0.06±0.22	-0.9	28	0.3
	Experimental	0.12±0.14			
WHR	Control	-0.002±0.003	-1.09	28	0.2
	Experimental	0.05±0.2			
Thickness of body fat(mm)	Control	0.54±0.35	0.3	28	0.7
	Experimental	0.51±0.26			
Vo2max (ml/kg/min)	Control	0.16±0.78	-5.4	28	*0.001
	Experimental	5.64±2.14			
Pmax	Control	-8.70±10.64	-13.7	28	*0.001
	Experimental	65.76±18.02			

$p \leq 0.05$

Discussion

It was revealed that three weeks of HIIT of boys could improve bioenergetic indices including aerobic and anaerobic power in both groups. Body composition including weight, BMI, and to measure thickness of body fat, the thickness of subcutaneous fat layer was measured with a caliper (SAEHAN, South Korea) on abdomen, chest and thigh showed reduction only in experimental group.

There are inconsistencies in the results of studies about the effect of HIIT on body composition variations. Some studies show no change [27,28] whilst others report significant changes [14, 24, 11].

According to Trapp et al. (2008), 15-week HIIT intervention had more effect on body composition than steady-state exercise training [11]. Gremeaux et al. (2012) observed a significant improvement in body composition after a long period of HIIT, too [14]. The study was conducted on overweight people posed exposed to a long-time intervention (9 full months) including nutritional counseling, HIIT and resistance training. Post-intervention results indicated significant decreases in all anthropometric indices expect muscle mass which showed no significant difference with baseline. They concluded that a combination of HIIT and resistance training with nutritional control can be an optimized way for maintaining muscle mass during fat loss. Another study revealed that two-week HIIT intervention resulted in significant loss of body composition and WHR [15]. However, it should be considered that the participants were obese, sedentary men, which may be a factor affecting the results of this study. Tremblay et al. (1994) found that long-time HIIT decreased subcutaneous significantly in both young men and women. They compared HIIT with steady-state exercise training and found that although total energy cost was lower (about half) in HIIT than in steady-state training, just HIIT changed body composition [23].

Trapp et al. (2008) examined normal-weight men and women and observed that 15-week HIIT intervention resulted in favorable changes in body composition. They compared interval training with steady-state training and control (no training). Total body mass and fat mass was significantly lower in HIIT group than in other two groups. They, also, stated that the trend of fat loss from legs was desirable in HIIT group. HIIT resulted in significant loss of central abdominal fat as compared to steady-state group. HIIT group showed significantly higher lean body mass. The changes in other lean tissues were not significant [11]. Also, shing et al. (2013) reported significant loss of body fat percentage after 4-week HIIT, whilst the subjects had good body shape. So, it is possible to have body composition change even after a short period of these trainings. They compared interval training with traditional resistance training and observed that interval training changed body composition significantly. Gender plays an important role in body composition so that the results of tests differ for men and women, so they should not be compared. The other aspects which should be considered in body composition studies include age and heritage because they both considerably influence body composition. For example, adipose tissue percentage depends on heritage and also, on exercise and nutrition [24].

Long-time exercise trainings usually impact body composition indices considerably. Most studies on HIIT show that the longer the exercise trainings are, the more effective they are on body composition indices. In fact, the inconsistencies in the results of the studies are likely to be associated with the differences in training durations and subjects. In the present study, since a short-time (3-week) HIIT intervention was administered, it did not significantly affect body composition indices [11, 23].

A significant difference was found in VO2max and Pmax between control and experimental groups in the present study. In general, VO2max is known as the best indicator of cardiovascular endurance and aerobic fitness. Whilst continuous training and other long-time trainings are widely used for improving VO2max and almost all athletes in most sports use them, recent studies show that the effects of HIIT on the improvement of aerobic power is similar to that of long-time trainings. It may be associated with high intensity of HIIT and the intervals between training sets. VO2max is reportedly increased by 5-14% after HIIT. The present study showed a similar increase (11.8%) in VO2max in experimental group (intervened with HIIT) as compared to control.

The results of the present study are in agreement with most previous studies. In this sense, Laursen et al. (2005) reported the increased VO2max among cyclists by 4-week HIIT intervention. They suggested that peripheral adaptations are more responsible for performance improvement than central adaptations. A mechanism for increasing aerobic power is the increased activity of oxidative enzymes as reported in some studies [25]. In a study on the effect of interval training at 95% and 100% of the velocity at VO2max on aerobic physiological indices and running performance, Denadai et al. (2010) found that post-training VO2max did not change in two groups and that VO2max performance was significantly increased in the group of 100% of VO2max [26]. Also, castagna et al. (2010) studied the physiological aspects of futsal-oriented HIIT and reported that aerobic velocity and threshold, maximum velocity, and VO2max were significantly related to training program [19]. Astorino et al. (2012) examined the impact of HIIT on cardiovascular performance, VO2max, and muscular power and observed a significant improvement in VO2max as compared to baseline [27]. In a study on the effect of skill-based maximal intensity interval training on aerobic and anaerobic performance of female futsal players, Karahan (2012) reported that mean aerobic power and VO2max of experimental group were improved by 10.7, 22.1 and 9.6%, respectively. It implied that skill-based HIIT influenced aerobic and anaerobic performance of female futsal players significantly [18].

On the contrary, some studies show that VO2max is not affected by HIIT. For example, Laursen et al. (2002) and Burgomaster et al. (2005) reported that 2-week HIIT did not increase VO2max significantly [29, 30]. The difference in results may be associated with the difference in subjects (trained and not-trained) as well as the difference in training program duration. Experiments have shown that HIIT improves blood pumping by heart. This finding may explain why VO2max is increased by HIIT as observed in some studies. Also, following the trainings, aerobic phosphorylation rate is increased. This adaptation may be brought about by the increase in the number and activity of oxidative enzymes in muscles which can be a likely mechanism for VO2max improvement. Interestingly, most studies on the impact of HIIT on physiological factors that affect aerobic capacity show good adaptations in spite of lower intensity of their interval training programs.

One another finding of the present study was the 13.8% improvement of anaerobic power in experimental group, whereas it showed a 2% decrease in control group. Other studies confirm these findings. Although most studies report the increase in anaerobic capacity following HIIT, the reported range of the increase varies. For example, Tabata et al. (1996) reported a 28% increase in anaerobic capacity after 6-week HIIT intervention [9]. One reason for inconsistent responses can be the duration of training program. Also, the effect of pre-training anaerobic fitness and the size of its response to training program can be another reason for the observed inconsistency. The improvement of aerobic capacity can be related to such factors as the increased concentration of phosphocreatine in muscles and its reproduction rate duration recovery, the activity of anaerobic enzymes, activation of motor unit, and the increase in buffer capacity of muscles. Low number of participants and the lack of nutritional control can be mentioned as the limitations of the study.

In conclusion, the present study examined the effect of 3-week HIIT intervention on body composition and bioenergetic indices of boy futsal players. It was found that HIIT increased aerobic and anaerobic powers significantly as compared to control. It seems that HIIT with the studied intensity and duration can be an effective training program for improving body composition and bioenergetic variables among boys. It is recommended to study the effect of similar trainings with longer durations on other indices in other sports in future studies.

Acknowledgement

The research was carried out by Rasht Branch of Islamic Azad University, Rasht, Iran.

Conflict of interest

The authors declare that there is no conflict of interest

References

1. Meckel and Yoav, et al. The effect of a brief sprint interval exercise on growth factors and inflammatory mediators. *The Journal of Strength & Conditioning Research*, 2009; 23(1): 225-230.

2. Gibala MJ and McGee SL. Metabolic adaptations to short-term high-intensity interval training: a little pain for a lot of gain? *Exercise and sport sciences reviews*, 2008; 36(2):58-63.
3. Hill-Haas SV, Coutts AJ, Rowsell GJ and Dawson BT. Generic versus small-sided game training in soccer. *International journal of sports medicine*, 2009; 30(9):636-42.
4. Burrows M and Bird SR. Velocity at VO2 max and peak treadmill velocity are not influenced within or across the phases of the menstrual cycle. *European journal of applied physiology*, 2005; 93(5):575-80.
5. Helgerud J, Hoydal K, Wang E, Karlsen T, Berg P, Bjerkaas M, et al. Aerobic High-Intensity Intervals Improve VO2max More Than Moderate Training. *Medicine and science in sports and exercise*, 2007; 39(4):665.
6. Barbero Alvarez JC and Castagna C. Activity patterns in professional futsal players using global position tracking system. *Journal of Sports Science and Medicine*, 2007; 6:208-209.
7. Doğramacı SN and Watsford ML. A comparison of two different methods for time-motion analysis in team sports. *International Journal of Performance Analysis in Sport*, 2006; 6(1):73-83.
8. Dupont G, Akakpo K, Berthoin S. The effect of in-season, high-intensity interval training in soccer players. *The Journal of Strength & Conditioning Research*, 2004; 18(3):584-9.
9. Tabata I, Nishimura K, Kouzaki M, Hirai Y, Ogita F, Miyachi M, et al. Effects of moderate-intensity endurance and high-intensity intermittent training on anaerobic capacity and VO2max. *Medicine and science in sports and exercise*, 1996;28(10):1327-30.
10. Helgerud J, Engen LC, Wisloff U, Hoff J. Aerobic endurance training improves soccer performance. *Medicine and science in sports and exercise*, 2001; 33(11):1925-31.
11. Trapp EG, Chisholm DJ, Freund J, Boutcher SH. The effects of high-intensity intermittent exercise training on fat loss and fasting insulin levels of young women. *International journal of obesity*, 2008; 32(4):684-691.
12. Gladden LB. lactate metabolism: a new paradigm for the third millennium. *The journal of physiology*, 2004; 558(1):5-30.
13. Barbero Alvarez JC, Castagna C. Activity patterns in professional futsal players using global position tracking system. *Journal of Sports Science and Medicine*, 2007; 6: 208-209.
14. Gremeaux V, Drigny J, Nigam A, Juneau M, Guilbeault V, Latour E, et al. Long-term lifestyle intervention with optimized high-intensity interval training improves body composition, cardiometabolic risk, and exercise parameters in patients with abdominal obesity. *American Journal of Physical Medicine & Rehabilitation*, 2012; 91(11):941-950.
15. Whyte LJ, Gill JM, Cathcart AJ. Effect of 2 weeks of sprint interval training on health-related outcomes in sedentary overweight/obese men. *Metabolism*. 2010; 31;59(10):1421-1428.
16. Sheikh Jafari M R, AghaAlinejad H. Effects of Progressive High Intensity Interval Training (HIT) on Aerobic and Anaerobic performance of male In-line speed Skating. *International Journal of Sport Studies,* 2014; 4(3): 297-303.
17. Bickham DC and Le Rossignol PF. Effect of High-Intensity Interval Training on the accumulated oxygen deficit of endurance-trained runners. *Journal of Exercise Physiology*, 2004 1; 7:40-47.
18. Karahan M. The effect of skill-based maximal intensity interval training on aerobic and anaerobic performance of female futsal players. *Biology of Sport*, 2012; 29(3):223-230.
19. Castagna C, Alvarez JC. Physiological demands of an intermittent futsal-oriented high-intensity test. *The Journal of Strength & Conditioning Research,* 2010; 24(9):2322-2329.
20. Castagna C, Belardinelli R, Impellizzeri FM, Abt GA, Coutts AJ, D'Ottavio S. Cardiovascular responses during recreational 5-a-side indoor-soccer. *Journal of Science and Medicine in Sport*, 2007; 10(2):89-95.
21. Silva G, Oliveira NL, Aires L, Mota J, Oliveira J, Ribeiro JC. Calculation and validation of models for estimating VO2max from the 20-m shuttle run test in children and adolescents. *Archives of Exercise in Health and Disease,* 2011; 3(1-2):145-52.
22. Moore R, Bullough S, Goldsmith S, Edmondson L. A systematic review of futsal literature. *American Journal of Sports Science and Medicine*, 2014;2(3):108-16.
23. Tremblay A, Simoneau JA, Bouchard C. Impact of exercise intensity on body fatness and skeletal muscle metabolism. *Metabolism*, 1994; 43(7):814-818.
24. Shing CM, Webb JJ, Driller MW, Williams AD, Fell JW. Circulating adiponectin concentration and body composition are altered in response to high-intensity interval training. *The Journal of Strength & Conditioning Research,* 2013; 27(8):2213-8.
25. Laursen PB, Shing CM, Peake JM, Coombes JS, Jenkins DG. Influence of high-intensity interval training on adaptations in well-trained cyclists. *The Journal of Strength & Conditioning Research*, 2005; 19(3):527-533.

26. Denadai BS, Ortiz MJ, Greco CC, de Mello MT. Interval training at 95% and 100% of the velocity at V O2 max: effects on aerobic physiological indexes and running performance. *Applied Physiology, Nutrition, and Metabolism,* 2006;31(6):737-743.
27. Astorino TA, Allen RP, Roberson DW, Jurancich M. Effect of high-intensity interval training on cardiovascular function, VO2max, and muscular force. *The Journal of Strength & Conditioning Research,* 2012;26(1):138-145.
28. Smith AE, Walter AA, Graef JL, Kendall KL, Moon JR, Lockwood CM, et al. Effects of β-alanine supplementation and high-intensity interval training on endurance performance and body composition in men; a double-blind trial. *Journal of the International Society of Sports Nutrition*, 2009; 11;6(1):1-10.
29. Laursen PB, Blanchard MA, Jenkins DG. Acute high-intensity interval training improves Tvent and peak power output in highly trained males. *Canadian Journal of Applied Physiology*, 2002; 27(4):336-348.
30. Burgomaster KA, Hughes SC, Heigenhauser GJ, Bradwell SN, Gibala MJ. Six sessions of sprint interval training increases muscle oxidative potential and cycle endurance capacity in humans. *Journal of applied physiology,* 2005; 98(6):1985-1990.

16

EFFECTIVENESS OF FOLK GAMES' APPLICATION IN FORMATION OF PEDAGOGIC SPECIALTIES GIRL STUDENTS' VALUE ORIENTATIONS ON PHYSICAL CULTURE

Mayevsky M.I.
Pavlo Tychyna Uman State Pedagogical University

Abstract. *Purpose:* to determine effectiveness of structurally meaningful model of formation of girl students' value orientations on physical culture. *Material:* in the research control group (28 girl students) and experimental group (30 girl students) participated. We used sociological questioning, testing of physical and theoretical fitness. *Results:* It was found that combination of four blocks (theoretical, methodic, practical and managerial) is optimal for technology of model realization. It ensures impact on physical and spiritual-intellectual sides of girl students. *Conclusions:* it is recommended to practice active immersion in folk traditions and customs of Ukraine with girl students. It permits to form girls' psychological and social readiness for conducting of cultural measures. Motor activity in personal and future professional functioning makes elements of such measures.
Key words: values, physical culture, model, girl students, customs.

Introduction

In modern pedagogic space of Ukraine the problem of non physical culture specialties students' orientation on physical culture values has still been unsolved. It is known that health condition of future pedagogues insistently signals about negative tendencies. Girls require special approaches to organization and building of physical culture trainings. In most cases they are rather far from systemic motor activity. Girls are the most critical in choice of forms and methods of trainings' organization. All these require from sports and physical culture specialists to find more effective approaches to increasing of young people interest to physical culture and sports, considering their desires.

Scientific researches of domestic scientists (N.A. Dedeliuk, S.V. Nikolayev, V.V. Zkhozhiy (2013) [19]; T.Yu. Krutsevych, G.V. Bezverkhnia (2010) [6]; V.O. Sutula, P.M. Kyzym, V.V. Shiteyev, Yu.O. Fishev, L.S. Lutsenko (2014) [11]; S.M. Futornoy (2015) [14]; A. Tsos, A. Shevchuk, O. Kasarda (2014) [16]) and foreign specialists (Chatzisarantis N.L.D., Hagger M.S. (2009) [18]; Standage M., Gillison F.B., Ntoumanis N., Treasure D.C.(2012) [21]; Aelterman N., Vansteenkiste M., VanKeer H., Vanden BergheL., DeMeyer J., Haerens L. (2012) [17]; How Y.M., Whipp P.R., Dimmock J.A., Jackson B. (2013) [20]; Koka A. (2013) [21]) point at demand in increasing of students' motor functioning through formation of their interest and stimulation of their demands and motives for physical exercises' practicing. In general, such approaches relate to value orientations on physical culture sphere.

Application of folk games in practice of students and pupils' physical education was tested by different authors (V.M. Vakulenko [3], T.I. Kulik, T.I. Kudriashova [7], O. Tkachenko [12]). But ethno-pedagogic potential of the mentioned scientists did not contain purposeful impact on formation of students' value orientations on physical culture. In the researches by M.M. Sainchuk effectiveness of folk games for solution of such tasks was proved on example of senior pupils. But by the present time there have been declared no works on formation of pedagogic specialties girl students' value orientations on physical culture by means of folk games. It conditioned the topicality of our research.

Purpose, tasks of the work, material and methods

The purpose of the work is to determine effectiveness of the author's structurally meaningful model of formation of pedagogic specialties girl students' value orientations on physical culture

The tasks of the research: registration of changes in physical and theoretical fitness indicators, in indicators of physical health, attitude to discipline "physical culture. Separately we registered indicators of independent sport-physical culture functioning after implementation of the offered model.

Results of the researches

Pedagogic experiment implied implementation of structurally meaningful model of value orientations' for physical culture formation in pedagogic specialties girl students in process of physical education by means of ethno-pedagogic (folk games). Pavlo Tychyna Uman State Pedagogical University was the base for those pedagogic researches. At the beginning of forming experiment we formed control group (CG – 28 girl students of pre-school education faculty) and experimental group (EG – 30 girl students of philological faculty).Both groups consisted of 2nd year students. By their health these girls related to main health group. They had no counter indications or any limitations to trainings.

In EG experimental work on formation of value orientations on physical culture was conducted in academic lessons during several semesters (3rd – 4th). At physical culture trainings special accent was made on inner setting of ethno-cultural values. It was realized through recreation of ethno-cultural system of values in process of physical exercises' fulfillment. It permitted to perceive life and spiritual experience of ancestors in aspect of modern cultural process. In CG the trainings were conducted according to traditional program.

Structurally meaningful model of formation of future Ukrainian philology teachers' value orientations on physical culture in physical education process consisted of the following blocks: theoretical, methodic and managerial. All blocks were analyzed in detail in one of the author's articles [8]. The games were selected so that they would influence on preservation and strengthening of girl students' health by opening their spiritual, mental and physical potentials. Thus, value orientations on physical culture on the base of folk motor culture were formed.

Effectiveness of realization of structurally meaningful model of value orientations on physical culture formation in philological faculty girl students was tested by comparison of indicators' changes before and after experiment6 in EG and CG): physical fitness; physical health; theoretical fitness; attitude to discipline "physical culture"; independent practicing of sport-physical culture activity.

Indicators of EG and CG girl students before experiment (see table 1) witness girls of non physical culture specialties have rather weak physical qualities (low level). These indicators were in one range of data. Before experiment difference in dexterity (CG – 11.20 ± 0.11 sec.; EG – 11.21 ± 0.11 sec.), flexibility (CG – 17.3 ± 0.78 cm.; EG – 17.1 ± 0.70 cm.) was not found. Results of test for quickness (CG – 6.14 ± 0.12 sec.; EG – 5.97 ± 0.09 sec.), power abilities (by dynamometry): CG – 19.8 ± 0.46 kg.; EG – 20.8 ± 0.49 kg.), power endurance (CG – 12.4 ± 0.77 times; EG – 14.2 ± 0.92 times) and explosive power (CG – 160.9 ± 3.77 cm.; EG – 158.4 ± 4.14 cm.) point also at close to each other values between both groups. EG girls showed better results (CG – 23.6 ± 1.55 times against 29.3 ± 1.86 times in EG) only in speed-power qualities (torso rising during 30 sec.).

After forming pedagogic experiment only in physical fitness EG girl students showed confident changes in some tests (dexterity and strength). In CG actual results remained on previous level. It witnesses that type structure of physical culture girl students' training does not facilitate improvement of physical fitness. In CG we also did not register any increment in physical qualities. The highest achievement (not confident) was registered in explosive power in comparison with previous values 160.9 ± 3.77 cm. Final increment was 5 cm (165.9 ± 2.95 cm.).

Thus, analysis of physical fitness indicators (before and after pedagogic experiment) showed significant improvement of EG girls' physical condition. Though, their physical fitness corresponds to average level of senior school pupils. In CG physical fitness remained on previous level.

After pedagogic experiment, there were registered some changes in physical health of EG girls. Before experiment there was no confident difference between CG and EG. After experiment, health level of CG girls remained at previous level (below average, 5 points). In CG no index changed confidently and noticeably. Actually their indices remained close to initial data. In EG (after experiment) physical health improved by 2 levels: from low (3 points) to average (9 points). It happened at the account of confident ($p < 0.05$) improvement of power index indicator and heart beats rate restoration (HBR). Power index increased from 35.8 ± 1.11% to 42.3 ± 1.23%. This result (improvement) correlates with previous data of physical fitness, where we detected undoubted growth of strength. In respect to HBR restoration: after 20 squats EG girls showed improvement of results from low level (3.11 ± 0.22 min.) to average (1.52 ± 0.36 min.). It witnesses about better functioning of cardio-vascular system.

Testing of theoretical fitness of EG and CG girl students (see table 2) at the beginning of pedagogic experiment showed that among EG girls low level dominates – 73.4%. This indicator exceeded twice CG group (32.1%). Most of CG girls demonstrated average level (67.9%) and only 23.3% EG girls showed the same. In EG only one girl (3.3%) had sufficient level of theoretical knowledge on physical culture.

Table 1. Physical fitness indicators of CG and EG girl students before and after pedagogic experiment

Physical quality		Indicators											
		Control group (n=28)						Experimental group (n=30)					
		Before experiment			After experiment			Before experiment			After experiment		
		$\overline{x}$	m	δ	$\overline{x}$	m	δ	$\overline{x}$	m	δ	$\overline{x}$	m	δ
Quickness (30 m. run), m/sec.		6.14	0.12	0.62	6.05	0.14	0.53	5.97	0.09	0.38	5.47	0.11	0.41
Dexterity (shuttle ruin 4 x 9 m.), sec.		11.20	0.11	0.59	11.16	0.12	0.52	11.21	0.11	0.59	9.31*	0.12	0.49
Power	Explosive power (long jump from the spot) cm.	160.9	3.77	20.9	165.9	2.95	11.9	158.4	4.14	26.3	171.3*	3.15	20.1
	Hand dynamometry, kg	19.8	0.46	2.28	20.5	0.41	2.91	20.8	0.49	2.39	25.6*	0.41	2.25
	Pressing ups, times	12.40	0.77	4.32	14.1	0.75	4.82	14.2	0.92	5.17	18.5	0.83	4.37
	Torso rising for 30 sec.	23.60	1.55	8.20	24.2	1.60	8.35	29.3	1.86	9.23	31.7	1.68	8.75
Flexibility (forward torso bending) cm.		17.30	0.78	4.41	17.8	0.71	4.32	17.1	0.70	4.11	19.01	0.65	3.94

Notes: *(P<0.05)

Table 2. Physical culture theoretical fitness in CG and EG

Levels of knowledge	Control group (n=28)				Experimental group (n=30)			
	Before experiment		After experiment		Before experiment		After experiment	
	n	%	n	%	n	%	n	%
Low	9	32.1	8	28.6	22	73.4	3	10
Average	19	67.9	20	71.4	7	233	17	63.3
Sufficient	–	–	–	–	1	3.3	10	26.7

After forming experiment theoretical fitness cardinally improved only in EG. In Cg there were practically no changes (only one girl student improved her level, passing from low level to average). Structurally meaningful model facilitated decreasing of part of girls with low level (in EG it reduced up to 10%), increasing of average level (up to 63.3%) and sufficient (up to 26.7%). Practical application of models stimulated independence and interest to physical culture knowledge. All these witness about serious rise of EG girls understanding of physical culture.

In attitude to discipline "physical culture qualitative changes took place only in EG. For them discipline "physical culture" became more interesting. Accordingly, lessons became more attractive (in this aspect girls improved their results from 1.9–2.0 points to 1.4 points). The best result implies 1 point. Physical education classes awakened demand in independent motor activity (from neutral mark 2.5 points – improvement to 1.6 points) and wish to train additionally in sport circle (from 3.4 points to at the beginning of experiment to 1.5 – after it). It also promoted systemic character of EG girl students practicing of physical exercises. EG girls joined to kinds of physical functioning of health related character. In particular it was aerobics and rhythmic gymnastic (from 3.3% to 16.7%), sport dances (6,7%), light athletic (from 13.3% to 20%). Such form as sport cultural leisure covered 23.3%. In CG involvement in systemic physical exercises' practicing did not practically change.

So, structurally meaningful model of formation of value orientations on physical culture enriched philological faculty girl students with motor experience of folk physical culture through received by them knowledge, skills of application of games in professional and independent activity.

Discussion

The received experimental data confirm results of other scientists (O.YU. Marchenko, Марченко, 2010; A.A. Bilichenko, 2014) [2, 9] concerning usage of stimulating and limiting factors in work with girl students for their motivation for physical culture. Also we confirmed results of V. Vakulenko, 2010; I. Kulyk, T.I. Kudriashov, 2009; N.N. Sainchuk, 2012; A. Tkachenko, 2013) about effectiveness of ethno-pedagogic means (folk games) in practice of pupils' and students' physical education for formation of their motivation-values settings on motor functioning [3, 7, 10, 12].

We supplemented and expanded scientific data of B.D. Bazilchuk [1], N.I. Turchina [13], I. Gonchar [4], A.G. Gladoshchuk [5], V.V. Tsybulskaya [15, who noted that formation of value orientations and positive motivation for systemic practicing of motor functioning and sports in extra-curriculum time are influenced by organizational-methodic conditions of HEE educational process.

For the first time structurally meaningful model of formation of girl students' value orientations on physical culture by means of ethno-pedagogic was theoretically substantiated and worked out. The model consisted of such blocks as: theoretical, methodic, practical and managerial. These block influence logically and consistently on physical and spiritual-intellectual spheres of personality. They cultivate students' positive holistic attitude to physical culture. Besides we determined limiting and stimulating factors, which influence of formation of value orientations on physical culture. As limiting factors, we determined: theoretical fitness, health condition, motivation for trainings and success in trainings. As positive factors we determined: axiological, orientation on healthy life style, image of physically cultural person, communicative factor, consideration of girl students' interests to different kinds of sports and physical exercises, reliance on game traditions of Ukrainians.

Conclusions

1. Realization technology of structurally meaningful model of formation of future Ukrainian philology teachers' value orientations on physical culture in physical education process was connected with optimal combination of four blocks – theoretical, methodic, practical and managerial. It permitted to ensure influence on girl students' physical and spiritual-intellectual sides. This influence was realized through activation of girl students' understanding of traditions and customs of Ukrainians as well as through strengthening of girls' psychological and sociological readiness for conducting of cultural measures with motor functioning elements. EG girl students changed their understanding of physical culture values. In particular they improved their marks on significance of "physical culture" discipline for future work by 0.8 points – from 24 points to 1.6 points (1 – implies the best mark). Qualitative dynamic (from 2.1 points to 1.5 points) was found in their recognition that physical culture can ensure development of general culture.
2. Structurally meaningful model of value orientations' on physical culture formation influenced on physical component of philological faculty girl students. Application of this model resulted in strengthening of their health (from low to average level) and better progressing of physical qualities (especially strength). Intellectual-spiritual side also was enriched with knowledge of organization of motor cultural measures in practical work. It is confirmed by girl students' theoretical fitness. It was facilitated by basic level of knowledge of healthy life style rules, methodic of training of physical qualities and self control methods for physical exercises' practicing, (at the beginning of experiment there were 36.7% of involved in different forms of sports and physical functioning; at the end of experiment there were 86.7%).

The prospects of further researches can be implementation of additional stimuli (self control of physical condition being the most important among them) in physical education process.

Conflict of interests

The author declares that there is no conflict of interests.

Reference:

1. Bazil'chuk VB. *Organizacijni zasadi aktivizacii sportivno-ozdorovchoi diial'nosti studentiv v umovakh vishchogo navchal'nogo zakladu. Cand.Diss.* [Organizational principles of activation of students' health-related sport functioning in conditions of higher educational establishment. Cand. Diss], LDUFK; 2004. (in Ukrainian)
2. Bilichenko OO. *Genderni osoblivosti formuvannia motivacii do zaniat' fizichnim vikhovanniam u studentiv. Cand.Diss.* [Gender peculiarities of formation of students' motivation for physical education classes. Cand. Diss.], Dnipropetrovsk; 2014. (in Ukrainian)
3. Vakulenko VM, Stiagunova OO. Rol' gendernogo aspektu u formuvanni cinnisnikh oriientacij na ideiakh narodnoi pedagogiki majbutnikh pedagogiv. [Role of gender aspect in formation of future pedagogues' value orientations on ideas of folk pedagogic]. *Dukhovnist' osobistosti: metodologiia, teoriia i praktika*, 2010; 2; 44–54. (in Ukrainian)
4. Gonchar GI. *Organizacijno-metodichni umovi formuvannia motivacii studentiv institutiv fizichnoi kul'turi do profesijno-prikladnoi fizichnoi pidgotovki. Cand.Diss*. [Orgnizational-methodic conditions of formation of physical culture students' motivation for professionally applied physical training. Cand. Diss.], Dnipropetrovsk; 2013. (in Ukrainian)
5. Gladoshchuk OG. *Pedagogichni umovi vdoskonalennia kul'turi zmicnennia zdorov'ia studentiv v sistemi fizichnogo vikhovannia u vishchomu navchal'nomu zakladi. Cand.Diss*. [Pedagogic conditions of improvement of students' health strengthening culture in system of physical education at higher education establishment. Cand. Diss.]. Kiev; 2008. (in Ukrainian)
6. Krucevich TIu, Bezverkhnia GV. *Rekreaciia u fizichnij kul'turi riznikh grup naselennia* [Recreation in physical culture of different population strata], Kiev: Olympic Literature; 2010. (in Ukrainian)
7. Kulik IG, Kudriashova TI. Ukrains'ki narodni rukhlivi igri iak zasib dosiagnennia fizichnoi doskonalosti studentstva. [Ukrainian motor games as method of achievement of students' physical perfectness]. *Pedagogics, psychology, medical-biological problems of physical training and sports,* 2009;3;85–87. (in Ukrainian)
8. Maievs'kij MI. Eksperimental'na model' formuvannia cinnisnikh oriientacij na fizichnu kul'turu studentok pedagogichnikh special'nostej. [Experimental model of formation of pedagogic specialties' girl students' value orientations on physical culture]. *Visnik Chernigivs'kogo nacional'nogo pedagogichnogo universitetu imeni T.G. Shevchenka,* 2015;129:210–213. (in Ukrainian)
9. Marchenko OIu. *Formuvannia cinnisnikh kategorij osobistoi fizichnoi kul'turi u students'koi molodi. Cand.Diss. [*Formation of students' value categories of personal physical culture. Cand. Diss.] Dnipropetrovsk; 2010. (in Ukrainian)
10. Sainchuk MM. *Formuvannia cinnisnikh oriientacij u sferi fizichnoi kul'turi i sportu uchniv starshikh klasiv u procesi fizichnogo vikhovannia. Cand.Diss*.[Formation of senior schoolchildren's value orientations in sphere of physical culture and sports in process of physical education. Cand. Diss.], Kiev; 2012. (in Ukrainian)
11. Sutula VO, Kizim PM, Shutieiev VV, Fishev IuO, Lucenko LS. Shliakhi optimizacii fizichnoi aktivnosti students'koi molodi [Ways of optimization of students' physical functioning], *Slobozhans'kij naukovo-sportivnij visnik,* 2014;6(44);106–111. (in Ukrainian)
12. Tkachenko O. Deiaki aspekti formuvannia igrovoi kul'turi pedagoga [Some aspects of formation of pedagogue's playing culture], *Naukovi zapiski.* 2013;120:286–288. (in Ukrainian)
13. Turchina NI. *Pedagogichni osoblivosti modelej fizichnogo vikhovannia studentiv VNZ na riznikh kursakh navchannia. Cand.Diss*. [Pedagogic features of models of HEEs students' physical education at different years of studying. Cand. Diss.], Kyiv; 2009. (in Ukrainian)
14. Futornij SM. *Teoretiko-metodichni osnovi innovacijnikh tekhnologij formuvannia zdorovogo sposobu zhittia studentiv v procesi fizichnogo vikhovannia. Cand.Diss*. [Theoretical-methodic principles of innovation

technologies of students' healthy life style formation in process of physical education. Cand. Diss.], Kyiv; 2015. (in Ukrainian)

15. Cibul's'ka VV. *Formuvannia motivacii do profesijno-prikladnoi fizichnoi pidgotovki studentiv pedagogichnikh special'nostej na riznikh formakh navchannia. Cand.Diss.* [Formation of motivation for professional-applied physical trainings of pedagogic specialties' students at different forms of studying. Cand. Diss.], Uman; 2014. (in Ukrainian)
16. C'os' A, Shevchuk A, Kasarda O. *Rukhova aktivnist' u motivacijno-cinnisnikh oriientaciiakh studentiv. [Motor functioning in students' motivation-value orientations], Fizichne vikhovannia, sport i kul'tura zdorov'ia u suchasnomu suspil'stv,* 2014;4;83–87 (in Ukrainian)
17. Aelterman N., Vansteenkiste M., Van Keer H., Van den Berghe L., De Meyer J., &Haerens L. Students' Objectively Measured Physical ActivityLevels and Engagement asa Function of Between-Class and Between-Student Differences in Motivation Toward Physical Education. *Journal of Sport & Exercise Psychology*; 2012;34(4);457–480.
18. Chatzisarantis N.L.D. and Hagger M.S. Effects of an intervention based on self-determination theory on self-reported leisure-time physical activity participation. *Psychology and Health*; 2009;24;29–48.
19. Dedeliuk N, Nikolayev S, Zakhozij V, Comparative analysis of female students physical fitness state and physical activity, *Human and Health*; 2013;7(2);3–7.
20. How YM, Whipp PR, Dimmock JA & Jackson B. The Effects of Choice on Autonomous Motivation, Perceived Autonomy Support, and Physical Activity Levels in High School Physical Education. *Journal of Teaching in Physical Education;* 2013;32(2);131–148.
21. Koka A. The effect of teacher and peers need support on students' motivation in physical education and its relationship to leisure time physical activity. *ActaKinesiologiae,* 2013;19:48–62. http://dx.doi.org/10.12697/akut.2013.19.0.
22. Standage M, Gillison B, Ntoumanis N & Treasure DC. Predicting students' physical activity and health-related well-being: a prospective cross-domain investigation of motivation across school physical education and exercise settings. *Journal of Sport & Exercise Psychology*; 2012;34(1);37–60.

THEORETICAL TRAINING IN PHYSICAL EDUCATION OF HIGHER EDUCATIONAL ESTABLISHMENTS' GIRL STUDENTS

Gordienko Y.V.
Poltava National Technical Yuri Kondratyuk University

Abstract. *Purpose:* testing and analysis of theoretical-methodic training of girl students at physical education classes. *Material:* in the research 45 2nd year girl students of 18-19 age, participated. One group dealt with power-lifting and volleyball. Second group – practiced trainings by usual academic program. *Results:* it was found that girl students' theoretical knowledge corresponds to middle level. It was also established that increase of motivation for acquiring and mastering knowledge facilitates effectiveness of physical education trainings' construction. *Conclusions:* absence of physical education theoretical knowledge or its low level in girl students sharply reduces effectiveness of training and education, weakens interest to physical exercises' and sports' practicing.

Key words: girl students, physical education, power-lifting, test, control.

Introduction

Physical culture in HEE is an academic discipline and important basic component of formation of youth's general culture. It is known that mastering only practical skills of physical perfection, without sufficient theoretical and methodic knowledge does not permit for students to correctly apply their skills in independent practicing of physical exercises [2-5; 9; 26; 32, 34-36; 40] и во время профессиональной деятельности [3; 8; 11; 15; 16; 20-26].

Studying this problem, scientists T. Krutsevich, O. Marchenko and A. Tomenko conclude that important place in perfection of physical education system belongs to formation of values through theoretical training and increase of pedagogic control's effectiveness [10; 19]. In works by V. Sorokina and V. Temchenko main components of students' personal education level have been found. With it the authors underline need in control of theoretical knowledge in physical education. The authors affirm that presence of objective information permits to find strong and weak sides of structure of preparedness, to realize proper planning and correction of training process [15; 16].

Increase of effectiveness of pedagogic control over students' fitness level is rather important in perfection of physical education [6; 22-25, 37, 38]. N. Moskalenko et al. substantiated innovative technologies of physical education. They are directed on strengthening of students' health with the help of theoretical training and cultivation of personal values and motives for trainings [12]. In researches by N. Zavidovskaya and P. Oksem it is noted that theoretical aspects of education in sphere of physical culture have declarative character in higher school and exist only on pages of program documents [7; 14].

Analysis of publications shows that in conditions of higher education's reforming problem of theoretical learning and control over students' progress in practical and theoretical skills and knowledge acquires special urgency and requires further researches.

Purpose, tasks of the work, material and methods

The purpose of the research is testing and analysis of theoretical-methodic training of girl students at physical education classes. *The methods of the research:* in the course of our work we used pedagogic observation for analysis and assessment of girl students' theoretical knowledge. Experimental researches were conducted on the base of Poltava National Technical Yuri Kondratyuk University (PoltNTU). In the research 45 2nd year girl students of 18-19 age, participated. First group dealt with power-lifting and volleyball. Second group – practiced trainings by usual academic program.

Results of the researches

As the main hypothesis of this research we assumed that theoretical knowledge indirectly facilitates significant increasing of purposefulness and effectiveness of physical education process. Proper organization of physical education trainings in university shall envisage compulsory lecture hours for theoretical course. In this case all material to be studied is distributed by semesters. Topics of lecture course shall contain main information about theory and methodic of physical education and sports, healthy life style, professional-applied physical fitness.

In PoltNTU rather interesting teaching modules on program "Physical education" are practiced. Alongside with practical part (trainings and practical-methodic classes) theoretical section is stipulated. This section forms students' world vision, scientific-methodic knowledge and facilitates formation of positive attitude to physical culture and sports. Every module envisages complex of compulsory lessons. It includes also theoretical and independent students' trainings. Theoretical course is delivered in the form of lectures (12 academic hours). The course offers independent studying of the subject with the help of recommended literature and Internet resources. Student's individual work implies profound studying of separate theoretical and methodic questions of physical fitness's perfection, health improvement, sport's perfection.

Lecture course includes the following topics:

Lecture № 1. Physical culture and sports as natural component of general culture of society. Physical culture (PC) as social phenomenon in life of society. Main means of PC. PC and sports in life of modern man. Factors, determining demand of modern man in practicing of physical exercises. PC and sports in system of higher school. Functioning of sport club (SC).

Lecture № 2. Natural-scientific principles of physical education. Human organism as uniform complex biological system. Motor functioning and its influence on functioning of human organs and organism. Physical inactivity and hypokinesia. Laws of human organs' and organism systems' development in process of physical; exercises' practicing. Physiological characteristic of motor functioning means.

Lecture № 3. Principles of healthy life style (HLS). Conception of health. Main components of HLS and their characteristics. Factors, influencing on quality of life and life span of an individual. Motor functioning as important component of healthy life style.

Lecture № 4. Principles of physical and sports training. The essence of training process. Methodic principles of training's and its components' construction. Sport competitions as mean and method of sportsmen's training. Specific features of organization and planning of sport trainings.

Lecture 5. Professional-applied physical trainings (PAPT). Content and main tasks of PAPT. Factors, determining importance and general orientation of PAPT. Formation of applied movements, motor skills. Cultivation of special physical qualities. Dynamic of human workability during day, week. Means of workability's rising; struggle with industrial fatigue; prevention of professional diseases. Tests and control normative of PAPT. .

Lecture № 6. Physical culture in scientific organization of work (SOW). Physical culture and sports in SOW. Purpose and main tasks of physical culture in SOW. Formation of system of knowledge, motor skills in purposeful application of physical culture and sports' means in work and leisure for prevention of industrial fatigue. Prophylaxis of professional diseases; rising of productivity; preservation and strengthening of health.

Independent classes are organized with the help of electronic library of the university. Students deepen their knowledge with manuals and methodic recommendations, Internet resources. For control of theoretical knowledge we conducted pedagogic experiment in the form of theoretical testing at the end of 2nd academic year.

For determination of students' theoretical knowledge questionnaire is used at department of physical education of PoltNTU. The questionnaire contains 50 questions. Every question has four alternative answers, from which one, correct, shall be chosen. The tests include questions about healthy life style, history of physical education and sports, specific features of physical exercises' practicing, planning of physical loads in independent trainings.

Criteria of students' knowledge assessment depend on quantity of correct answers. Every correct answer brings 1 point: 50-40 points – "excellent"; 39-30 points – "good"; 29-20 points –satisfactory"; 19 points and less – "unsatisfactory".

For experiment we formed three groups of girl students. Two experimental groups: EG1 (girl students practiced power-lifting by the author's methodic); EG2 (girl students trained volleyball). One control group CG consisted of girl students, who were trained as per traditional academic program of PoltNTU. Quantity of girl students in every group was 15 persons. By mean group indicators of physical condition and physical fitness all girl students did not confidently differ. We carried out experimental substantiation of training process's methodic. Effectiveness of the offered methodic was assessed by results of girl students' performances at competitions and by control over their emotional and physiological status.

Analysis of testing of girl students' theoretical knowledge in all directions of physical trainings showed that it corresponds to middle level. More detail results of the researches showed low level of theoretical knowledge of girl students, who were trained by traditional physical education program (CG) (see table 1). Girl students from volleyball group (EG2) had higher level of knowledge. The highest indicators belonged to girl students – power lifters (EG1).

Table 1

Assessment of knowledge in "Physical education" subject of PoltNTU second year girl students

№	Mark	EG1		EG2		CG	
		quantity	*%*	*quantity*	*%*	*quantity*	*%*
1	Excellent	8	40	6	30	4	20
2	Good	7	35	6	30	2	10
3	Satisfactory	5	25	6	30	12	60
4	Unsatisfactory			2	10	2	10

Comparing of inter group indicators showed that the highest level of theoretical preparedness is observed in EG1. In this group mean indicator was 35.85% of correct answers. These results are significantly higher than in CG. In Egl this result was 33.65%. In CG we registered only 28.85% of correct answers. Nearly all indicators of "Power-lifting" and "Volleyball" girl students' theoretical preparedness correspond to middle and high levels.

Testing results permit to affirm that EG1 girl students mastered theoretical knowledge in physical education better than EG2 and CG girl students. The best results of testing were demonstrated by "Power-lifting" girl students. It witnesses about higher scope of knowledge and higher quality of these girl students' thinking.

Also we can affirm that EG1 girl students paid more attention to independent work with subject. In their independent classes the girl students see possibility to achieve certain aim of learning cognitive activity in training process. In EG2 group we did not observe interest to subject "Physical education". This group's girl students received theoretical knowledge only from academic material oriented on curriculum. The presented results of the researches witness about insufficient "Physical education" theoretical knowledge of CG girl students.

Absence or low level of girl students' theoretical knowledge in physical education sharply reduce effectiveness of training, weaken interest to physical exercises' practicing; hinder cultivation of students' positive attitude to systemic independent physical culture trainings.

Discussion

Results of the conducted experiments are confirmed by other researches [29-31, 33-40]. The authors affirm that scope of knowledge about physical culture is in direct proportion to level of motor functioning's mental component. It results in better progress in mastering of skills when practicing physical exercises.

Also we confirmed the data about unsatisfactory level of girl students' theoretical-methodic preparedness in physical education (S. Berezka [2]; N. Moskalenko, T. Sycheva [12]). Results of the researches permitted to supplement the data about effectiveness of physical education trainings' construction by choice of students that facilitate increase of motivation for acquiring and mastering of knowledge (G.V. Vlasov [4], V.A. Temchenko [18]). We supplemented also information that increasing of physical fitness is accompanied by rising of students' theoretical knowledge level (T. I. Dukh[6]).

The data about positive influence of power lifting program on girl students' interest in theoretical course of physical education and improvement of their knowledge of this subject are the novelty of the researches.

Conclusions:

Results of the researches permit to affirm that author's model of formation of modern HEE girl students' harmonious personalities under influence of power-lifting trainings can be considered in working out of new conception of governmental physical education program. With it, for increasing of cognitive activity and girl students' interest in self education it is necessary to perfect teaching of theoretical section, involving new informational technologies, effective and modern teaching methods.

Acknowledgement

The research has been fulfilled in compliance with plan of scientific research works of Ministry of education and science, youth and sports of Ukraine by topic 3.6 "Scientific-theoretical principles of innovative technologies in physical education of different population strata" (state registration number 0111U001169).

Conflict of interests

The author declares that there is no conflict of interests.

References:

1. Afanas'iev VV, Gavrilova NM, Mikhajlenko VM. Fizichne vikhovannia u zhitti studentok [Physical education in girl students' life]. *Pedagogics, psychology, medical-biological problems of physical training and sports*. 2008; 10: 13−16. (in Ukrainian)
2. Berezka SM. Teoretichni ta metodichni znannia studentiv z navchal'noi disciplini «fizichne vikhovannia» [Theoretical and methodic knowledge of students in discipline "physical education"]. *Pedagogics, psychology, medical-biological problems of physical training and sports.* 2011; 3: 12–14. (in Ukrainian)
3. Bilogur VIe. *Teoretiko-metodichne zabezpechennia fizichnogo vikhovannia u vishchikh zakladakh osviti. Cand. Diss*. [Theoretical-methodic provisioning of physical education in higher educational establishments. Cand Diss.], Rivne, 2002. (in Ukrainian)
4. Vlasov GV. Vivchennia dinamiki sportivnikh upodoban' studentiv vishchikh medichnikh navchal'nikh zakladiv [Study of sport bents' dynamic of students of higher medical establishments]. *Naukovij visnik Donbasu.* 2011;1(13):45-50. (in Ukrainian)
5. Volkov V. Problema rozrobki tekhnologii upravlinnia fizichnoiu pidgotovkoiu suchasnoi students'koi molodi [Problem of working out of technology of modern students' physical trainings' control]. *Teoriia i metodika fizichnogo vikhovannia i sportu,* 2008;2:41–46. (in Ukrainian)
6. Dukh TI. *Teoretiko-metodichna ta fizichna pidgotovka studentiv iz zastosuvanniam vzaiemonavchannia u processi fizichnogo vikhovannia. Cand. Diss*. [Theoretical-methodic and physical training of students with application of peer learning in physical education. Cand. Diss.], Lviv, 2014. (in Ukrainian)
7. Zavidivs'ka NN. *Pedagogichni zasadi formuvannia zdorovogo sposobu zhittia studentiv vishchikh zakladiv osviti ekonomichnogo profiliu. Cand. Diss*. [Pedagogic principles of formation of higher economic educational establishments students' healthy life style. Cand. Diss.], Lviv, 2001. (in Ukrainian)
8. Klimakova TA. Analiz stanu fizichnogo vikhovannia u vishchikh navchal'nikh zakladakh [Analysis of physical education status at higher educational establishments]. *Pedagogics, psychology, medical-biological problems of physical training and sports*. 2011; 8: 36−39. (in Ukrainian)
9. Koval'chuk V. Suchasni pidkhodi do ociniuvannia navchal'nikh dosiagnen' iz fizichnogo vikhovannia studentiv [Modern approaches top assessment of educational progress in students' physical education]. *Fizichne vikhovannia, sport i kul'tura zdorov'ia u suchasnomu suspil'stvi.* 2012;4:285–289. (in Ukrainian)
10. Marchenko O.Iu, Krucevich T.Iu. Vliianie vneshnikh i vnutrennikh faktorov na formirovanie cennostnykh orientacij fizicheskoj kul'tury studentov [Influence of external and internal factors on formation of value orientation of students' physical culture]. *XII Mezhdunarodnyj nauchnyj kongress "Sovremennyj olimpijskij i paralimpijskij sport i sport dlia vsekh"* [XII International scientific congress "Modern Olympic and para-Olympic sports and sports for all"], Kiev, 2008; T.1:89–90. (in Russian)

11. Merkulova ZIa. Poshuk diievikh shliakhiv formuvannia rukhovoi kul'turi u procesi fizichnogo vikhovannia studentiv vishchikh tekhnichnikh navchal'nikh zakladiv [Searching of practical ways of motor culture formation in physical education of technical higher educational establishments' students]. *Pedagogics, psychology, medical-biological problems of physical training and sports.* 2008;6:54–56. (in Ukrainian)
12. Moskalenko N, Sichova T, Anastas'ieva Z. Innovacijni tekhnologii fizichnogo vikhovannia spriamovani na zmicnennia zdorov'ia studentiv [Innovative technologies of physical education, oriented on strengthening of students' health]. *Sportivnij visnik Pridnistrov'ia*, 2012;2:10–12. (in Ukrainian)
13. Muntian VS. Fight-fitness v programme fizicheskogo vospitaniia studentov vysshikh uchebnykh zavedenij [Fight - fitness in program of higher educational establishments' students]. *Physical education of students*, 2011;1:94-98. (in Russian)
14. Oks'om P, Berezhna L, Shmatkova A. Stavlennia studentok vishchogo pedagogichnogo navchal'nogo zakladu do fizichnogo vikhovannia [Attitude of higher educational establishments' girl students to physical education]. *Teoriia i metodika fizicheskogo vospitaniia,* 2008;2:11–14. (in Ukrainian)
15. Okhrimenko OV, Vereshchagina OP. Zavdannia vikladacha – vikhovannia moral'nikh iakostej u students'koi molodi na zaniattiakh z fizichnoi kul'turi i sportu [The task of teacher – cultivation of moral values in students at physical culture and sport trainings]. *Pedagogics, psychology, medical-biological problems of physical training and sports.* 2008;11:130–133. (in Ukrainian)
16. Prisiazhniuk S. Kriterii ociniuvannia uspishnosti studentiv z predmeta „Fizichne vikhovannia" [Criteria of students' progress assessment in discipline "Physical education"]. *Fizichne vikhovannia v shkoli*, 2003; 2: 35–38. (in Ukrainian)
17. Sorokina VM, Sorokin DIu. Formirovanie otnoshenij k zdorovomu obrazu zhizni kak professional'noj cennosti u studentov [Formation of attitude to healthy life style as students' professional value]. *Sovremennye problemy nauki i obrazovaniia,* 2009; 6: 52–56. (in Russian)
18. Temchenko VA. *Sportivno orientirovannoe fizicheskoe vospitanie v vysshikh uchebnykh zavedeniiakh s primneniem informacionnykh tekhnologij. Cand. Diss.* [Sport oriented physical education in higher educational establishments with application of information technologies. Cand. Diss.], Kharkov, 2015. (in Russian)
19. Tomenko O, Krucevich T. Konceptual'na model' nespecial'noi fizkul'turnoi osviti uchnivs'koi molodi [Conceptual model of students' and pupils' not special physical education]. *Sportivnij visnik Pridniprov'ia*, 2011;2:164–167. (in Ukrainian)
20. Alekseev N, Kutergin N, Kulinichev A, Gorbatenko A. Integrated method development of general and special students stamina involved in the fight. *Physical Education of Students*. 2014;3:3–8.
21. Bichescu A. Leisure Time Sport Activities of the Students at Resita University. *Procedia - Social and Behavioral Sciences*. 2014;117:735–40.
22. Brown GTL. Self-regulation of assessment beliefs and attitudes: a review of the Students' Conceptions of Assessment inventory. *Educational Psychology*. 2011;31(6):731–48.
23. Buckworth J, Nigg C. Physical Activity, Exercise, and Sedentary Behavior in College Students. *Journal of American College Health*. 2004;53(1):28–34.
24. DiGironimo N. What is Technology? Investigating Student Conceptions about the Nature of Technology. *International Journal of Science Education*. 2010;33(10):1337–52.
25. Dudnyk IO. Formation of positive motivation as the basis of students will qualities' perfection in physical culture practicing. *Physical Education of Students*, 2015;3:3-9. http://dx.doi.org/10.15561/20755279.2015.0301
26. Ennis CD. Implementing meaningful, educative curricula and assessments in complex school environments. *Sport Educ Soc*, 2012;18:115–120.
27. Fomenko E. Practical recommendations for the implementation of health technologies to enhance physical fitness of students in extracurricular classes during non-traditional gymnastics. *Pedagogics, psychology, medical-biological problems of physical training and sports.* 2014;7:31–6.
28. Iermakova TS. Peculiarities of forming health culture of pupils in Poland: historical aspect. *Pedagogics, psychology, medical-biological problems of physical training and sports.* 2014;.6:16-20. http://dx.doi.org/10.6084/m9.figshare.1004090

29. Kozina ZL, Iermakov SS. Analysis of students' nervous system's typological properties, in aspect of response to extreme situation, with the help of multi-dimensional analysis. *Physical Education of Students*, 2015;3:10-19. http://dx.doi.org/10.15561/20755279.2015.0302
30. Lobko VS. Psycho-physiological characteristics of students-powerlifters of different training experience, who have affections of muscular skeletal apparatus. *Pedagogics, psychology, medical-biological problems of physical training and sports.* 2015;5:22-26. http://dx.doi.org/10.15561/18189172.2015.0504
31. Martyniuk OV, Vilyanskiy VN. Assessment of students' health condition by indicators of adaptation potential, biological age and bio-energetic reserves of organism. *Physical education of students*, 2015;3:20-28. http://dx.doi.org/10.15561/20755279.2015.0303
32. O'Leary N, Wattison N, Edwards T, Bryan K. Closing the theory–practice gap Physical education students' use of jigsaw learning in a secondary school. *European Physical Education Review*, 2015; 21: 176–194.
33. Olkhovy OM, Petrenko YM, Temchenko VA, Timchenko AN. Model of students' sport-oriented physical education with application of information technologies. *Physical Education of Students*, 2015;3:29-37. http://dx.doi.org/10.15561/20755279.2015.0304
34. Pichurin VV. Psychological and psycho-physical training as a factor of personal anxiety at students. *Pedagogics, psychology, medical-biological problems of physical training and sports.* 2015;3:46-51. http://dx.doi.org/10.15561/18189172.2015.0307
35. Serorez T, Navka P. Methodical features dispensing exercise, used in extracurricular activities to improve health students. *Pedagogics, psychology, medical-biological problems of physical training and sports.* 2014;5:60–66.
36. Serorez T. The indicators of the physical health of students on the characteristics of the physical fitness, aerobic and anaerobic productivity of their body. *Pedagogics, psychology, medical-biological problems of physical training and sports.* 2014;9:54–59.
37. Standal ØF, Moen KM, Moe VF. Theory and practice in the context of practicum: The perspectives of Norwegian physical education student teachers. *European Physical Education Review*, 2014; 20: 165–178.
38. Ward P. The role of content knowledge in conceptions of teaching effectiveness in physical education. *Res Q Exerc Sport*, 2013; 84: 431–440.
39. Yermakova TS. Individualization of forming health culture in schoolchildren of Polish schools. *Pedagogics, psychology, medical-biological problems of physical training and sports.* 2015;1:29-33. http://dx.doi.org/10.15561/18189172.2015.0106
40. Zepke N, Butler P, Leach L. Institutional research and improving the quality of student engagement. *Quality in Higher Education*. 2012;18(3):329–47.

18

THE RELATIONSHIP BETWEEN BIORHYTHM (PHYSICAL CYCLE) AND SPORTS PERFORMANCE IN WOMEN'S BASKETBALL

Shafiee Shahram[1], Rahim Ramezaninezhad[1], Hakime Afrouzeh[1], Vahid Rabbani[2]
[1]University of Guilan, Iran
[2]Allameh Tabataba'i University, Tehran, Iran

Abstract. *Purpose*: Despite many researches that have been done in the field of biorhythm and due to lack of single view among scholars, as well as importance of forecasting of athletes' performance to improve their results, the purpose of this study is to determine relationship between biorhythm (physical cycle) and sports performance of Iranian Super League women basketball players. *Material*: This is a descriptive-correlational study. Statistical population was women basketball players in 1394-95 women's Super League and the statistical sample included all of the players of the teams, qualified as semi-finalists (44 players). The tool, used in this research, was athletes' performance questionnaire (Charbonneau, 2001) containing five questions by a Likert scale from 1 (poor) to 5 (excellent) points. Biorhythm software and descriptive tests and also inferential statistical test including Chi-Square, independent T-test and one way ANOVA at significance level of ($\alpha \leq 0.05$) in SPSS software were used for analyzing the collected data. *Results:* results showed that there was no significant relationship between physical energy and performance of athletes ($p = 0.85$). Also the results of one way ANOVA test showed that there was no significant difference between performance of athletes at three levels (positive, negative and critical) and physical cycle ($p = 0.96$). The value of Chi-Square was equal to 2.63 that showed there was no significant relationship between different levels of physical cycle and the results (win or lose) of match ($p = 0.026$). *Conclusion*: The results of this study revealed that physical performance did not depend on 23-day cycle, stated in the Biorhythm theory, and there was no evidence proving existence of these cycles. It can be concluded that there is no justifying reason to use the Biorhythm software in hard exercises.
Keywords: biorhythm, performance, sports, physical cycle, women's sport.

Introduction

Biorhythm is one of the newest topics in the area of mind ergonomics identification, which can be very effective in reducing work related accidents and any mistakes without apparent reasons through identifying intellectual, physical and emotional aspects of a person [4, 7]. Today, there is too much emphasis on attending different aspects of human resources, both physical and non-physical in order to maximize individual and organizational productivity and the prerequisite for this is identifying human resources accurately in terms of physical and intellectual ergonomics. One of the most essential elements in this kind of identification is using biorhythm, which represents their intellectual, physical and emotional characteristics in different days of their lives [10, 9].

The changes in stamina and ability to carry out everyday activities, such as exercising and participating in a party, feeling healthy or sick, dealing with problems and even intellectual order or critical moments of life that an individual experiencing his/her worst or best conditions in terms of energy are categorized in three alternating cycles, namely physical, emotional and intellectual, which altogether form the individuals` biorhythm [13]. Awareness about the situation of physical, emotional and intellectual energy can help increase individual`s productivity. For example, when the physical energy is in its peak, it is the best time for doing heavy works, sports, surgical practices and making vital decisions. In the course of positive thinking and perception, one must act more carefully and avoid risky activities, because there is a high possibility of error and making mistakes in this period [21].

The word "Biorhythm" has been derived from the Greek words "bios", meaning life, and "rhythmus", meaning regular and thoughtful move. From the perspective of Biorhythm theory, humans are being influenced by physical, emotional and intellectual cycles from the day they are born and continuing until death [19, 6]. These cycles include 23-day physical cycle, 28-day emotional cycle and 33-day cognitive cycle, each of which has the following features [11, 5]:

a. A high-level or positive phase;
b. A low-level or negative phase;
c. A critical day.

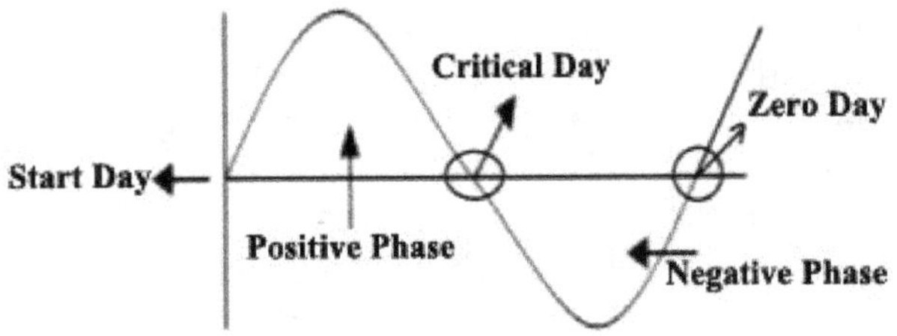

Fig. 1. Different parts of biorhythm cycle.

As it is seen in figure 1, the top part of the curve shows the positive phase. A positive phase includes those days when the body releases its energy and is likely to be at its peak. The lower part of the curve shows the negative phase in which the body returns the released energy in the positive phase and is likely to have a below normal performance. The number of days in this phase is equal to the number of days in positive phase. The body tends to instability on critical days. The critical point is an almost neutral point belonging to one of the positive or negative cycles or it does not belong to any of them at all [11].

It seems that half of the time period of each cycle is positive and the other half is negative. In other words, in each first 11.5 days, physical activity is associated with mobility, energy, high physical strength, accurate and effective work together with endurance and stability. Weakness, fatigue, lack of stored energy and lack of ability are observed in the next 11.5 days. Optimism, willingness to work and live and active participation in works are observed in the first 14 days of emotional cycle. The second 14 days are associated with bad temper, irritability, impatience and moroseness. Similarly, for intellectual cycle, after the first 16.5 days, intelligence, understanding, high analytical spirit and creativity will be replaced by second 16.5 days and its features such as forgetfulness, laziness of thought and difficulty in focusing and decision making [8, 12].

Physical cycle

Phyllis believed that physical cycles originate from muscle tissues. This cycle refers to the masculinity of people and affects their physical conditions. It is believed that there is a concurrence between adrenal gland and physical cycle in the body. This cycle continues for 23 days and associates with strength, mobility, determination, endurance and innovation. When the physical cycle is above the baseline (2nd to 11th day), the physical condition of person is charged and will be discharged gradually. In such a situation, the person is able to do better in physical works and feels stronger and more enthusiastic than before. There is a low probability of the person becoming ill and he/she can also endure and handle more pressure. Some doctors believe that between the second and ninth days, when the patient's physical cycle is well placed in positive area, is the best time to do surgery. On the other hand, when the physical cycle is placed below the baseline (13th to 23rd day), the released energy will be charged gradually. In such situations, the person simply gets tired and is susceptible to cold and other diseases [2, 3, 15 & 13].

Emotional cycle

This cycle dominates in nervous system. It is more related to femininity of a person and affects a person's feelings. In fact, all women feel the existence of this cycle in their bodies. This is a 28-day cycle which controls sensitivity, emotional issues, temperament, moods, nervous system and creativity. As long as this cycle remains above the baseline (2nd to 4th days), individual`s creativity, emotions, love and spirit of cooperation is in a good condition and he/she is more optimistic and happier than before. On the contrary, people feel bored, grumpy and depressed when this cycle is placed below the baseline (the 16th to 28th days). Also people become more cantankerous and irritable than before in such situations [1, 4].

Perceptual or Intellectual cycle

This cycle continues for 33 days and affects individual`s learning ability, analytical thinking, reasoning, judgment and decision-making. When this cycle is placed above the baseline (2nd to 16th days) people are able to think more intelligently, solve the problems more effectively, perform more successfully in the exams and make decisions more accurately. This is an appropriate time for creative thinking and producing novel ideas. But when the cycle is placed below the baseline (18th to 33rd days), individual`s thinking capacity is reduced. They show a poor judgment and memory performance falls off. They may find it hard to focus or may take wrong decisions. This period may be a good time to review previous known ideas (Moemeni Piri et al, 2012). Biological foundation of some of body cycles is completely recognized. The most well-known cycle is the menstrual cycle of women which follows a certain time rhythm and regularly repeats every 28-35 days. The researchers believe that even the most complex human functions such as intelligence, emotions and physical skills follow such cycles that start from the birth and are repeated regularly throughout the life [9].

Rabiei and Khatami No (2011) showed a significant relationship between biorhythm and job satisfaction. Also Hosseini and Mahdi Zadeh (2009) indicated in their study that there is a significant relationship between biorhythm and academic performance.

A handful of studies have been done about Biorhythm theory in sports some of which confirmed the theory while some showed inconsistency in their results. In a research conducted by Faria and Elliott (1980), the maximum consumed oxygen of vo2max by female gymnasts in the critical days of physical biorhythm cycle was tested and the result showed that physical biorhythm cycle does not have a significant effect on aerobic capacity of athletes. Maura (2009) in study examined the relationship between the biorhythm cycles and sports performance of 61 students from four teams in three phases in football final matches and the results showed a significant relationship between performance and biorhythm cycles.

Shaebani Bahar et al. (2013) examined the relationship between competition results and physical, intellectual and emotional cycles in a student's Olympiad. They concluded that there is a significant relationship between physical, intellectual and emotional cycles with the competition results. Moldovan et al. (2011) studied the performance of gymnasts and biorhythm and the results showed that gymnasts had a better performance in positive phase. Souatra and Wiyor (2002) in a 15-month study showed that people`s critical days of biorhythm has been the primary cause of work-related accidents. Taylor's research (2004) on employees of the UK electricity company revealed that there is a significant relationship between biorhythm and reduction of work-related accidents and that there is a significant relationship between more accurate decisions of senior managers and their good and bad days. Willey & Farnkoni (2003) mentioned lack of attention to biorhythm of people, especially its emotional aspect, as the primary cause of reduction in efficiency or employees` quality of work in administrative jobs.

In fact, the purpose of studying biorhythm cycles or identifying and calculating people`s rhythmic cycles is to determine the impact of these rhythms on individual`s conditions, calculate the optimal and critical days, perform activities optimally, predict weakness and strength times and not to perform some activities in critical days (Dehghan, 2008). Researchers believe that knowing about the athletes` positive and negative phase or critical days of physical cycle by the coach or other people, who are in contact with them, can increase productivity, prevent sports injuries, improve performance and other factors influencing physical performance of athletes (Zareian et al., 2014). However, there are very limited and conflicting results about the application of Biorhythm theory in sports. Some supporters of Biorhythm theory refer to the relationship between success of athletes and the days when their biorhythm is in a positive condition and others believe that there is no relationship between biorhythm and athletes' success. Lack of research in this field either overseas or local has induced researchers to try to answer the following questions: Is there any relationship between the performance of athletes and their biorhythm?

Hypothesis: This study tries to evaluate the relationship between physical dimension of biorhythm and performance of the players at the professional level in the women's tournament so that we could approve or reject this influence and provide valuable information for the coaches about the players` condition at the day of the match or even weeks of training. This can greatly contribute to success of the players.

***Purpose*:** Despite many researches that have been done in the field of biorhythm and due to the lack of a single view among scholars, as well as the importance of forecasting the performance of athletes to improve their performance, the purpose of this study is to determine the relationship between biorhythm (physical cycle) and sports performance in Iranian Super League women's basketball players.

Material and methods

Participants: The statistical population was women's basketball players in 1394-95 women's Super League and the statistical sample included all of the players of the teams qualified as semi-finalists (44 players).

Procedure: This study is an applied research and is a descriptive correlational study in terms of nature. The tournament was held in the form of home and international matches. The tool, used in this research, was athletes` performance questionnaire (Charbonneau, 2001) containing five questions on a Likert scale of 1 (poor) to 5 (excellent) points. This questionnaire was delivered to the coaches after each match so that they could evaluate the players` performance with answering its questions based on the day of the match, comparing to previous matches and other days and their knowledge and expectations of the players. The results of the competition were recorded in which code 1 denoted a win and code 2 denoted a loss.

Biorhythm software and a form to collect information were used in order to determine the athletes` biorhythm. Data on age and date of birth of the athletes were collected through a demographic information form. Athletes who were in their menstrual cycle, as well as those who were injured or psychologically damaged by being faced with some bad news before the match were excluded for integration purpose. The Farsi version of Biorhythm software was employed to draw athletes' biorhythm. The software drew players` biorhythm by entering their date of birth. [21].

After revealing the athletes` biorhythm through Biorhythm software, all of their cycles were examined.

Based on the physical cycle of biorhythm in each course of collecting questionnaire`s data, three different phases were distinguished:

1. Cycle is located above the zero line (positive phase).
2. Cycle is located below the zero line (negative phase).
3. Cycle is located in the zero and critical range (48-hour).

Statistical analysis: Inferential statistics such as Pearson correlation coefficient, independent two-sample T-test, Chi-Square test, one-way analysis of Variance (ANOVA) and Tukey post hoc test were used to investigate the hypotheses. It should be noted that all statistical analyses were performed by using SPSS software at the significance level of ($P \geq 0.05$).

Results of the researches

The results given in table 1 show that there is a positive relationship between physical energy and athletes` performance, but this relationship is not significant (r= 0.02, p= 0.851).

Table 1. Relationship between biorhythm (physical cycle) and sport performance

index / Variable	N	Pearson Correlation Coefficient	p-value
Relationship between biorhythm (physical cycle) and sport performance	88	0.02	0.851

The results of table 2 show that there is no significant difference between the energy average in two groups of win and loss (p= 0.851).

Table 2. Independent T results of mean physical energy with match results

cycle	Groups	N	Mean±SD	df	t	p-Value
Physical	Winner	47	51.83±26.38	86	0.188	0.851
	Loser	41	52.95±29.48			

The results of table 3 show that there is no significant differences between athletes` performance in three levels (positive, negative and critical) of physical cycle (p= 0.96).

Table 3. One-way ANOVA results of Athletes` performance with different levels physical cycle

	Sum of Squares	df	Mean Squares	F	P-value
Between Group	64.8	2	32.4		
Within Group	59900	75	798.68	0.041	0.96
Totla	59964	77	-		

Based on the results of table 4, the value of Chi-Square is 2.63 showing a significant relationship between different levels of physical cycle and match results (win or loss) (p= 0.26).

Table 4. Relationship between match results with different levels physical cycle

Physical cycle		match results		Total
		Winner	loser	
Positive	Frequency	17	24	41

	percent	41.5	54.5	100
Negative	Frequency	13	14	27
	percent	48.1	51.9	100
critical	Frequency	7	3	10
	percent	70	30	100
Total		37	41	78
Chi-squared test	x^2=2.63	df =2		p-value =0.268

Discussion

According to the Biorhythm theory, people face internal changes at different times, which may be the cause of different behaviors and performances at different times. Biorhythm can determine good and bad of people's performance in different days. In fact, according to biorhythm in critical days, people inherently tend to be inaccurate and if they do some risky works at this period, this inaccuracy may cause them some problems. Interpretation of different conditions of biorhythm physical cycle in different situations can be a great help to justify and evaluate physical conditions and performance of athletes. Also according to biorhythm, knowing the physical condition of athletes can help to plan for getting the best results (Shaebani Bahar, 2013). This is the question that needs to be answered here: is there any relationship between biorhythm and performance of athletes?

The results of this study showed that there is no significant relationship between physical energy and performance of athletes. This means that increasing the level of physical energy has no effect on increasing or decreasing the performance of athletes on the day of the match. This is consistent with findings of Reilly et al. (1983) about the impact of the biorhythm on the performance of professional women athletes, and with findings of Wolcott et al. (1977) about professional hammer throw. Also this is consistent with the findings of Connor & Molly (1991), and Ezanlou et al. (2007) who investigated the biorhythm experimentally and concluded that biorhythm cycle has no effect on people`s performance. Perhaps one of the reasons of these consistencies is the professional level of the studied tournament. However, the results were inconsistent with the findings of the Biorhythm theory by Willis (1972), Wallerstein and Roberts (1973), Wilhelm Felix (1928) and Alfred Teleshter (1920) which all believed that the performance is improved when the biorhythm cycle is located at the top of the baseline. Also this is inconsistent with the findings of Shaebani Bahar et al. (2013). However, these studies evaluated the performance of novice athletes in training and student matches and perhaps the differences in the level of competition and maintaining physical and intellectual fitness of athletes in professional events are the cause of these different results. We can also mention the difference in performance in practices and matches as a reason in this regard. Because an athlete can control many factors in a practice, but the performance in a match will be very different from practice and its conditions. However, we cannot certainly acknowledge the inefficiency of this software, because it has increased the performance on positive days of physical cycle in some cases, such as factories, staff and students. This increase was proved to be significant based on the findings of Rabiei & KhatamiNo (2011) and Hosseini & Eshraghi (2010). Also based on the findings of Vazifedoust et al. (2013), the biorhythm has an impact on the quality of managers' decision-making. Perhaps this software works fine when it comes to the people who do not need permanent intellectual, emotional and physical fitness.

The results of the study did not show any significant difference between the performance of athletes at three levels of physical cycle (positive, negative and critical) (p= 0.96). These results are consistent with findings of Jenkins et al. (2011), Lester (1990), Pilianidis et al. (1993), Quigley (1982), Faria and Elliott (1980), and are inconsistent with the findings of Moemeni (2012), Rabiea and KhatamiNo (2011), Hosseini and Mehdi Zadeh (2009), Singh and Sharma (2011), Parikh et al. (2010), Maura (2009) and Taylor (2004). So, it can be concluded that awareness of positive, negative and critical situations of physical cycle is not effective in achieving desirable results for athletes` performance. Therefore, it is not possible to predict the athletes` best time to do the match when their physical cycle is in positive condition. In fact, there are many factors affecting the quality of performance in a match, such as physical condition, having no injuries, good condition of training before the match and getting enough rest and sleep before the match.

With regard to relationship between match results (win or loss) and different conditions of physical cycle, the findings showed that positive and negative conditions of athletes have no effect on their wins or losses. This is inconsistent with the findings of Moldovan (2011) which showed that the performance of athletes is higher in positive conditions of biorhythm cycle. This is also inconsistent with the findings of Ehsani and Parsa (2010), who revealed a decrease in employees` performance on critical days and an increase on positive days, and findings of Taylor (2004) on the reduction of work-related accidents in the positive phase of the cycle. It can be concluded that the conditions and situations that happen in a match such as key players being sent off, biased referee judgments, unfavorable conditions of safety and security and even bad weather conditions all may affect a team`s winning and losing. Therefore, the positive condition of the team is not a reasonable predictor for its winning chance.

With regard to receiving many stimuli by the athletes during the matches and the ability and experience of professional athletes in competition with controlling intellectual and emotional conditions as well as maintaining physical fitness at desirable level for major events, it can be concluded that using biorhythm in sports and for athletes in a major event could be effective in increasing athlete`s motivation provided that it is in a positive phase. It should also be noted that the coach should not use this software fraudulently for increasing motivation of the athletes. Otherwise, for professional athletes who need to keep their physical conditions and energy at the best level during matches, the negative phase of this theory could implicate some undesirable intellectual effects during the competitions. However, the coaches can use biorhythm in practices for increasing athletes` performance, motivation and self-confidence at the best condition of physical cycle, but this software does not cause any increase or decrease in performance for match conditions. Of course, more researches need to be done in this area.

Conclusions

So any long-term planning to use biorhythm as a basis for competition and training is a bit unwise. Although knowing intellectual features and physical conditions of the athletes could help coaches to select players for important matches, but this software is hardly helpful for the coaches in this case. It should be noted that professionalism requires athletes to maintain their intellectual, emotional and physical fitness to compete in the best conditions. This could be one of the most important factors indicating why Biorhythm theory does not apply to professional athletes.

Conflict of interests

The authors declare that there is no conflict of interests.

References:

1. Singh R & Sharma R. The influence of "biorhythm" on the incidence of injuries among Agra foundry workers. *International Journal*, 2011;3: 20-25.
2. Raut TS, &.Kaware SHH. Comparative study of Biorhythms with Various physical fitness components. *International Referred Research Journal,* 2011;4:32-33.
3. Faria IE, & Elliott TL. Biorhythm patterns of maximal aerobic power of females. *The Journal of sports medicine and physical fitness,* 1980; 20(1): 81-86.
4. Ehsani A, Parsa Y. *Biorhythm based on the theory of industrial management decision-making process for the implementation of automation in production units*. 2nd International conference on industrial Automation. 2011; P. 11-16. (Article in Farsi)
5. Parikh RH, Askhedkar RD, Singh MP. Biorhythms for accident prevention. *International Journal of Multidisciplinary Research and Advances in Engineering,* 2010; 2(1):217-232.
6. Zareian E, Rabbani V, Saeedi F. The Effect of Physical Biorhythm Cycle on some Physical Fitness Factors of Adolescent Volleyball Players. *Annals of Applied Sport Science,* 2014; 2(1): 11-20.
7. Ezanloo B, Ebrahimi S, Ghavam Habibi M, Asgarabad. *The Investigation of the Validity of Intellectual Cycles of Biorhythm through Cognitive Functions. Research in Psychological Health*. 2007;1(3):38-50. (Article in Farsi)
8. Javaherdashti R. The *Management of Man's Physiological Behavior*. TADBIR. 2001; 11(109):58-60. (Article in Farsi)
9. Hoseini SM, Mehdizadeh A, Ashrafi. Biorhythm and Educational Performance: (Students of Islamic Azad University, Firoozkuh Branch. Pajouheshgar). *Journal of Management,* 2009;6(13):70-6. (Article in Farsi)
10. Rabiee A, Khatamino F. Study of the Relationship between Biorhythm and Staff's Job Satisfaction (Case study: Nargan Company). *Quarterly Management & Human Resurces in Oil Industry,* 2011; 2(8):29-52.
11. Buttery, T.J. The influence of biorhythm on human physical, emotional, and intellectual behavior. *Education.* 1977; 98(2), 117-121.
12. Sha'bani Bahar GR, Samadi A, Momeni Piri S. The relationship between Intellectual and Emotional cycles with respect to Biorhythm Theory and athletes' sport performance. *Journal of Sport Psychology Studies*, 2013; 2(3):13- 28. (Article in Farsi)
13. Moemeni Piri S, Shabani Bahar G. *The Determination of Relationship between Biorhythm (Physical Cycle) and Sport Performance in Athletes of Individual Sports in Hamadan Province*. Master thesis Physical Education, Bu-Ali Sina University of Hamedan; 2012.
14. Willey P & Farnkoni A. Scientific tests of biorhythmology do not support its claims. In: Frazier (ED.) *Science confronts the paranormal.* Buffalo, NY: Prometheus; 2003. 219-221.
15. Dehghan AM. The psychological factors affecting investment in stock. *A Monthly Magazine TADBIR on Management.* 2008;196: 60-63. (Article in Farsi)

16. Maura S. *Bio-periodicity and its influence on the football results obtained by the student teams during the "university spring" sport competition*. Citius Altius Fortius; 2009.
17. Moldovan E, enoiu RS, ruxanda RA, & leibovici A. The influence of the human biorhythm in the performance sport activity. *Gymnasium*, 2011; 12: 34-46.
18. Talor CG. *The structure & dynamics of the biorhythm, collected works, 8, R.F.C hull, (trans.)*. Bollingen series XX, pantheon books; 2004.
19. Zollitsch HG. Biorhythms and management. *Industrial management,* 1976;11: 1- 4.
20. Reilly T, Young K & Seddon R. Investigation of biorhythms in female athletic performance. *Applied Ergonomics,* 1983; 14(3), 215-217.
21. *Bio-chart. Biorhythms -Some History*. Available from: http://www.bio-chart.com/geschichte.html. 2014 (accessed 22.05.2016).
22. Joncas SX, Carrier N, Nguyen M, & Farand P. Biorhythm Theory Does Not Predict Admission for Acute Myocardial Infarction. *The Journal of Alternative and Complementary Medicine*. 2011; 17(2): 143-146.

19

DETERMINATION OF FUTURE DESIGNERS' PROFESSIONALLY IMPORTANT COORDINATION QUALITIES

Chernovsky S. M., Kolumbet A. N.
Kiev National University of Technology and Design

Abstract. *Purpose:* to find out girl students' motor abilities, influencing to the largest extent on successfulness of designer's professional functioning. *Material:* 210 girl students of 18-22 years' age participated in experiment. *Results:* it was found that all indicators of future designers' professional qualities are closely connected with indicators of definite coordination abilities. High interconnection with kinesthetic indicators and girl students' professional skillfulness were noted. It was determined that quickness, concentration and re-switching of attention were closely connected with attention, operative memory, accuracy of reproduction of received information. *Conclusions:* for girl students-designers' successful professional progress it is necessary to develop kinesthetic, responding and orientation coordination qualities. These qualities are required for quick and effective solution of professional tasks, connected with accurate perception in the shortest possible time and keeping great volume of space information in memory.
Key words: students, designers, specialized physical education, professional-applied physical training.

Introduction

Scientific-technical progress and wide implementation of computer information technologies result in further intensification and complication of studying at HEE. More and more increasing volume of information to be perceived requires student's high psychological tension and physical efforts. Such transformation of functioning can not but reflect in specific features of adaptation processes and health condition of people, dealing with mental work and spending much time with computer.

Formation of future designers' professional qualities in technical HEE is one of the most important tasks. The process of specialist's training at HEE includes a number of pedagogic aspects. They include professional-applied physical training. At HEE discipline "Physical education" contains such part as professional-applied physical training. But this part does not have clear, scientifically substantiated methodic instructions on organization of trainings of different specializations students. Besides, there is no software maintenance of this part.

It should be noted that the problem of formation of motor skills and abilities in professional training is connected with condition of certain coordination mechanisms. The basis of professional training is control and assessment of motor system's condition and its sub-systems [3, 8, 13, 14, 17, and 23]. This is really existing problem and it is connected with working out of effective methodic of physical education teaching, considering future professional functioning. Its solution in educational process is closely connected with physical trainings of girl students-designers. In these trainings development of basic coordination qualities, which are the basis for further formation of professionally important coordination qualities, take place.

Training of coordination qualities have always been paid great attention. The works of a number of authors are devoted to perfection of youth's coordination qualities [4, 7, 11, 12, and 20]. Some works elucidate professional-applied physical training of technical HEEs' students [8, 10, 16, 21, and 22]. However, there are quite a few researches, devoted to specialized physical training of designers [1]. It proves the importance of this problem.

Purpose, tasks of the work, material and methods

The purpose of the work is to find out girl students' motor abilities, influencing to the largest extent on successfulness of designer's professional functioning.

The methods and organization of the research: 210 girl students of 18-22 years' age from Kiev technical HEE were tested.

Results were received with usage of methodic and with the help of motor-coordination analyzer ADKR-2. This device is a plate, on which there are four carved tracks of different configuration (every track of 450 mm length). At the beginning and at the end of each track there are special contacts. Electric probe touches these contacts in initial position and at the end of task. In response to light bulb (0.45W) ignition the tested, trying not to touch walls, shall move probe from the beginning to the end of track. Before test instructions were given. These instructions were repeated in the course of movement: do quicker, not neglecting accuracy in favor of speed. Considering high scope of tests, light irritators were given to every tested with interval of 10-15 sec. It excluded influence of previous reaction. Before testing, short training in the form of simple measurements of the tested time parameters, was carried out with each tested. With multiple repetitions variation of indicators reduced and stabilized.

The level of girl students' *accuracy* was assessed with the help of the following tests: 1) accuracy of reproduction of pre-set effort value was determined with hand dynamometer; 2) accuracy of reproduction of pre-set amplitude of arms' movements was determined with kinematic meter of M.I. Zhukovskiy.

Responding qualities were registered with the following tests: 1) for quickness of reaction (test "Catching rule" [6]); 2) test for reaction to moving object. For this test computer program "Prognoz", worked out by Institute of physiology, named after A.A. Bogomolets of AS of Ukraine, Kiev; 3) test for quickness of visual-motor reaction (simple and complex) with computer program "Prognoz"; 4) Test for quickness of reaction ("Catching stick" 1]); 5) complex coordination test for determination of multidirectional speed-power movements per definite time (computer program "Prognoz".

Orientation in space was assessed with the help of test "Labyrinth" [5].

Assessment of girl students-designers' *professionally important abilities* was conducted with the following tests: 1) distribution of attention (test "Finding of numbers" [15]); 2) scope of mechanic memorizing (test "Quantity of men figures" [15]); 3) distribution of attention and quickness of operative thinking (test "Assembly of puzzles for definite time" [1]); 4) quickness of operative thinking (Koss's cubes" [2]); 5) quickness, re-switching and concentration of attention and accuracy of task's fulfillment were registered with special device [9].

Static balance was studied with Romberg's test (posture of "Stork"); 2) *dynamic balance* was assessed with test "Turns on gymnastic bench" [18].

Results of the research

Having fulfilled multiple correlation analysis we built correlation matrix. In this matrix information was analyzed, considering character, quantity and density of the received correlations. Attention was paid only to statistically significant indicators. It was found that all indicators of future designers' professional qualities were interconnected with indicators of definite coordination abilities. Alongside with it, the conducted analysis showed ambiguous character of correlations by different kinds of future designers' professional qualities.

Correlation analysis showed dependence of attention distribution indicator on indicator of orientation in space, quickly and accurately fulfill task. In this case correlation coefficient was 0.67. It reflects moderate correlation of the tested indicators. It should be noted that in test "Labyrinth" time and accuracy of task's fulfillment were assessed. In the same way, when fulfilling test "Finding numbers" time and attention were assessed. Activity of such character takes place in professional functioning of designers (for example when making fine and precise movements with brush, when preparing markup and drawing).

In table 1 we present analysis of parameters' correlation matrix. These parameters show dependence of indicator "Quantity of men figures" on indicators of tests "Labyrinth", complex visual motor reaction, "Catching rule". Analysis of test "Quantity of men figures" correlation with indicators of tests for responding (orientation and kinesthetic qualities) permits to think that development of coordination facilitates progress of professional skills. Degree of density of the tested parameters was moderate. It is witnessed by correlation coefficients (0.61-0.77).

The determined character of correlations witnesses about significance of responding, orientation and kinesthetic qualities of girl students. These qualities are required for quick and effective solution of professional tasks, connected with accurate perception in the shortest time and keeping great volume of space and other information in memory.

One of the most important disciplines at design faculty is "Painting". When assessing progress in this subject the following moments are considered: naturalistic level of drawing (observance of volume, plan; presence of fine details); proportionality of figure in the picture; correctness of composition; fulfillment of sketch by lines or by spot with the help of fine and thick brushes. Analysis of progress in their professional discipline "Painting" correlation with indicator of test "Reproduction of pre-set amplitude of arm's movement" showed moderate degree of the tested parameters' density (correlation coefficient was 0.61).

Table 1. Correlations of indicator, reflecting attention, operative memory, quickness of memorizing and accuracy of the received information reproduction with indicators of orientation, responding and kinesthetic qualities

Indicators	Correlation coefficient
Orientation ability (accuracy of reproduction of pre-set movement's trajectory, test "Labyrinth")	0.61
Responding ability (test CVMR)	0.72
Responding ability (test "Catching rule")	0.64
Responding ability (test "Catching stick")	0.63
Responding ability (test SVMR)	0.68
Responding ability (reaction to moving object)	0.74
Distribution of attention (test "Finding numbers")	0.77
Dynamic balance	0.68
Static balance	0.63
Complex coordination test	0.72

Notes: CVMR – complex visual motor reaction; SVMR – simple visual motor reaction.

In discipline "Drawing" ability to build objects, to model volume; quality of shading, ability to locate drawing on paper correctly are assessed. Drawings are fulfilled by pencils and other soft materials (for example with coal). These materials are very fragile. That is why it is necessary to feel arms' pressure on them. We analyzed indicators of progress in discipline "Drawing". This analysis showed dependence with indicators of kinesthetic qualities and ability of orientation in space. Density of correlations was moderate (0.61-0.77). It witnesses that it is important to perfect girl students' basic kinesthetic and orientation, coordination qualities for their future professional functioning.

We also determined correlation of test "Assembly of puzzles" (which reflects fine motor abilities of working arm) with indicators of test "Koss's cubes" (quickness of operative thinking, ability to constructive praxis). Degree of density of the tested parameters was moderate (0.75). Test for quickness of operative thinking is a complex one. It reflects development of girl students' moor skills and shows component of mental processes (ability to observe composition: presence of composition center, ability to distinguish tints, to reproduce shape of the depicted object), which is rather important for future designers. It witnesses that it is necessary to improve girl students' coordination: ability to constructive praxis, quickness of operative thinking, ability to quickly and accurately react to the received task and fulfill it exactly in compliance with the set purpose.

General level of girl students-designers was determined with points. These points reflected relation of accuracy of standard drawing fulfillment to time of its fulfillment. Correlation analysis showed interconnection of this indicator with indicators of kinesthetic and responding qualities (test "Reaction to moving object"); test "Reproduction of pre-set amplitude of arm's movements"). Analysis of the found dependences' character (between assessment points and kinesthetic level) witnesses about presence of expressed correlation (correlation coefficient was 0.80). Correlation of indicator of girl students' professionalism with indicator of responding qualities (test "Reaction to moving object") can be estimated as moderate. Correlation coefficient was 0.62.

In table 2 we render analysis of parameters' correlation matrix. This analysis opens dependence of indicator of *attention re-switching and concentration and accuracy of task's fulfillment* (test "Balls) on indicator of other tests. Analysis of indicators' correlation in test "Balls" with development of *responding, orientation and kinesthetic* qualities showed their influence on progress of professional skills. Parameters' density was moderate and high (correlation coefficients were 0.55-0.86).

Thus, correlation analysis of girl students-designers' professional qualities and indicators of coordination qualities showed at their close interaction.

Discussion

Results of our experiments proved the works of other authors about training of professional qualities by physical education means [19, 24-28].

The fulfilled researches continue the series of experiments on professional (specialized) physical training of students. If earlier we tested girl students of Ukrainian pedagogic HEEs, then in our present works girl students of technical HEEs participated.

It was found that by most of indicators characteristic of the tested indicators is nearly equal. Differences concern only professional skills (different tests, assessment scales and parameters). Varying of correlation coefficients (±5.0) is not significant.

Table 2. Correlations of indicator, which characterizes quickness of attention re-switching, attention concentration and accuracy of fulfillment (test "Balls"), with indicators of orientation, responding and kinesthetic qualities

Indicators	Correlation coefficient
Responding ability (test CVMR)	0.76
Responding ability (test "Catching rule")	0.85
Responding ability (test "Catching stick")	0.86
Responding ability (test SVMR)	0.79
Responding ability (reaction to moving object)	0.82
Distribution of attention (test "Finding numbers")	0.63
Dynamic balance	0.58
Static balance	0.55
Scope of mechanical memorizing (test «Quantity of men figures")	0.67
Distribution of attention and quickness of operative thinking (test "Assembly of puzzles")	0.77
Quickness of operative thinking (test "Koss's cubes")	0.69
Accuracy of reproduction of pre-set effort	0.75
Accuracy of reproduction of pre-set movement's amplitude	0.74

Notes: CVMR – complex visual motor reaction; SVMR – simple visual motor reaction.

Further researches will be devoted to testing of future economists, engineers of light industry, future pharmacists and chemists.

Conclusions

The data, received in correlation analysis permit to make the following conclusions:

1) For successful professional progress of girl students-designers it is necessary to train mainly kinesthetic, responding and orientation coordination qualities. However, correlations were found not with all kinds of coordination qualities. We did not find correlation of professional skills and ability to keep static balance. It can be explained by the fact that it is well developed and is habitual for the girl students. But keeping one posture in work (for example standing at easel or sitting at computer) is very difficult.

2) When working out program maintenance for professional-applied physical training it is necessary to pay attention exactly to perfection of the above listed coordination qualities. It is still more important that the fulfilled correlation analysis of kinesthetic, responding and orientation qualities showed negative dynamic in period from 1st to 4th year of study. Already in 1st year girl students-designers test indicators were lower average age standards ("Catching of vertically falling object", "Reaction to moving object", complex coordination test).

3) Pedagogic influence shall be started from the 1st year. Then, by the graduation girl students-designers will acquire required professionally important skills and abilities to the highest extent.

Acknowledgements

The work has been fulfilled in compliance with topical plan and general problem of scientific researches of physical education and health department of Kiev national university of technology and design "Social-pedagogic aspects of healthy life style formation in students by physical education means". The work is a part of scientific direction of researches of physical education and martial arts department of physical education and sports

Faculty of National pedagogic university, named after M.P. Dragomanov "4.6.3.1. "Formation of youth's physical perfection in educational system".

Conflict of interests

The authors declare that there is no conflict of interests.

References:

1. Afanas'eva IV. *Metodika sovershenstvovaniia professional'no znachimykh koordinacionnykh sposobnostej u budushchikh specialistov dizajnerov. Cand. Diss.* [Methodic of perfection of professionally important coordination abilities of future specialists-designers. Cand. Diss.]: Omsk; 2008. (in Russian)
2. Burlachuk LF. *Psikhodiagnostika* [Psycho-diagnostic], Sankt Petersburg: Peter; 2006. (in Russian)
3. Vilenskij MIa, Il'inich VI. *Fizicheskaia kul'tura rabotnikov umstvennogo truda* [Physical culture for mental workers], Moscow: Knowledge; 1987. (in Russian)
4. Vilenskij MIa, Safin MIa. *Professional'naia napravlennost' fizicheskogo vospitaniia studentov pedagogicheskikh special'nostej* [Professional orientation of pedagogic specialties' students' physical education], Moscow: High school; 1989. (in Russian)
5. Gorskaia IIu, Suiangulova LA. *Bazovye koordinacionnye sposobnosti shkol'nikov s razlichnym urovnem zdorov'ia* [Basic coordination abilities of schoolchildren with different level of health], Omsk: SibGUFK; 2000. (in Russian)
6. Dushanin SA. Bal'naia sistema kompleksnogo vrachebno-pedagogicheskogo kontrolia na zaniatiiakh massovymi formami fizicheskoj kul'tury [Points' system of complex medical-pedagogic control at classes of mass forms of physical culture]. *Teoriia i praktika fizicheskoj kul'tury* 1978;4:49-52. (in Russian)
7. Il'inich VI, Golovina VA, Masliakova VA, Korobkova AV. *Professional'no-prikladnaia fizicheskaia podgotovka* [Professional-applied physical training], Moscow: High school; 1983. (in Russian)
8. Kabachkov VA, Polievskij SA. Razrabotka professional'no-prikladnoj fizicheskoj podgotovki i opyt ee vnedreniia v uchebnykh zavedeniiakh proftekhobrazovaniia [Development of professional-applied physical training and experience of its implementation in vocational education establishments]. *Teoriia i praktika fizicheskoj kul'tury,* 1980;7;30-34. (in Russian)
9. Kirichenko SI. *Professional'no-prikladnaia fizicheskaia podgotovka studentov ekonomicheskogo fakul'teta. Cand. Diss.* [Professional-applied physical training of economic faculty students. and. Diss.], Maikop; 1998. (in Russian)
10. Kolumbet OM. Psikhofizichni osoblivosti trudovoi diial'nosti vchiteliv-naochnikiv [Psycho-physical characteristics of work of teachers, using visual aids]. *Pedagogics, psychology, medical-biological problems of physical training and sports* 2012;8:48-53. (in Ukrainian)
11. Kolumbet OM. *Rozvitok koordinacijnikh zdibnostej molodi* [Development of youth's coordination abilities], Kiev: Education; 2014. (in Ukrainian)
12. Kolumbet A.N. Influence of stimulated plasticity training method on coordination indicators of high pedagogic educational estableshments' girl students. *Physical Education of Students*, 2015;6:31-37. http://dx.doi.org/10.15561/20755279.2015.0604
13. Korobejnikov GV. *Psikhofiziologicheskie mekhanizmy umstvennoj deiatel'nosti cheloveka* [Psycho-physiological mechanisms of human mental functioning], Kiev; 2002. (in Russian)
14. Korovin SS. *Teoreticheskie i metodologicheskie osnovy professional'noj fizicheskoj kul'tury uchashchejsia molodezhi* [Theoretical and methodological principles of students' professional physical culture], Moscow: VNIIFK; 1997. (in Russian)
15. Sizanov AN. *Testy i psikhologicheskie igry* [Tests and psychological games], Minsk; 2008. (in Russian)
16. Raevskij RT. *Professional'no-prikladnaia fizicheskaia podgotovka studentov tekhnicheskikh vuzov* [Professional-applied physical training of technical HEEs' students], Moscow: High school; 1989. (in Russian)
17. Gorelov AA, Kondakov VL, Usatov AN. To the question about the use of independent physical training in educational space of modern higher institute. *Physical Education of Students*, 2013;1:17-26. http://dx.doi.org/10.6084/m9.figshare.156351
18. Hirtz P. *Koordinative Fahigkeiten im Schulsport* [Coordinative abilities in school sports], Berlin: Volk und

Wissen, Volksseigener Verlag; 1985. (in German)
19. Khripunova LD. To the question of the formation of personal qualities of future doctors by means of combat sports. *Physical Education of Students*, 2014;5:43-47. http://dx.doi.org/10.15561/20755279.2014.0508
20. Kolumbet AN. Physical education for the students of pedagogical specialities. *III international research and practice conference Science "Technology and Higher Education", Westwood, Canada*. 2014. P. 34-42.
21. Kolumbet AN. Development of coordination abilities of young people. *V international research and practice conference "Science and Education"*, Munich, Germany. 2014. P. 54-62.
22. Kondakov VL, Kopeikina EN, Balysheva NV, Usatov AN, Skrug DA. Causes of declining interest of students to employment physical education and sports. *Physical education of students*, 2015;1:22–30. http://dx.doi.org/10.15561/20755279.2015.0104
23. Korobeynikov G. Psychophysiological Peculiarities of Sexual Dimorphism in Athletes. *Psychologe Research*, 2012;2(6):336-342.
24. Otravenko OV. Formation of student personality's physical culture as subject of professional functioning. *Physical Education of Students*, 2015;6:50-55. http://dx.doi.org/10.15561/20755279.2015.0607
25. Pichurin VV. Resilience of students and their readiness for professional functioning. *Physical Education of Students*, 2015;3:38-43. http://dx.doi.org/10.15561/20755279.2015.0305
26. Radchenko AV. Professional self-assessment of future health basics teachers as professionally important quality. *Pedagogics, psychology, medical-biological problems of physical training and sports*, 2015;12:87-90. http://dx.doi.org/10.15561/18189172.2015.12013
27. Stepanchenko NI. Structure and state of the university of physical culture students' professional-pedagogical motivation. *Pedagogics, psychology, medical-biological problems of physical training and sports*, 2013;3:62-68. http://dx.doi.org/10.6084/m9.figshare.644799
28. Voitovska ON. Computer diagnostics of level of professional competence formation of future physical culture teachers in the biological disciplines study. *Pedagogics, psychology, medical-biological problems of physical training and sports*, 2013;3: 11-17. http://dx.doi.org/10.6084/m9.figshare.644905

20

FACTORIAL ANALYSIS OF MASS MEDIA INFLUENCE ON ACADEMIC SPORTS DEVELOPMENT

Benar Noshin[1], Emami Mina[2], Eftekhari Ozra[3], Yeganeh Far Nastaran[4], Khan Mohammadi Ali Mohammad[5]
[1]Associate Professor at University of Guilan, Iran
[2]Master in Sport Management, University of Guilan, Iran
[3]Master in Sport Management, University of Shomal, Iran
[4]Lecturer at Islamic Azad University Bandar Anzali Branch, Iran
[5]Master in Sport Management, University of Guilan, Iran

Abstract. *Purpose:* Main objective of this research was factorial analysis of mass media influence on academic sports development. *Material:* Methodology of the research was descriptive- correlation. Population of the research was composed of all referees, coaches and athletes participating in students' sports Olympiad of Iran Payam e Noor Universities in year 2014. Statistical sample of research was chosen randomly and consisted of 176 persons. Data gathering tool was a researcher made questionnaire; its superficial and content validity was approved by academic professors and media experts; also the stability of research tool was reported to be at an acceptable level. SPSS 23 software was used to analyze research data and also AMOS 24 software was used to analyze structure validity. *Results:* Findings showed there is a significant difference between current situation and desirable situation in all research dimensions. Also, factorial analysis of all research variables showed improvement of coaches' technical performance (0.86), improvement of referees' technical performance (0.85), and promotion of academic sport managers' awareness (0.83) respectively are mostly influenced by mass media. *Conclusion*: It should be kept in mind that academic sports development is one of the factors of the entire country sports development. Hence, it is crucial to attend to different dimensions of student sport's aspects such as human, financial, planning and etc., especially in championship area to be able to further macro objectives of country's sports development. Considering current conditions, mass media should have a new perspective on academic sports in order to be able to attend to their responsibilities to further the excellence of country's sports.
Key words: Mass Media, Sports Development, Academic Sport, Women's Sport.

Introduction

Sports development requires attention to several dimensions at macro, middle, and micro levels. One of the most important components of sports is academic sport which is, based on evidence, highly influential on students' mental and physical health [12] and its main objective is to create the required context and appropriate opportunities for the pervasive stratum of college students, in order to attain healthy competitive and entertaining environment [5]. Physical activity and participation at university's sport programs can have a significant share in promotion of academic community's social, mental and physical health [8]. One of the main factors in cultural development is mass media [1, 6]. The most essential objective of mass media in support of each country's national agenda could be sports development, which itself has several dimensions and axes [13].

Traditionally researchers have divided mass media into published and electronic. Published media includes newspapers and journals while electronic media includes radio, television, cinema, and internet (as modern media) [3, 10 and 11], all of which render direct influence on values and norms of the society since span of their activities includes a great number of the population of society [2]. Due to this reason, in most countries different media have established especial channels for sports [1].

Based on the discussion above, one of the important and influential factors in academic sports development is mass media. It is evident that effort to increase presentation of sport matches and programs as well as news coverage of women's sport in different sub-parts such as academic sport will be highly influential on more enhancement of participation and quality of performance of athletes, coaches and referees and will also result into development of other components of women's sport in the country. In this research, influence of television, radio, and press on academic sport development has been analyzed.

Analysis shows the existing distance between current situation in mass media and favorable situation of cultural development has a significant difference and this weakness is also observed in sports domain [1]. In their research Emami and Mallaei (2013) [4] have also reported that share of women's sport in TV news coverage wasvery minimal. Mahdavian Mashhadi (2008) [7] claimed mass media to play significant role in activating public, educative, championship, and technical sports especially in respect to women's sport. Ghasemi et al. (2008) described media role, particularly of the entire country TV, as important in development of championship sport and explained the importance of paying attention to all sport components in television. Academic sport has always been studied and analyzed from different aspects; but in Iran it still has not reached the necessary dynamics as a study domain. On the other hand, importance and necessity of attention to influential factors on academic sport development and lack of professional studies in this area make the significance of this research more obvious. As a result, in this research, to analyze the influence of television, radio, and press (as mass media) on academic sport development, athlete students participating in Iran's sports Olympiad of Payam e Noor Universities' students has been approached.

Purpose

The purpose of this research was factorial analysis of mass media influence on academic sports development.

Material and methods

Participants: population of the research consisted of all participating referees, coaches, and athletes in Iran sports Olympiad of Payam e Noor Universities, 2014. Statistical sample of research consisted of 176 persons who were selected randomly.

Research Design: methodology of this research is descriptive - correlation. To gather research data a researcher made questionnaire was utilized. In order to determine superficial and content validity of research tool, the questionnaire was approved by academic professors and media experts. Questionnaire's stability was reported to be α=0.91.

Statistical Analysis: to analyze research data, descriptive statistics (frequency, frequency percentage) and inferential statistics (Kolmogrov-Smirnov test and Wilcoxon) using SPSS 23 software were performed; also to analyze structure validity and to present measurement models of research variables AMOS 24 software was used.

Results of the research

Demographic findings of the participating athletes are summarized in table 1.

Table 1. Description of Personal Characteristics of Respondents

Percentage	Frequency	Variable		Percentage	Frequency	Variable	
78.7	137	Less than 1	Time Spent Watching Sport Programs on TV (Hour)	32.8	57	18-21	Age (Year)
16.7	29	1-2		48.9	85	22-26	
2.9	5	3-4		13.2	23	27-31	
1.7	3	More than 4		5.2	9	32-36	
69.4	120	Less than 1	Time Spent Listening to Sport Programs on Radio (Hour)	52.6	92	Physical Education	Field of Education
20.2	35	1-2		47.4	83	Other than Physical Education	
5.2	9	3-4		6.3	11	Associate Degree	Educational Attainment
5.2	9	More than 4		85.1	148	Bachelor	
36.6	63	Less than 1	Time Spent Reading Sports Press (Hour)	8.6	15	Master and Higher	
41.4	72	1-2		27.5	46	1-6	Sport Background (Year)
14.4	25	3-4		46.7	78	7-12	
8.6	15	More than 4		22.2	37	13-18	
				3.6	6	19-24	

Using Kolmogrov-Smirnov test, hypotheses of abnormal distribution of data was disapproved; hence to compare current situation and desirable role of mass media in academic sport development Wilcoxon test was used (Table 2).

Table 2. Comparison of Current Situation and Desirable Role of Mass Media in Female Academic Sports Development

Overall Result	Significance Level	Z Statistics	Variable
Existence of Difference	0.001*	-9.151	Promotion of Public Awareness of Academic Sport
Existence of Difference	0.001*	-9.201	Athletes' Performance Improvement
Existence of Difference	0.001*	-9.538	Identification of Sports Talents
Existence of Difference	0.001*	-9.128	Improvement of Coaches' Technical Performance
Existence of Difference	0.001*	-9.516	Improvement of Referees' Technical Performance
Existence of Difference	0.001*	-9.732	Promotion of Academic Sports Managers' Awareness
Existence of Difference	0.001*	-9.110	Determining Academic Sports Strategies
Existence of Difference	0.001*	-10.088	Fair Allotment of Academic Sport Facilities
Existence of Difference	0.001*	-9.527	Increased Research on Academic Sport
Existence of Difference	0.001*	-9.836	Increasing Allocated Budget for Academic Sport
Existence of Difference	0.001*	-9.452	Increasing Sponsors and Public Investment
Existence of Difference	0.001*	-9.804	News Coverage of Academic Sport
Existence of Difference	0.001*	-9.826	Increased Employment and Entrepreneurship at Students' Olympiads
Existence of Difference	0.001*	-9.951	Increased Audiences for Academic Sports
Existence of Difference	0.001*	-9.431	Familiarity with Academic Sport Champions

*:$p<0.05$

Table 3 demonstrates the factor analysis of role of television, radio, and press, separately, on sports development.

Table 3. Factor Analysis of Role of Television, Radio, and Press on Academic Sport Development

		Standard Regression Weight of TV Influence on Research Items	Standard Regression Weight of Radio Influence on Research Items	Standard Regression Weight of Press Influence on Research Items	Significance Level
Promotion of Public Awareness of Academic Sport	<---	.677	.644	.643	***
Athletes' Performance Improvement	<---	.715	.748	.715	***
Identification of Sport Talents	<---	.667	.672	.707	***

Improvement of Coaches Technical Performance	<---	.805	.810	.675		***	
Improvement of Referees' Technical Performance	<---	.727	.718	.740		***	
Promotion of Academic Sports Managers' Awareness	<---	.850	.737	.723		***	
Determining Academic Sport Strategies	<---	.768	.778	.690		***	
Fair Allotment of Academic Sport Facilities	<---	.785	.793	.679		***	
Increased Research on Academic Sports	<---	.737	.612	.641		***	
Increasing Allocated budget for Academic Sport	<---	.651	.593	.575		***	
Increased Sponsors and Public Investments	<---	.642	.587	.563		***	
News Coverage of Academic Sports	<---	.553	.474	.549		***	
Increased Employment and Entrepreneurship in Students' Olympiads	<---	.581	.557	.513		***	
Increased Audiences for Academic Sport	<---	.596	.530	.600		***	
Familiarity with Academic Sport Champions	<---	.621	.479	.603		***	
RMSEA	CFI	IFI	NFI	AGFI	GFI	CMIN/DF	Fit Indices
0.055	0.97	0.97	0.92	0.88	0.92	1.537	Factor Analysis of TV's Role
0.059	0.96	0.96	0.91	0.86	0.91	1.604	Factor Analysis of Radio's Role
0.064	0.95	0.95	0.90	0.85	0.90	1.713	Factor Analysis of Press's Role

***:p<0.05

From table 3, it is evident that factors of promotion of academic sports managers' awareness, improvement of coaches' technical performance, and improvement of referees' technical performance respectively take the highest influence from television, radio, and press.

Table 4. Fit Indices of Measurement Model for Level of Influence of Mass Media on Academic Sport **Development**

RMSEA	CFI	IFI	NFI	AGFI	GFI	CMIN/DF	Fit Indices
0.062	0.97	0.97	0.93	0.86	0.91	1.673	Factor Analysis of Role of Mass Media

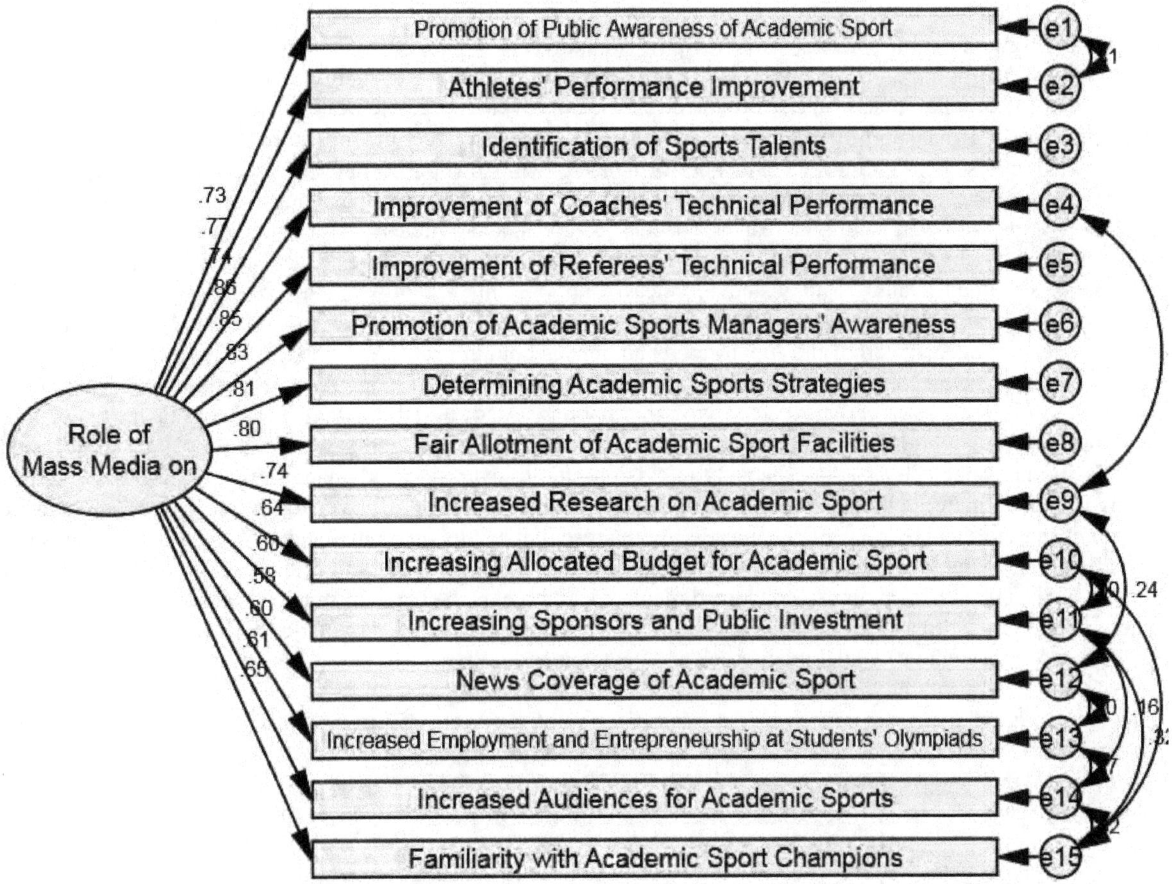

Figure 1. Measurement Model for Level of Influence of Mass Media on Iran's Female Academic Sport Development

Based on measurement model for level of influence of mass media on Iran's female academic sport development (figure 1), improvement of coaches' technical performance (0.86), improvement of referees' technical performance (0.85), and promotion of academic sport managers' awareness (0.83) respectively are the mostly influenced variables by mass media.

Discussion

Results of the research clarified that there is a significant difference between current situation and desirable situation of influence of media under investigation in all research variables. In other words, mass media does not perform appropriately on their designated roles. Hence, media is expected to enhance their effort to achieve their prophecy regarding academic sport development. Rahimi Ajdadi (1996) [9] had indicated television, radio, and press have had a crucial and significant role in progression and development of women's sport in society and had been able to expand people's beliefs to criticize as well as make progress in the society. It is worth mentioning despite conduction of several studies over different periods of time on influences of mass media on different sport areas, yet there are still deficiencies in achieving the relevant objectives in case of media most especially in terms of women's sport. This represents a gap between mass media performance in broadcast of women's sport and results of the conducted researches.

Results of factorial analysis of this research showed that television renders respectively the most influence on promotion of academic sport managers' awareness (0.85), improvement of coaches' technical performance (0.80), and fair allotment of academic sport facilities (0.78). Based on results of research, it seems those engaged in different TV channels should pay much more attention to their performance in terms of sports; since television is amongst the most influential media on development of different sport areas which is, based on the related factor analysis, influential on development of dimensions of academic sport.

Results of factor analysis on radio demonstrated that this media is respectively influential on improvement of coaches' technical performance (0.81), fair allotment of academic sports facilities (0.79), and determining academic sports strategies (0.78). In other part, factor analysis of extensible variables that are influenced by press respectively include improvement of referees' technical performance (0.74), increasing academic sport managers' awareness (0.72), and improvement of athletes' performance.

Finally, overall factorial analysis of mass media influence on academic sport development showed improvement of coaches' technical performance (0.86), improvement of referees' technical performance (0.85), and increasing academic sport managers' awareness (0.83) are respectively the most influenced variables by mass media. Based on research findings, technical performance in women's sport events and matches is one of the most essential factors that is influenced by mass media. In other words, presentations and media reports of women's events will play significant role in increasing coaches, referees, and athletes' performance quality. This might be due to lack of visibility of valuable efforts of women in sports. Therefore, based on research results and respondents' comments, audio and visual broadcast and presentation of women's sports on mass media is motivational sign to increase women's performance quality to even higher levels in sports fields. Motivation to being seen, encouraged, cheered, and supported by audiences both in sport arena and media is amongst important reasons to enhance women's performance quality in sports. Therefore, mass media such as television, radio, and press have a crucial and effective role to make this happen. Also, based on final measurement model of this research, media has a high influence on increasing academic sports managers' awareness especially in terms of women's sports. Since mass media especially television, due to extensive audience coverage, are important and effective tools to increase awareness and to direct beliefs and cultures, all over the world a great amount of attention is paid to them by audiences. Considering the research results, mass media due to this serious role, shall exert effort to transfer information and awareness such as sending messages and criticisms of those involved in sports as well as people of society to concerned managers and others in charge as much as possible. As it has been argued, one of the indirect communication channels of athletes or non-athlete people in society with concerned high officials is through influential media such as television and radio.

Other results of the final factor analysis of research demonstrated that determining academic sport strategies, increased academic sport research, identification of sport talents, promotion of public awareness about academic sport, fair allotment of academic sport facilities, increased budget allocation to academic sport, increased sponsors and public investment, increased employment and entrepreneurship in students' Olympiads, and increased audiences for students' sports are also variables highly influenced by mass media in Iran.

Conclusions

It is evident that information dissemination role of media could be utilized as a tool for increase of public awareness level in respect to academic sport as well as to attract college students toward sports. Media, by taking advantage of advertising, information dissemination and education about sport and its advantages, can cause more active participation of female college students in different fields of public sports as well as championships in universities. At the same time, if women's sport is broadcasted by media, it probably would increase investment and financial supports both from public and private sectors in terms of women's sport; since, one of main objectives of financial supporters is to be introduced to public and attract even more consumers. This would be possible in shadow of media's higher supports from women's sport. Another dimension of academic sport development by mass media is increased employment and entrepreneurship; this means support and introduction of entrepreneurs and others engaged in the field by mass media would perform as a motivational force for others to be creative and innovative at students' sport events and Olympiads.

Conflict of interests

The author declares that there is no conflict of interests.

References

1. Afroozeh MS, Hamidi M, & Elahi A. Identification of Vantage points of Universities' Sports Council Members Regarding Media Approach to Sports. *Journal of Research Communication*, 2012; 19(1): 55-70.
2. Asadi A, & Rezaee Soufi M. Analysis of current situation and desirable role of mass media in development of volleyball sport field amongst students of sports sciences. *Communication Management in Sports Media*, 2014; 2(5): 59-63.
3. Black J & Bryant J. *Introduction to Media Communication* (4th ED) Dubuque. IA: Brown & Benchmark; 1995.
4. Emami M, & Mallaei M. Analysis of Sports News Content: Case Study of Channel 3. *Communication Management in Sports Media*, 2013; 1(3): 15-24.
5. Ghasemi H, Tejari F, Kohandel M, & Khodayari A. *Media activities on sport*. Bamdad e Ketab; 2008.
6. Hamidi M, Elahi A, Akbari Yazdi H, & Hamidi M. Students Sport of Islamic Republic of Iran, View and Development Strategy. *Sports Management Studies*, 2011; 12: 13-26.

7. Mahdavian Mashhadi M. Comparison of Current Situation and Desirable Role of Mass Media in Women's Sport. *First National Conference of Sport Management of Shomal University*, 2008; P. 24-26.
8. Mehdizadeh R, & Andam R. Solutios for Public Sport Development in Iran's Universities. *Sports Management Studies*, 2014; 22: 15-38.
9. Rahimi Ajdadi F. *Analysis of content of women's role in mass media mediums* (Unpublished master's thesis). Islamic Azad University, Tehran, Iran; 1996.
10. Roberts R & Olson JS. *Wining is the Only Thing: Sport in America Since 1945*. Baltimore, MD: Johns Hopkins university press; 1989.
11. Sage GH. *Wining is the Only thing: Sport in America Since 1945*. Baltimore, MD: Johns Hopkins university press; 1998.
12. Sotiriadou K, Shilbury D. The Attraction, retention, Transation, and Nurturing Process of Sport Development: Some Australian Evidence. *Journal of Sport Management*, 2008; 22: 247-272.
13. Zarifi M, & Davoudi K. National Media and Development of Public Sports. *Journal of Communication Research*, 2012; 19(69): 119-134.

21

ANTHROPOMETRICAL PROFILE AND BIO-MOTOR ABILITIES OF YOUNG ELITE WRESTLERS

Rahmat Ali Jafari[1], Arsalan Damirchi[1], Bahman Mirzaei[1], Hadi Nobari[2]
[1]Department of Exercise Physiology, Faculty of Sport Sciences, University of Guilan, Iran
[2]PhD student of Biochemistry and Exercise Metabolism, University of Isfahan, Iran

Abstract. _Aim:_ This study investigated the association between motor performance and somatic type, anthropometric, body composition, physiologic and physical fitness profile in young wrestlers.
Material: 16 young wrestlers aging 16–19 with a 4–year–experience of taking part in national championships were selected for the study. Following the standard methods in the testing center of Alborz province some tests like aerobic power, muscular endurance, flexibility and agility speed tests and 1RM were taken to integrate the participants. Also, it should be noted that the participants' height, weight, the girth of thigh, elbow, calf and arm and skin thickness were measured.
Results: Somatotype, Somatotype Attitudinal Distance (SAD), Height Weight ratio (HWR) were calculated according to Carter and Heath anthropometric method. Body Fat Percentage (%BF), HWR and SAD resulted in 10.90±1.64, 43.27±0.87 and 0.94±0.87 respectively. Somatotype Standard Deviation and mean regarding endomorphic, mesomorphic and ectomorphic components were 2.16±0.46, 5.20±0.77 and 2.88±0.64 respectively. Physiologically, wrestlers VO_{2MAX} (kg/min) were 49.31±4.22 and their Resting Heart Rate (bpm) were 68.31±6.64.
Conclusion: As the present study illustrates, Somatotype of the Endomorphs, Mesomorphs and Ectomorphs were the same. As a result, coaches can plan wrestlers' training programs and review of techniques based on anthropometric and physiologic data driven from their sports performances.Besides, wrestlers could be well-informed about their performance. Moreover, aforesaid information could be beneficial to wrestling federations and all other organizations contributing the wrestling federation while holding talent identification programs and recognizing young wrestlers.
Key words: somatotype, wrestling, talent, test, physical.

Introduction

Wrestling is one of the most challenging competitive and anaerobic sports because of its stress on metabolic systems [1]. Therefore, the intensity of the wrestling match can determine muscle energy resources and the amount of all three resources consumed. Anthropometric and Physiologic features are considered as crucial concepts regarding athletes' performances among all sports [2]. The obtained capabilities and distinctive features could indicate the athlete's current condition and also could facilitate the comparison process of his previous and current results [3].

Physical fitness test results mark wrestles' weak points, strengths through wrestling matches and all the requirements for their future accomplishments. High capacity of aerobic and anaerobic, strength, power, agility, and flexibility in upper body and lower body are all considered as the most important physical fitness factors required to succeed in wrestling competitions [4,5].

Nowadays one of the most distinctive issues in sports is the process of discovering talented athletes. In other words recognizing, training and evaluating talented athletes at their early ages would help them constitute impressive future achievements. Sports instructors should dedicate the whole majority of their time and energy to elite athletes since they have potentials to succeed otherwise the presence of instructors would be inefficient. Thus most talented athletes with special aptitudes should be considered as the target goal of the instructors [6].

Following Carter and Heath, Somatotype provides significant information on special sports achievements [7]. Also Bloomfield et al. believe that Somatotype data can predict athlete's success in all fields of sport [8]. According to the analysis of the athletes' performance through international matches and Olympic Games, in order to succeed in competitions athletes should be equipped with bio-motor, anthropometry, structure and body compositions. By virtue of the data driven from the analysis, the evaluations on Somatotype features and comparing them with elite athletes' test results are regarded as a method to predict prominent athletes' success [9, 10]. Interestingly, the information achieved through aptitude and anthropometric tests play a crucial role in screening process [6, 9].

One of the most important criteria through the process of talent identification is the evaluation of somatotype information. Due to its variety, there have been several studies done on somatotype criteria. According to the analysis done on studies, there is a close relationship between the somatotype information of young and adult athletes' similarities and consistency of their somatotype features through all their lives [7]. Regarding the point that somatotype features are greatly influenced by genetic factors rather than other factors such as practice and diet [2, 11, 12]. The obtained information are so eminent in identifying talented athletes. The key factors to achieve success in various athletic fields are anthropometry, structure evaluation, and physical features [13].

The present study aims at providing anthropometric features, body composition, somatotype, physiologic and body fitness factors contributing to young wrestlers' performance. The result of the study would provide a profile for young wrestlers in the different age range in order to devalue the comparison of adult wrestlers' talent aptitude test results and young wrestlers' results.

Material and methods:

Participants: The present study follows a field descriptive method. Also, the aim of the present research is categorized as a functional and practical research. The subjects were 16 young elite wrestlers aging 16–19 years old. It is necessary to mention that the participants had the experience of practicing wrestling and being the champion for 4 years.

Research Design

All the tests and measurements were done during the same time in 6 days. In order to homogenize participants and measure their aerobic power, a physical fitness tests including Bruce test, Trunk lift flexibility, Shoulder flexibility, Sit and Reach Test, Muscle Endurance (Curl up, Pull up), Bench Press Maximum Strength, Squat based on Brzycki [14] formula, speed (36 m) and agility (4×9 m Test) were held.

The Brzycki (1993) equation is as follows while recording anthropometric measurements, the number of practice sessions was reduced. All the measurements over anthropometric features, body structure, and other variables were taken according to an international association of ISAK while the wrestlers were resting. Somatotype was analyzed and calculated with Somatochart software (version 1.2). Body density (BD) was estimated using the method of Jackson and Pollock [15]. BD was transformed to %BF by the Brozek's equation [16].

Statistical Analysis

To analyze the data, descriptive statistic methods were used.

Results

Table 1 the results of the present research on Anthropometric features and body composition are presented; in table 2 Somatotype and table 3 bio-motor ability among of young elite wrestlers are shown.

Table 1. Anthropometric and body composition characteristics of young elite wrestlers

Variable	Mean	Std. Deviation	Maximum	Minimum
Age (years)	17.43	1.15	19	16
Experience (years)	4.21	1.35	7	2
Anthropometric				
Weight (kg)	66.70	8.48	87.50	57.40
Height (cm)	173.25	5.79	184	165
BMI (kg/cm^2)	22.14	1.68	25.84	20.44
Sitting height (cm)	88.53	3.79	94	81
Skin-fold (mm)				
Chest	2.50	1.83	5	3
Axilla	3.76	2.65	7	5
Triceps	4.32	3.23	10	5
Subscapular	5.89	4.39	15	8
Abdomen	5.11	4.04	14	6
Suprailium	5.04	4.47	16	4
Front thigh	6.12	4.48	11	5
Biceps	2.03	1.43	4	2
Calf	3.55	2.70	8	4
Sum of 9 skin-fold (mm)	38.32	2.80	54	29
Body fat (%)	10.90	1.64	15	7.90
Lean body mass (kg)	58.96	7.10	73.90	50.20
Lengths (cm)				
Arm span	174.40	6.18	185	166
Humerus	74.06	4.58	85	64
Femur	105.75	8.71	118	93
Girths (cm)				
Flexed arm	28.79	1.90	33	26
Waist	73.75	5.06	87	67
Hip	91.40	4.39	101	86.20
Calf	35.35	2.26	40.50	32

Table 2. Somatotype variables of young elite wrestlers

Variable	Mean	SD	Maximum	Minimum
Endomorphy	2.16	0.46	2.9	1.4
Mesomorphy	5.20	0.77	6.5	3.3
Ectomorphy	2.88	0.64	3.7	1.8
SAD*	0.94	0.87	2.03	0.13
HWR*	43.27	0.87	44.1	41.53

* SAD (Somatotype Attitudinal Distance); HWR (Height to Weight Ratio).

Table 3. Bio-motor ability of young elite wrestlers

Variable	Mean	Std. Deviation	Maximum	Minimum
		physiologic		
Aerobic power				
VO_{2MAX} (kg/min)	49.31	4.22	59	42
VO_{2MAX} (l/min)	3.17	0.49	4	2.39
MET*	14.05	1.19	16.80	12
Heart Rate (bpm)				
Resting Heart Rate	68.31	6.64	78	57
Maximum Heart Rate	198.68	8.63	218	186
Flexibility (cm)		**Physical fitness**		
Sit and reach	41.93	5.45	55	35
Trunk	46.81	7.72	58	31
Shoulder	29.56	7.70	47	16
Muscular endurance (number of repetitions)				
Poll ups	11.18	3.31	18	6
Sit and reach	49.25	5.25	60	40
Maximal strength (kg)				
Bench Press	72.88	13.73	103.64	50.63
Squat	100.27	18.07	145.18	77.14
Speed (seconds)				
36 m.	4.26	0.26	4.91	3.93
Agility (s)				
4×9 m	8.86	0.48	9.72	8.10

*Metabolic Equivalent

The calculated somatotype was achieved through anthropometric features of height, weight, femur breadth, elbow breadth, calf girth, flexed arm girth, body composition. Also, their triceps skinfold, subscapular, suprailium and calf skinfold were calculated in two- dimensional based on Heath – Carter's method [2]. In order to do the analysis, the researcher used the Somatochart software (version 1.2) which is presented in figure 1. As the schematic figure illustrates, the mean is 2.2 – 5.9 – 2.9.

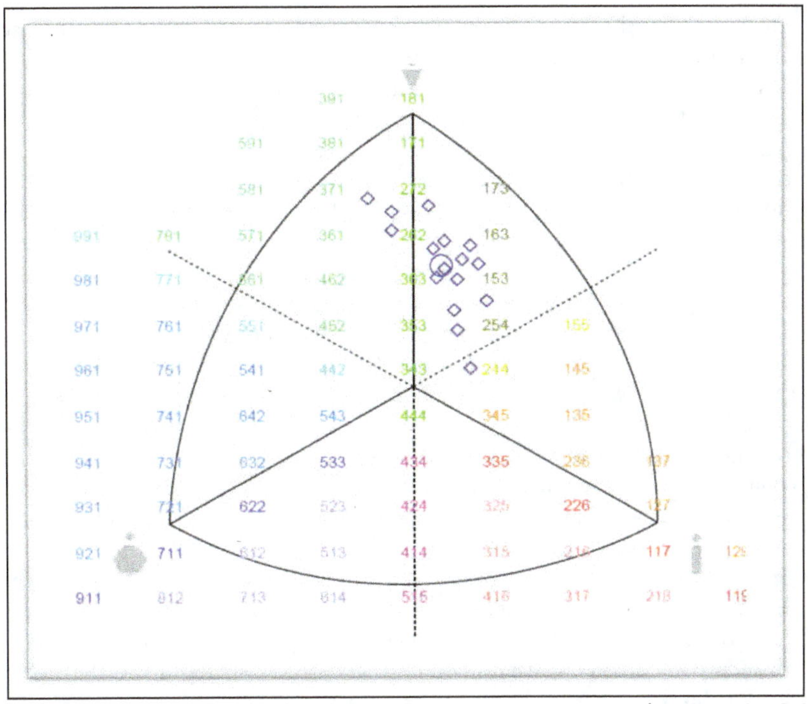

Figure 1. Somatotype features of young elite wrestlers. O = somatotype mean (2.16 – 5.9 – 2.9)

Discussion

One of the scientific aims of training is to use laboratory experiments to predict the athletes' performances. It has been proven that when athletes have the minimum amount of Body Fat %, they have the highest amount of Oxygen intake [13]. Mirzaei and Sadeghi did a study on the introduction to the state of physical fitness among adult wrestlers in freestyle wrestling national team. Based on their findings, VO_2Max was 50.6 ± 5.7 ml/kg/min and the amount of body fat% was 11.5±5.3 [17]. According to all researches done on wrestlers, one of the most important criteria that wrestling coaches should consider is Cardio Vascular Endurance. Additionally, the wrestler should have anaerobic power, agility, flexibility endurance and 1Repitation Maximum. Besides all these factors, the anthropometric variables increase as wrestlers aging 10–14 grow older and it would lead to advance in physical fitness records of the wrestlers [18].

Therefore, it is better to consider the age range of wrestlers while the talent identification process is being held since the obtained results would be more generalizable to evaluate the profiles. Robinson Ramirez-Velez reported VO_2Max as 49 ml/kg/min [19]. Also through other fact-findings VO_2Max counted as 45.9 ml/kg/min [12, 20], and 41.2 ml/kg/min among American wrestlers [3]. The concordance failure might be due to variety of athletes' practicing methods, body weight and fitness level of their body while doing the test or even because of environmental differences such as height, temperature and so forth [19].

The present study measured wrestlers' resting heart rate (68.31 bpm). The mean of resting heart rate was 60-100. Arslanoglu Erkan conducted a research on Turkish young wrestlers' resting heart rate. However, Arslanoglu's report on resting heart rate (63.2 bpm) did not concur with the result achieved by the present study [21]. On the other hand, according to Yoon's research, the maximum amount of elite wrestlers' heart rate was 197.5 [22] which was concurrent with the findings of the present study (198.68).

Based on the results achieved through the present study, the mean amount for the sit and reach test was 41.93 cm which follows the national norm of Iranian wrestlers [17]. Mirzaei et al. stated that the flexibility record among various weight range was very close to each other [3]. However, in a case study Mirzaei et al. reported the sit and reach test as 45cm [23]. In contrast, some experimental researches concluded that when the wrestlers' muscle strength increases, their flexibility does not decrease [22]. Following the statement mentioned above, many types of research done on wrestlers' physical fitness, the most prominent factor is muscle strength [17]. One of greatest features of wrestlers is the strength of upper and lower body (1RM) chest press and squat were 72.88 and 100.27 kg respectively. All the aforesaid amounts were less than Mirzaei et al.'s findings [23] and followed the national norm of Iran [3].

In the present study 4×9 m test, the agility was 8.86 seconds which was in accordance with the national norm of Iran. Based on researchers' agility is one of the most influential features of a successful wrestler. Due to the point that wrestling is associated with fast directional changes, body performance, and frequent flounce, what is required to fulfill the goal is a sharp reaction in the meantime [4].

A wrestler's anthropometric feature plays a crucial role in determining his/her potentials to succeed in matches. Specific physical features and anthropometric profiles are required in order for the maximum performance of the athletes in special sports. In addition to physiologic features mentioned through the present research, young elite wrestlers' anthropometric features, somatotype features, and body composition should be perused. According to Yoon, the appropriate amount of body fat % for wrestlers is 7 to 10 and in order to balance this measurement the wrestler must go on a specific diet and do suitable aerobic exercises [22]. Zakani also studied Italian national team wrestlers anthropometric features and their body compositions. There were 32 wrestlers aging 18-33 taking part in his study. Through his study some variables such as anthropometric weight, height, sitting height, some girth and body composition were measured and the minimum amount of body fat % was 5 [1,18]. Mirzaei et al. described the freestyle young elite wrestlers' profile and calculated their body fat % as 10.6±3.8 [3]. They resulted in the agreement between Iranian young elite wrestlers' physiologic profile and young elite wrestlers physiologic profiles of other countries. Sterkowize et al. studied the somatotype of heavyweight and finally they concluded that heavyweight wrestlers are either mesomorph or endomorph [24]. However, through this research, the somatotype of young wrestlers weighing about 66.70 ± 8.48 was considered as a mesomorph. Based on their findings it is clear that weight classes among lighter wrestlers were more like mesomorph and their body fat % were lower.

Robinson Ramirez-Velez did a research on 21 national Colombian wrestlers Mesomorph – ectomorph – somatotype mean (3.8– 5.3–1.6) of the wrestlers were analyzed by a related software which is shown in Figure 2 [19]. Data- driven from diagram 2 do not concord with the results of the present study. It is obvious that the mesomorphy is dominant and endomorph and ectomorph are equal (or the measured difference is only half a unit). In order to identify each body composition and compare various factors, the researcher must take special anthropometric girth into account and also include data mentioned in present research as a reference. Additionally, the present study would be advantageous for practical purposes as well as electing elite wrestlers and design their practicing plans through future researches and talent identification programs.

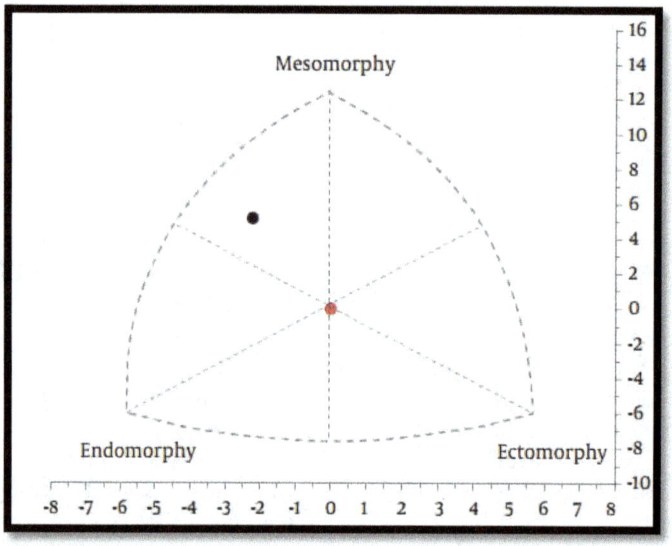

Figure 2. Somatotype average characteristics of Columbia wrestlers' national team. O = somatotype mean (3.8 – 5.3 – 1.6), [19].

Conclusion

The results of the present study would provide wrestling coaches with anthropometric features, body composition and somatotype profile of elite wrestlers. Such information including relative physiologic factors and body fitness could help wrestling coaches to balance wrestlers' practice schedules based on anthropometric profile and their sports performances. It is important not to ignore the role of energy resource in wrestling matches since they are more anaerobic but energy producer especially while wrestlers' recovery through taking aerobic system pathway. Therefore, information such as high VO_{2MAX}, low resting heart rate, agility, 1RM, high speed and flexibility would be beneficial.

Also considering anthropometric characteristics of lightweight tend to be more mesomorph, medium height and have low BMI and low body fat % could help young wrestlers to analyze performance information and appropriate practicality of such information themselves. Moreover, sports associations and wrestling federation could use driven information from the present study for talent identification plans and identification of elite wrestlers at their early ages.

Acknowledgment

All researchers who took part in the procedure of the present study would highly appreciate all wrestling coaches and wrestlers of Alborz province because of their time, consideration and cooperation.

Conflict of interests

The authors declare that there is no conflict of interests.

References:

1. Demirkan E, Kutlu M, Koz M, Özal M, Favre M. Physical fitness differences between freestyle and greco-roman junior wrestlers. *Journal of human kinetics*, 2014;41(1):245–251.
2. Eston R, Reilly T. Kinanthropometry and exercise physiology laboratory manual: tests, procedures and data: volume two: physiology. *Routledge*; 2013;1:23–30.
3. Mirzaei B, Curby DG, Rahmani-Nia F, Moghadasi M. Physiological profile of elite Iranian junior freestyle wrestlers. *The Journal of Strength & Conditioning Research,* 2009;23(8):2339–2344.
4. Rahmani-Nia F, Mirzaei B. The comparison of Oxygen consumption maximum among nominated young wrestlers in Guilan in the morning round and evening round. *The Journal of Olympics*, 2000;9(2-1):93–98.
5. Sharratt MT, Taylor AW, Song TM. A physiological profile of elite Canadian freestyle wrestlers. Canadian journal of applied sport sciences. *Journal canadien des sciences appliquées au sport*, 1986;11(2):100–105.
6. Kamali S. Talent identification in sports. *Proceedings of the National Conference of Sports Talent*, 2007. P. 100–104.
7. Ackland TR, Elliott B, Bloomfield J. *Applied anatomy and biomechanics in sport*. Human Kinetics; 2009.
8. Bloomfield J, Ackland TR, Elliot BC. *Applied Biomechanics and Anatomy in Sport*. Wiley–Blackwell; 1995.
9. Pieter W, Bercades LT, Center O. Somatotypes of national elite combative sport athletes. *Brazilian Journal of Biomotricity*, 2009;3(1):21–30.
10. Ratamess NA. *ACSM's foundations of strength training and conditioning.* Wolters Kluwer Health/Lippincott Williams & Wilkins; 2012.
11. Bompa TO, Haff GG. *Periodization: Theory and methodology of training.* Human Kinetics Publishers; 2009.
12. Qankqya C. Examination of Young Wrestlers' Leg Reaction Times and Their Relationships with Explosive Power. *World Appl. Sci. J.* 2013;16:189–197.
13. Arrese AL, Ostáriz ES. Skinfold thicknesses associated with distance running performance in highly trained runners. *Journal of sports sciences*, 2006;24(1):69–76.
14. Brzycki M. Strength testing—predicting a one-rep max from reps-to-fatigue. *Journal of Physical Education, Recreation & Dance*, 1993;64(1):88–90.
15. Jackson AS, Pollock ML. Generalized equations for predicting body density of men. *The British journal of nutrition*. 2004;91(1):161–168.
16. Brožek J, Grande F, Anderson JT, Keys A. Densitometric analysis of body composition: revision of some quantitative assumptions. *Annals of the New York Academy of Sciences*, 1963;110(1):113–140.
17. Mirzaei B, Mansour Sadeghi M. The profile of physical fitness of the adult wrestlers taking part in national team of freestyle wrestling preparation expeditions. *The Journal of Olympics*, 2006;15(38):81–89.
18. Shahed A, Khakpour B. The analysis of the contribution of some anthropometric features and physical fitness among teenage wrestlers aging 10–14 in Tabriz. *Third national athletic talent identification forum*, Iran, 2013.
19. Ramirez-Velez R, Argothyd R, Meneses-Echavez JF, Sanchez-Puccini MB, Lopez-Alban CA, Cohen DD. Anthropometric characteristics and physical performance of colombian elite male wrestlers. *Asian journal of sports medicine*, 2014;5(4):100–105.
20. Häkkinen K, Alen M, Komi PV. Neuromuscular, anaerobic, and aerobic performance characteristics of elite power athletes. *European journal of applied physiology and occupational physiology*, 1984;53(2):97–105.
21. Arslanoglu E. Physical profiles of Turkish young Greco-Roman wrestlers. *Educational Research and Reviews*. 2015;23;10(8):1034–1038.
22. Yoon J. Physiological profiles of elite senior wrestlers. *Sports Medicine*, 2002;32(4):225–233.
23. Mirzaei B, Curby DG, Barbas I, Lotfi N. Anthropometric and physical fitness traits of four-time World Greco-Roman wrestling champion in relation to national norms: A case study. *Journal of Human Sport and Exercise.* 2011;6(2):406–413.
24. Sterkowicz-Przybycień K, Sterkowicz S, Żarów R. Somatotype, body composition and proportionality in polish top greco-roman wrestlers. *Journal of human kinetics*, 2011;28:141–154.

22

SPECIFIC FEATURES OF TEAM KINDS OF SPORTS SPORTSMEN'S INDIVIDUAL CHARACTERISTICS

Liashenko V.N., Tumanova V.N., Hatsko E. V.
Kiev University Boris Grinchenko

Abstract. *Purpose:* to study individual characteristics of personalities of team kinds of sports sportsmen, specializing in football. *Material:* in the research football players (n=28, age 18 – 20 years) participated. Psycho-diagnostic testing by methodic 16PF of Kattel was used. *Results:* we found high correlation between factors, which were conditioned by caution in choosing partners for communication and active contacts. Such sportsmen express their emotions expressively. It facilitates improvement of relations in conditions of co-operation in little group. It was also found that one of personality's leading characteristics in sportsmen is their activity in social contacts. The higher is courage the more active is communication. It promotes discussion of common interests and targets for the given group of people. *Conclusions:* Sportsmen, who have many emotional interests and are ready to risk (or having bent to adventures) have to face non understanding of other players. In such case conflict can be inevitable. Especially it manifests, if opposite side has the same indicators in this factor. Just courage, risk and adventurism push them to conflict solution of problem situations.
Key words: conflictness, expressiveness, conservatism, self-control, team, football.

Introduction

Any sport team in every kind of sports is a kind of "little" social group [4, 14], the structure of relations in which corresponds to known psychological schemas and pedagogic plan. Success of human activity in social organizations depends on people's consolidation, co-operation, compatibility and conflict-free relations [12, 22, 32, 43]. According to some authors [9, 11, 21, 30], sport team is a special kind of contact community. Team is consolidated by common target of mutual sport activity, the main kinds of which are training and competitions.

It was found that the most typical for sportsmen features of character are: emotional stability, strive for leadership, bent to risk, pragmatism, and inventiveness, and self-control, communicability [25, 26, 35]. In other works [2, 29] authors stress on bent to risk. The authors found that risk is connected with probability of traumas. That is why individual characteristics play great role and reflect dynamic side of a personality. The temper of personality is a complex system of logically interconnected properties with great potentials for inter-compensation of some properties by other. Just correlation of properties determines sportsman's reaction to extreme situation. It was determined that only compensation of "negative" features by "positive" ones can influence on sports functioning [33].

Sport functioning is rather specific in team kinds of sports. It implies solution of current tasks in non-stationary medium. Leading specialists in sports psychology [3, 27] think that in such activity sportsman personality's certain properties will realize. These properties optimize behavior in conflict situations and in struggle with opponent. Therefore, it is necessary to study the most important individual properties of personality for successful competition functioning.

In other studies it was found [27, 28, 31], that efficiency of sport functioning to large extent is determined by personality's individual characteristics. Sportsmen have high aggressiveness, high motivation for achievements, high self-assessment and self-assurance; they also have extraversion and firm character. Operational-functioning characteristics in individual kinds of sports [5, 7] point at sportsmen's high self-assurance, high self-assessment, communicability and expressiveness [8, 10, 19]. However, in game kinds of sports specific of training and competition functioning is different. That is why it is necessary to pay attention to social-psychological features of a personality, whose influence on results is the most probable exactly in team kinds of sports [13, 15, 17]. That is why, in our work, among sportsmen's multiple and different characteristic features we regarded the following: communicability (demand in communication); credulity-suspiciousness, straightness, conformity (ability to quickly change opinion, under influence of collective pressure), authority (bent to dominate), self-control and discipline [20].

Hypothesis: it was assumed to mark out and study the most significant individual characteristics of sportsmen's personality in team kinds of sports, considering specificity of co-operation for achievement high sport results.

The purpose of the research: to study individual characteristics of personalities of team kinds of sports sportsmen, specializing in football.

Material and methods

Participants: in the research sportsmen, specializing in football, participated. The age of participants was 18 – 20 years; the quantity – 28 persons. When forming the group of sportsmen we considered criterion of uniformity of the tested (variation coefficient did not exceed 10%).

Organization of the research: the research took the period of 2013-2014. Psycho-diagnostic testing by methodic 16PF of Kattel was used [18, 34].

Statistical analysis: for every indicator we found mean arithmetic, mean square deviation S (standard deviation) and variation coefficient (V). Sample testing for normality was fulfilled with the help of test χ^2. Besides, Pearson's correlation analysis was used. The presence of correlations was considered to be confident at significance level of $p \le 0.05$; 0.01.

Results of the research

Sports have distinctive features in comparison with other kinds of activity. Sport is activity, implying overcoming different obstacles. That is why cultivation of sportsman's features is a natural component of sportsman's psychological training.

For determination of football players' tested psychological qualities' significance of priority we conducted correlation analysis between indicators of psychological qualities: «A», «C», «E», «G», «H», «I», «L», «M», «N», «O», «Q1», «Q2», «Q4», «B», «F».

The highest quantity of correlations was found between factor "H": "shyness-courage" and "F": "carelessness – conflictness".

In our research mean group value of this factor was related to pole of courage and is interpreted as courage in social contacts. This factor positively correlates with conflictness (r=0.48) as well as with factors: A "communicability" (r=0, 42); E "obedience - dominance" (r=0.44); F "restraint – expressiveness" (r=0.70); Q1 "conservatism – radicalism" (r=0.56); Q3 "low self-control – high self-control" (r=0.45). There is negative correlation with factor M "practicality – daydreaming" (r=-0.45), $p<0.05$.

There was also great correlation of factors H and A (r=0.42): "isolation – communicability". Mean group value by this pole is closer to positive (to communicability). These factors, in the whole, supplement each other.

Sportsmen with expressed communicability are expected to be easy in contacts with partners and in co-operation [23]. Such sportsmen strive for inter-personal contacts, empathize what is happening and expect the same emotions from other people. These sportsmen do not endure "overloading" of communication with many partners. They manage to orient in game situation and in inter-personal contacts.

Sportsmen's communication in game functioning implies situations of "forced co-operation", in which sportsman shall switch in rather active communications with partners. Serious practical problem [15, 16] emerges when non communicative sportsman shall support contact with partners and even control their behavior.

Non-coincidence of communicative demands can be also rather a problem for partners' co-operation in team. In such situation one sportsman wants to actively communicate and discuss what is happening. He emotionally responds to what is happening. Other sportsman is irritated by this and distracts from functioning. He thinks it is unnecessary and excessive. In some cases such differences can result in serious misunderstanding and even conflicts between sportsmen.

In the whole, communicability, openness, easiness in direct inter-personal contacts are characteristics of this factor with positive pole. Their correlation with courage in social contacts is mutually caused.

The highest correlation was observed between factors H and F - (r=0.70). Factor F was defined as "restraint- expressiveness". It is emotional expressiveness of personality [44]. It is interesting that with years impulsiveness and carelessness reduce. It can be regarded as an evidence of certain emotional maturity. Mean group value of this factor is "5". It means combining of two poles with correlation with factor "H".

In general factor F is oriented on measuring of emotional coloring and dynamic in the process of communication. Among tested football players such characteristics as "caution" (reasonability in choosing of partner for communication, bent to worry about future) and cheerfulness (impulsivity, expressiveness, enthusiasm, emotional brightness in communication with other people) are equally blended. Correlation of these factors is evident. On the one hand the sportsmen cautiously choose partners for communication and worry about their future. On the other hand they actively make contacts and expressively show their emotions. It facilitates improvement of relations in conditions of co-operation in little group.

The next correlation is H and Q1 - (r=0.56). Here Q1 is «conservatism-radicalism". This factor determines radical, intellectual, political and religious attitude. Mean group value is "6". It is in the center, between two poles of this factor, but closer to "+". In the whole team consists of players with combination of different qualities. They are: conservatism; stable attitude to traditions; bent to moralization and sermons; resistance to changes; orientation on definite real functioning. Other players have opposite qualities: free-thinking; perception of changes and new ideas; distrust in authorities; bent to analytical and theoretical functioning. However, sportsmen with orientation on new prevail. Desire to experiment is encouraged in sports [24, 46].

Optimal combination of the factor's poles permits for sportsmen to communicate with each other. Sportsmen share individual and mutual interests. It permits for them to work successfully in one group.

Moderate correlation is observed between indicators H and Q3 - (r=0.45). Here Q3 –is "low self-control – high self-control". This factor measures internal control of behavior and personality's integration.

People with high values by this factor are bent to organizational activity. They achieve success in professions, where objectiveness, decisiveness and balance are required [20, 36, and 38]. This factor characterizes human awareness in regulation of "Self" force (factor C) and "Super-Self" force (factor G). The factor determines expressiveness of personality's will. This factor is one of the most important for prognostication of success. It is positively connected with frequency of leader's election as well as with activity in solution of group problems.

Two poles of this factor are expressed in the following:

- "-" – low discipline, following own desires; dependence on emotions; inability to control own emotions and behavior;
- "+" – commitment, strong will; ability to control own emotions and behavior.

Mean group value by this factor is "6". It means approaching "+" pole. Low degree of this factor points at weak will and bad self-control. Such people's activity is disordered and impulsive. Person with high values by this factor has socially welcomed characteristics: self-control, insistence, consciousness, bent to follow ethics [37]. To correspond to these standards personality shall have distinct principles, beliefs and consideration of social opinion. This factor is important when solving group problems, characteristic for football team.

Now let us regard negative correlation with this factor: M - (r= -0.45), p <0.05, where M is "Practicality –daydreaming". This factor is rather complex. In general personalities with M have bright internal intellectual life with intensive feeling of ideas and emotions. In their behavior they can be "Bohemian", non-conforming. High degrees of this factor are intrinsic to artists, poets, researchers, experimenters, managers of high rank, editors. Low degrees are in persons, who deal with monotonous calculations (required attention and concentration). Such persons are characterized by inner balance and reasonability. However, in sudden situations they often feel deficit of imagination and inventiveness. In general this factor is oriented on measuring imagination features, reflecting in personality's actual behavior: practicality; "earthiness", some "head in clouds"; romantic attitude to life.

Mean group value of M factor is "6". This contingent of sportsmen is characterized by bent to intellectual life and deficit of concentration and attention. For sport collective it is characteristic to all its members in active work on solution of collective tasks. In such group high mutual demands, deep respect to every member exist. In such case personal interests of its members coincide with team's interests [40]. If in the group persons with expressed positive pole of this factor prevail there will be no need to seek mutual understanding. In this case in-team life will replace demand in inter-personal relations. It causes difficulties in collective's work on achievement team's targets.

The next factors with the highest quantity of correlations are conflictness – factor F (restraint-expressiveness); factor E (obedience- dominance); factor Q2) conformism – non-conformism) and factor Q4 "relaxation – tension).

The least quantity of correlations is observed in the following factors: B "intellect"; N "straightness – diplomacy"; O "calmness-anxiety"; G "low normative behavior – high normative behavior"; I "firmness – sensitivity"; C "emotional imbalance – emotional balance".

Discussion

Many authors note that for more effective functioning of sport team it is necessary to know the following: demands and motives of team members; requirements of current situation. Besides, it is necessary to consider such factors as: sportsmen's compatibility in team; identity of thinking; motivation; values' system [2, 15]. We found that the most developed in football players are such qualities as: courage in social contacts; communicability; expressiveness; conservatism; self-control. In this aspect our results well coincide with other authors' data [10, 12]. For fruitful communication sportsmen shall be prepared for actions in life situations, which would require communicative abilities [5, 14].

Self-control is of not less importance for football players [3, 20]. Acquiring and mastering of self-control skills imply general discipline of a person, internal culture and high professional fitness. In this context it is evident that self-control algorithms are fixed under influence of person's self-assessment and his assessment by other people [1, 3, 4, and 13].

It can be assumed that human self-control is included in integral structure of the most important personality's characteristics; self-respect [11, 39]. In its integral manifestations, self-control permits to control own behavior and behavior of collective. That is why self-control is an important professional quality for sportsmen of team kinds of sports [30]. In this context team is characterized by inter-personal relations of its members [3]. Between team members non-formal, friendly relations can exist as well as perfect game understanding, worked out by years of training. In such case these relations will serve as the basis of interaction during match [5, 45]. Emotional feeling of sport situation, expressiveness of sympathy or dislikes, degree of realization of non-formal friendly relations can be a criterion of interaction [11, 41]. Thus, specific of kind of sports or competition exercise requires co-operation from participants and personal contribution into team's success [42]. Specific of team kind of sports also requires interaction of players. The main condition of such interaction will be team's organization and personality's properties of every team member.

Conclusions

It has been determined that factor H is one of the main indicators. This factor characterizes degree of activity in social contacts. It reflects organism's activity and features of temper. We think that this factor is of substantial importance in structure of personal characteristics of team kind of sports sportsmen. The more courage sportsman has the more active and communicative he is. It facilitates improvement of contacts in team discussion of mutual interests and targets for the given group of people. With it, it is evident that it has strong correlation with conflictness. Sportsmen with many emotional interests and readiness to risk (or bent to adventurism) have to face misunderstanding of other players. In such case conflict is inevitable. Especially it is possible if other side has the same indicator in this factor. Exactly courage and adventurism push sportsmen to conflict solution of problem situations.

Conflict of interests

The authors declare that there is no conflict of interests.

References:

1. Abramova GS. *Obshchaia psikhologiia* [General psychology], Moscow: Academic Project; 2003. (in Russian)
2. Barinov VV. *Vliianie individual'nykh osobennostej lichnosti basketbolista na uspeshnost' sorevnovatel'noj deiatel'nosti. Kand. Diss.* [Influence of individual features of basketball player's personality on success of competition functioning. Cand. Diss.], Moscow; 2001. (in Russian)
3. Bermudes Torres Ankheolina. *Osobennosti samokontrolia v processe sorevnovatel'noj deiatel'nosti. Kand. Diss.* [On self-control in the process of competition functioning. Cand. Diss.], Leningrad; 1983. (in Russian)
4. Bondarchuk EI. *Osnovy psikhologii i pedagogiki* [Principles of psychology and pedagogic], Kiev: MAUP; 2001. (in Russian)
5. Vasiura SA. *Psikhologiia kommunikativnoj aktivnosti cheloveka* [Psychology of human communicative activity], Izhevsk: Udmurt State University; 2006. (in Russian)
6. Vasiura SA. Kommunikativnaia aktivnost' predstavitelej komandnykh i individual'nykh vidov sporta [Communicative activity of representatives of team and individual kinds of sports]. *Chelovek. Soobshchestvo. Upravlenie,* 2012;2:72 – 81. (in Russian)
7. Gogunov EN, Mart'ianov BI. *Psikhologiia fizicheskogo vospitaniia i sporta* [Psychology of physical education and sports], Moscow: Academy; 2000. (in Russian)
8. Gordeeva TO, Sychev OA. Vnutrennie istochniki nastojchivosti i ee rol' v uspeshnosti uchebnoj deiatel'nosti [Internal sources of insistence and its role in educational progress]. *Psikhologiia obucheniia*, 2012;1:33-48. (in Russian)
9. Il'in EP. *Psikhologiia sporta* [Psychology of sports], Sankt Petersburg: Peter; 2009. (in Russian)
10. *Introvert i ekstravert. Enciklopediia prakticheskoj psikhologii «PSIKhOLOGOS»* [Introvert and extravert. Encyclopedia of practical psychology "PSYCHOLOGOS"]. [Internet]. 2016 Oct 06 [cited 2016 Oct 06]; Available from: http://www.psychologos.ru/articles/view/introvert_i_ekstravert
11. Zeer EF. *Psikhologiia professij* [Psychology of professions], Moscow: Academic Project; 2008. (in Russian)
12. Il'in AB. Psikhologicheskij analiz prichin konfliktov v sportivnykh komandakh [Psychological analysis of reasons of conflicts in sport teams]. *Sportivnyj psikholog,* 2004; 3:27 - 30. (in Russian)
13. Il'in EP. *Psikhologiia sporta* [Psychology of sports], Sankt Petersburg: Peter; 2016. (in Russian)
14. Ishchenko V, Lisenchuk G, Daragan V. Sravnitel'nyj analiz fizicheskoj podgotovlennosti futbolistov komand raznoj kvalifikacii [Comparative analysis of physical fitness of different qualification teams' football players], *Nauka v olimpijskom sporte*, 2003;1:50 - 56. (in Russian)
15. Zagajnov R. *Psikhologiia sovremennogo sporta vysshikh dostizhenij* [Psychology of modern elite sports], Moscow: Soviet sport; 2012. (in Russian)
16. Zagajnov R.M. Psikhologicheskaia atmosfera kak psikhologicheskij fenomen [Psychological atmosphere as psychological phenomenon]. *Sportivnyj psikholog*, 2005;2:10 - 27. (in Russian)
17. Kardialis K, Aleksandravichiute B. Konfliktnost' i splochennost' sportivnykh komand [Conflictness and consolidation of sport teams]. *Psikhologicheskij zhurnal*, 2005;26(1):71 - 78. (in Russian)
18. Karelin AA. *Bol'shaia enciklopediia psikhologicheskikh testov* [Great encyclopedia of psychological tests], Moscow: Eksmo; 2007. (in Russian)
19. Kondrat'ev MIu, Kondrat'ev IuM. Social'no-psikhologicheskij fenomen avtoriteta i otnosheniia avtoritetnosti v gruppe [Social-psychological phenomenon of authority and authority relations in group]. *Mir psikhologii,* 2006;4:67 - 76. (in Russian)
20. Korableva EV. *Ustojchivost' samokontrolia v ekstremal'nykh usloviiakh v sviazi s emocional'no-volevymi osobennostiami lichnosti. Kand. Diss.* [Self-control balance in extreme situations in respect to personality's emotional-will characteristics. Cand. Diss.], Moscow; 1993. (in Russian)
21. Krys'ko VG. *Social'naia psikhologiia* [Social psychology], Moscow: Vlados-Press; 2004. (in Russian)
22. Kuznecov VV. *Psikhologicheskij analiz proiavleniia sub"ektno-lichnostnykh svojstv sportsmenov kak pokazatelia uspeshnosti ikh deiatel'nosti. Kand. Diss.* [Psychological analysis of sportsmen's subjective-

personalities qualities' manifestations as indicator of their functioning successfulness. Cand. Diss.], Kazan; 2004. (in Russian)

23. Labunskaia VA. *Social'naia psikhologiia obshcheniia kak osnova organizacii peregovorov* [Social psychology of communication as a base of negotiations' organization], Rostov on Don: UFU; 2010. (in Russian)
24. Lozhkin GV. Konceptual'nye predstavleniia o psikhologicheskom potenciale kvalificirovannogo sportsmena [Conceptual ideas about elite sportsman's psychological potential]. *Nauka v olimpijskom sporte*, 2007;1:87-93. (in Russian)
25. Lukina TA. *Ocenka pokazatelej, kharakterizuiushchikh lichnost' sportsmenov, i ikh dinamika v godichnom makrocikle. Kand. Diss.* [Assessment of indicators, characterizing sportsmen's personalities, and their dynamic in annual macro-cycle. Cand. Diss.], Moscow; 1997. (in Russian)
26. Liashenko VM, Tumanova V. Vivchennia psikhologichnikh osoblivostej kvalifikovanikh sportsmeniv [Study of elite sportsmen's psychological characteristics]. *Mizhnarodna naukovo-praktichna konferenciia "Fizichna kul'tura i sport u suchasnomu suspil'stvi", 20 listopada 2015r.* [International scientific-practical conference "Physical culture and sports in modern society"< November 20th, 2015], 2015. P. 130-134. (in Ukrainian)
27. Liashenko VN, Tumanova VN, Hatsko EV. Study of personality's temperament and self-assessment of higher educational establishments' students. *Physical Education of Students*, 2016;20(2):19-23. doi:10.15561/20755279.2016.0203
28. Liashenko VN, Tumanova VN, Mariskina TV. Features of manifestation of self-trained athletes specialized in jumping. *Physical Education of Students,* 2012;6:70-73.
29. Nogina EV. *Kommunikativnaia kompetentnost' kak faktor uspeshnoj sportivnoj deiatel'nosti regbistok vysokoj kvalifikacii. Kand. Diss.* [Communicative competence as a factor of successful sport functioning of elite female rugby players. Cand. Diss.], Malakhovka; 2005. (in Russian)
30. Sopov VF. *Teoriia i metodika psikhologicheskoj podgotovki v sovremennom sporte* [Theory and methodic of psychological training in modern sports], Moscow; 2010. (in Russian)
31. Tolkunova IV, Liashenko VN. Individual'no – psikhologicheskie razlichiia kvalificirovannykh legkoatletov i ikh vliianie na rezul'tativnost' sorevnovatel'noj deiatel'nosti [Individual psychological distinctions of elite light athletes and their influence on efficiency of competition functioning]. *Physical Education of Students*, 2009;2:97-100. (in Russian)
32. Khudiakov VP, Kishchenko SE. Psikhologicheskaia podgotovka sportsmenov v komandnykh vidakh sporta k trenirovochnomu processu i sorevnovaniiu [Psychological preparation of sportsmen for training process and competitions in team kinds of sports]. *Innovacionnye proekty i programmy v obrazovanii*, 2014;2:57 - 62. (in Russian)
33. Shustikov GB, Fudimov VV. Vliianie sportivnoj deiatel'nosti na formirovanie lichnostnykh kachestv zanimaiushchikhsia [Influence of sport activity on formation of trainees' personality qualities]. *Uchenye zapiski universiteta imeni P.F. Lesgafta,* 2012;1(83):163-167. (in Russian)
34. Iurov IA. *Psikhologicheskoe testirovanie i psikhoterapiia v sporte* [Psychological testing and psycho-therapy in sports], Moscow; 2006. (in Russian)
35. Amon AH. *Individual strategies of decision under uncertainty*. Unpublished doctoral dissertation, University of California: Berkeley; 1962.
36. Anderson CR, Schneier CE. Locus of control, leader behavior and leader performance among management students. *Academy of Management Journal,* 1978;21:690-698.
37. Zunaira Javed, Soulat Khan, Rukhsana Kausar. Group Cohesion, Decision Making Styles and Group Performance in University Students. *Psychological Abstracts,* 2012;14:81-82.
38. Hopper C, Fisher B, Munoz KD. *Physical activity and nutrition for health.* Champaign: Human Kinetics; 2008.
39. Ludovici-Connoly AM. *Winning Health Promotion Strategies*. Human Kinetics; 2010.

40. *Physical education and sport, healthy lifestyle boosts factors*. International scientific session (Bucharest, April 6th 2012). Ministry of education, research, youth and sport. Bucharest: BREN; 2012.
41. Rudenko R, Mahliovanyy A, Shyyan O, Prystupa T. Physical rehabilitation and thermoregulatory processes in athletes with disabilities. *Journal of Physical Education and Sport*, 2015; 15 (4): 730–735.
42. Ohromiy GV, Makarova NU, Kasyuha AM. Psychophysiological methods and criteria for the selection of individual metered loads in athletes of taekwondo section. *Physical Education of Students*, 2014;6:54-62. doi:10.15561/20755279.2014.0611
43. Schoeneman TJ. Reports of the Sources of Self-knowledge. *J. of Personality*. 1981;49(3):284-293.
44. Zion LC. Body concepts as it relates to self-concept. *Research Quarterly*, 1965;1:490-495 p.
45. Sharp RH. Viewing time and occluded time as determined of ball catching success. *British Journal of Physical Education*, 1974;5(6):22-24.
46. Whitting HTA. An oprerational analysis of a continuous ball throwing and catching task. *Ergonomics* 1975;13(4)" 445-454.

23

DEVELOPMENT OF GIRL-STUDENTS' PHYSICAL QUALITIES AT EXTRACURRICULAR CHEER-DANCE CLASSES (CHEER-DANCE SHOW)

Pyatnickaya D.V.
Kharkov Humanitarian Pedagogical Academy

Abstract. *Purpose:* to work out and substantiate methodic of cheer-dance means' usage in extracurricular trainings of girl students. *Material:* in experiment 450 girl-students of 17-20 years' age participated. *Results:* we generalized theoretical knowledge and practical experience in selection, content and organization of girl students' physical education. We presented the data of comparative analysis of girl students' physical condition and (sportswomen and not sportswomen). We noted significant interest to physical education, in which the offered methodic is used. It was found that demands in health strengthening can be formed by means of dance kinds of cheer-leading (cheer-dance and cheer-dance show). *Conclusions:* We have found prospects of girl students' physical education perfection. It permits to work out different variants of realization of educational health related strategy.
Key words: girl students, higher educational establishments, fitness, cheer-dance, cheer-dance show, physical qualities, health.

Introduction

Recent time in Ukraine there have been being observed steady tendency for reduction of health of population and students in particular. It is also paid attention to in governmental document, regulating physical education in higher educational establishments (HEE). It is studied by specialists in physical culture and sports.

For example, in researches [1, 7, 9, 11, 18, 30, 34] it was established that in period of studying in higher educational establishments quantity of special health group students increases up to 5.3% in the first year and up to 14.4% in the forth year. Accordingly, we can observe reduction of quantity of main group students: from 84.0% to 70.2%.

Besides, researches of other authors [11-13, 19-21, 27, 38-44] witness about low level of physical conditions, physical fitness and workability of students. Authors note insufficient level of solution of main physical education tasks. As a result (after graduation) most of graduates are not physically able to fulfill professional duties with proper quality and intensity. So working potential of youth reduces, though social and economical welfare of our country depends on it.

In this connection, one of the most important tasks of physical education in higher educational establishment is strengthening of health, rising of physical fitness and physical condition of students.

A number of authors [6, 10, 19, 20, 25, 26, 28] note decrease of motivation and interest to physical education classes. Results of these researches point at monotonous character of training material, insufficient effectiveness of existing methodic and forms of physical culture trainings. That is why the problem of upgrading of HEE physical education by implementation of innovative approaches to organization of training process, considering students' motivation, is rather important and urgent. Besides new, modern kinds of motor functioning, which would encourage students for physical exercises, require their implementation. That is why urgency of this problem is evident and requires explanation and analysis.

Purpose, tasks of the work, material and methods

The purpose of the research: is to work out and substantiate methodic of cheer-dance means' usage in extracurricular trainings of 1st-2nd year girl students.

The tasks of the research:

1. To generalize theoretical knowledge and practical experience in selection, content and organization of higher educational girl students' physical education in process of extracurricular classes.

2. To determine girl students' physical condition and physical fitness.

3. To carry out comparative analysis of girl students' physical condition and fitness: group of not sportswomen and group of cheer-dancers (cheer-leading).

4. To work out and experimentally prove methodic of application of cheer-dance means in extracurricular trainings of girl students.

5. To work out practical recommendations for physical culture teachers on implementation of the offered cheer-dance methodic in physical education process.

The object of the research: physical education of higher educational establishments' girl students in process of extracurricular trainings.

The subject of the researches: methodic of cheer-dance means' application in extracurricular trainings of 1st-2nd year girl students of higher educational establishments.

The methods of the research: analysis and generalization of literature data on this topic; generalization of advanced experience of specialists in physical education and coaches with the help of talks and questioning; pedagogic observations over competition and training functioning; pedagogic testing (determination of motor skills' level), functional testing of cardio-vascular and respiratory systems; pedagogic experiment; methods of mathematical statistic.

The contingent of the tested: first and second year girl students of Municipal establishment "Kharkov Humanitarian Pedagogical Academy" of Kharkov regional council. In experiment 450 girl students of 17-20 years' age participated.

We formed experimental and control groups. Each group consisted of 27 girl students. Distribution of girl students into groups was fulfilled by results of questioning, devoted to choosing of motor functioning at physical education classes. That is why trainings of experimental group included dance kinds of cheer-leading: cheer-dance and cheer-dance show [22, 34]. Control group was trained by traditional academic program for HEEs of Ukraine of III-IV accreditation. The research was conducted in stage-by-stage way.

At first stage we realized the following: pedagogic testing; initial testing of physical condition and physical fitness; analysis and generalization of scientific-methodic literature; determination of purpose, tasks, object and subject of the researches; selection of methods of the researches; working out of experimental methodic of training. Experimental methodic of trainings was oriented on reduction of body mass, normalization of metabolism, giving up of harmful habits, improvement of physical condition and general state, on propaganda of healthy life style (HLS) and motivation for physical exercises' practicing. Content of cheer-dance trainings included dance block. This block was built on the base of cheer-leading's basic elements: pirouettes, splits, waving, cheer-jumps, leaps. There were no elements of acrobatics, supports of partner, pyramids. That is why this methodic was quite accessible for girl students. Cheer-dance exercises included movements and musical fragments of different dance styles (jazz, funk, pop, rap, lyrical dance and so on). That is why this kind of cheer-leading facilitates not only physical development of girl students' motor skills but also their aesthetic education.

At second stage we conducted pedagogic experiment. It implied that application of cheer-dance means in extracurricular trainings stimulated interest to physical exercises. They were oriented on formation and strengthening of health, perfection of physical condition and fitness.

At third stage we processed the received results and fulfilled comparative analysis of them. It permitted to determine effectiveness of methodic of cheer-dance means' application in extra curricular trainings of higher educational establishments' girl students.

Results of the research

A number of authors dealt with perfection of physical education in HEEs of different profiles at the account of implementation of training material's optimal content, new forms and means. For example Barybina L.M., Semashko S.A., Kriventsova H.V. [5] worked out system of aerobic trainings with application of individual approach. Mishchenko V.S., Kuehne T., Vinogradov V.E., Melnik L.J., Niewiadomska A. [24] implemented 8- weeks' program of physical exercises, mainly of power character in combination with vibration impact of rotational type. The purpose of such researches is increasing of girl students' power potentials. Zaharova L.V., Lyulina N.V. [15] worked out aerobic experimental methodic with usage of imitation exercises of different kinds of sports. Uskov S.V. [31] regarded problems of preservation and strengthening of schoolchildren's and students' psychic health with the help of martial arts' trainings on example of karate-do. Yasko G.V., Kashuba E.V. [17] implemented Hatha yoga methods in students' learning process. Balamutova N.M., Babadganjan V.V. [4] applied hydro-pedagogic and hydro-kinesio-therapy as mean of students' suffering form scoliosis rehabilitation. Kozina Z.L. et al. [19] implemented game-oriented aqua-fitness with application of special technical devices. Voronov M.P., Stolyarenko O.M. [8] studied health related influence of gymnastic exercises with usage of modern computer technologies, oriented on formation of students' correct carriage. Bala T.M. [2, 3] researches influence of cheer-leading exercises on secondary schoolchildren's physical health and motor fitness. Loutsenko L.S. et al. [23] regarded construction of sportsmen's training process in cheer-leading at stage of specialized basic training. Ilnitskaya A.S. et al. [16] studied methodic of physical exercises' training on the base of body-flex and pilates. Fomenko E.V. [32] used innovative methodic of application of non-traditional kinds of gymnastic in extracurricular girl students' trainings and so on.

However, we have not found works, devoted to methodic of cheer-dance trainings and their influence on HEE students' physical condition and physical fitness.

With it, it should be noted that cheer-leading is modern, progressive, spectacular kind of motor functioning. It is becoming still more popular in our country.

This term resulted from English cheer-leading, where "cheer" – call and "lead" – means guide. One of its kinds is cheer-dance (cheer-dance show). It means call for dance (presenting of plot in dance). This is the simplest kind of cheer-leading because it does not require special equipment and large site for trainings. It excites by its movements and attracts modern youth by its show character. It can be practiced both by girls (cheer dance) and by boys (cheer-dance show).

In our opinion usage of specially selected cheer-dance exercises in physical education process will positively reflect on indicators of students' physical condition and physical fitness, increase their interest to physical trainings. That is why there is an urgent demand in working out of methodic of cheer-dance means' usage in girl students' physical education.

The largest reserves of application of such means belong to effective organization of health related physical culture functioning of girl students, especially in extracurricular classes [21, 29, 33]. However, physical education trainings with usage of modern technologies (in particular cheer-dance) differ from traditional. These trainings require provisioning of students with the newest modern information about health; lead to increased organism's energy losses. Results of the researches determine dominating preferences of students to training of different kinds of physical exercises.

Practical significance of our research is in working out of methodic of cheer-dance movements' usage, their rational application in girl students' extracurricular trainings. It permits to improve their physical condition, physical fitness and interest to physical culture trainings. Besides, the received materials can be used for formation and preparation of students' cheer-dance (cheer-dance show) teams for competitions of different levels.

Discussion

Results of testing of experimental group's girl students witness about their higher indicators in comparison with control group (see table 1).

Table 1

Confidence of indicators of first and second year girl students of experimental group

№	Indicators	17-18 years' age (n=27)	19-20 years' age (n=27)	p	t
Indicators of physical condition					
1	Mass, kg	56.4±2.6	60.7±2.9	< 0.05	2.13
2	Vital capacity of lungs (VCL), cm^3	2950±96.3	2770±101.7	< 0.05	1.28
3	Heart beats' rate (HBR) b.p.m.	69.1±1.46	69.6±1.84	< 0.05	0.25
Physical fitness					
1	Quantity of jumps per 20 sec, times	61.4±2.81	59.2±3.12	< 0.05	0.3
2	Flexibility, cm	13.32±1.84	9.97±2.03	< 0.05	1.22
3	Speed of motor response, sec.	9.86±0.86	13.2±1.02	< 0.05	2.51

Implementation of new kind of motor functioning (cheer-dance) resulted in girl students' higher load on cardio-vascular and respiratory systems. In experimental group's students pulse insignificantly increased. In control group HBR was much higher. Speed of motor response was assessed with test for speed of seizing of falling stick with stronger hand. The test's results showed that quality of this test's fulfillment reduced quicker in experimental group (19-20 years' age). In first group this indicator was 9.86 ± 0.86 sec. In older group it was 13.2 ± 1.02 sec. (t = 2.51). Change of flexibility was assessed by forward torso bent from sitting position. Speed-power endurance was measured by maximal quantity of jumps from the spot during 20 sec. In older group this indicator was less a little (see table 1).

Thus, comparative analysis of experimental group girl students' physical condition and physical fitness showed significant changes in their organisms in comparison with girl students of control group.

In our work we supplement and specified results of researches of V.P. et al. [14, 45], Iermakov S.S. et al. [11], Kozina Zh.L. et al. [19], Fomenko E.V. [32], Adashevskiy V.M. et al. [35], Buultjens M. и Robinson P. [36], Highstreet V.D. [37] et al. about advantages of physical education trainings with application of modern technologies in comparison with traditional trainings. Such trainings are accompanied by higher interest of students. They give students information about health and means of increasing of organism's energy consumption.

The received results showed girl students' dominating preferences of different kinds of physical exercises. Besides, we supplemented data base about specificities of cheer-dance exercises' training.

In our research conception of Krucevich T.I. [21] about importance of development and application of innovative technologies in students' physical education is further developed as well as conceptions of Kozina Z.L. and Iermakov S.S. [20] about purposefulness of working out and application of non-traditional systems in students' physical education.

Conclusions:

1. Implementation of substantiated methodic of cheer-dance trainings permits for girl students to significantly improve physical fitness, physical conditions and functional state of their organisms.
2. The worked out practical recommendations can be used in educational process of physical culture institutions, physical education faculties of pedagogic universities, higher physical culture establishments especially in studying of disciplines: theory and methodic of aerobic training, sport-pedagogic perfection, and as an independent component. Besides they can be used as a supplement to existing educational systems, working out of learning and methodic manuals.

It is recommended to direct further researches to finding of changes in girl students' physical condition after application of the offered cheer-dance methodic. Besides, they shall be pointed at studying of comparative characteristics of physical condition and physical fitness of 3rd and 4th year girl students, practicing cheer-dance.

Acknowledgement

The researches have been conducted in compliance with "Combined plan of scientific-research works in sphere of physical culture and sports for 2011-2015" by topic 2.4 "Theoretical-methodic principles of individualization in physical education and sports" (state registration number 0112U002001). The researches were fulfilled in compliance with scientific-research works at the account of governmental budget of Ministry of education and science of Ukraine for 2014-2015 "Theoretical-methodic principles of application of informational, pedagogic and medical-biological technologies for formation of healthy life style" (state registration number 0113U002003) and "Theoretical-methodic provisioning of formation of personality's healthy life style in conditions of educational establishment in context of European integration" (state registration number 0114U001781).

Conflict of interests

The author declares that there is no conflict of interests.

References:

1. Arefiev VG. Modeling of differentiated physical fitness in school children. *Pedagogics, psychology, medical-biological problems of physical training and sports*, 2014;1:3-8. http://dx.doi.org/10.6084/m9.figshare.894383

2. Bala TM. The influence of cheerleading exercises on the schoolchildren's physical health of 5-9th forms. *Pedagogics, psychology, medical-biological problems of physical training and sports*, 2012;4:12 - 16.
3. Bala TM. *Kompleksna ocinka vplivu vprav cherlidingu na fizichne zdorov'ia ta rukhovu pidgotovlenist' shkoliariv serednikh klasiv. Cand. Diss.* [Complex assessment of cheer-leadin exercises' influence on physical health and motor fitness of secondary schoolchildren. Cand. Diss.]. Kharkov, 2013.
4. Balamutova NM, Babadganjan VV. Hydro aerobics as means for physical state improvement of female students. *Pedagogics, psychology, medical-biological problems of physical training and sports*, 2013;3:3-6. http://dx.doi.org/10.6084/m9.figshare.644731
5. Barybina LM, Semashko SA, Kriventsova HV. Features of organization of sport mass work at the technical higher institution. *Physical Education of Students*, 2011;1:18-22.
6. Bubka SN. The role of Alexey Butovsky in the development of physical education, sport and Olympic Movement. *Pedagogics, psychology, medical-biological problems of physical training and sports*, 2012;9:5-8.
7. Vas'kov YV. Acmeological approach to physical education of students of secondary schools in the aspect of personality-oriented training. *Pedagogics, psychology, medical-biological problems of physical training and sports*, 2015;3:3-9. http://dx.doi.org/10.15561/18189172.2015.0301
8. Voronov MP, Stolyarenko OM. Influence of physical exercises on students with violation of organs of sight. *Physical education of students*, 2010;6:13-15.
9. Gryban GP. The evaluation of the efficiency of introducing the model of the methodical system of physical education of agrarian students. *Pedagogics, psychology, medical-biological problems of physical training and sports*, 2012;11:27-30. http://dx.doi.org/10.6084/m9.figshare.97350
10. Dovhanyk MS, Chychkan OA, Sirenko RR. Parameters of alpha - rhythm in the students who practise curative running. *Pedagogics, psychology, medical-biological problems of physical training and sports*, 2012;5:59-62.
11. Iermakov SS, Apanasenko GL, Bondarenko TV, Prasol SD. Physical culture as the main tool of health's culture. *Pedagogics, psychology, medical-biological problems of physical training and sports,* 2010;11:31 - 33.
12. Iermakova TS. Forming a health culture of future teachers in Polish educational establishments. *Physical Education of Students*, 2014;5:14-19. http://dx.doi.org/10.15561/20755279.2014.0503
13. Iermakova TS. Education of children in Polish family in a context of forming health culture. *Pedagogics, psychology, medical-biological problems of physical training and sports*, 2014;11:17-22. http://dx.doi.org/10.15561/18189172.2014.1104
14. Zajcev VP, Iermakov SS., Prusik Kr. Physical recreation in structure of students' active rest. *Physical education of students,* 2011;1:68-77.
15. Zaharova LV, Lyulina NV. Basis of integrated approach to sports and recreational activities of students of special medical groups. *Physical Education of Students*, 2014;1:17-21. http://dx.doi.org/10.6084/m9.figshare.903688
16. Ilnitskaya AS, Kozina ZL, Lakhno EG, Ilnitskaya LV, Cieślicka Mirosława, Stankiewicz Błażej, Pilewska Wiesława. Students' attitude to the possibility of applying modern information and communication technologies in the educational process in physical education. *Physical Education of Students*, 2014;2:18-24. http://dx.doi.org/10.6084/m9.figshare.906369
17. Yasko GV, Kashuba EV. Innovation sports and health areas in universities supporting basis orientation. *Physical education of students*, 2011;3:116-118.
18. Kozhevnikova LK. Professional-applied pedagogical teaching of junior school future teachers to working activity. *Physical Education of Students*, 2012;3:49-52.
19. Kozina ZL, Iermakov SS, Bazilyuk TA, Voloshina E. Innovative technologies of aquafitness of playing orientation with the use of technical devices in physical education of students. *Physical education of students*, 2012;1:42-46.

20. Kozina ZL, Iermakov SS. Analysis of students' nervous system's typological properties, in aspect of response to extreme situation, with the help of multi-dimensional analysis. *Physical Education of Students*, 2015;3:10-19. http://dx.doi.org/10.15561/20755279.2015.0302
21. Krucevich TI, Bezverkhnia GV. *Rekreaciia u fizichnij kul'turi riznikh grup naselennia* [Recreation in physical education of different population groups], Kiev: Olympic Literature; 2010. (in Ukrainian)
22. Lisickaia TS. *Aerobika na vse vkusy* [Aerobics to all tastes]. Moscow: Education, 1994. (in Russian)
23. Loutsenko LS, Zinchenko IA, Luchko OR, Shepelenko TV. Construction of annual cycle of preparation of sportsmen, specialized in cheerleading. *Physical education of students*, 2011;6:62-66.
24. Mishchenko VS, Kuehne T, Vinogradov VE, Melnik LJ, Niewiadomska A. The effects of health-related physical training combined with whole body vibration (vibration platform) on strength capacities of young females. *Physical Education of Students*, 2012;1:75-83.
25. Moskalenko NV, Kovtun AA. Influence of physical culture and sport on the psychophysiological state of students. *Physical Education of Students*, 2012;3:83-86.
26. Nosko MO, Iermakov SS, Garkusha SV. Theoretical and methodological aspects of strengthening physical health of pupils and students. *Visnik Chernigivs'kogo nacional'nogo pedagogichnogo universitetu*, 2010;76:243-247. (in Ukrainian)
27. Popichev M.I. Complex diagnostics and estimation of health of students level. *Physical Education of Students*, 2011;3:71-76.
28. Roters TT. Physical improvement of students during interactive physical and aesthetic education. *Physical Education of Students*, 2013;4:72-76. http://dx.doi.org/10.6084/m9.figshare.663624
29. Serhiyenko LP, Lyshevska VM. Soles dermatoglyphics in the prognosis of sports endowment: differences of soles dermatoglyphics in sportsmen of different sport kinds. *Pedagogics, psychology, medical-biological problems of physical training and sports*, 2013;3:57-61. http://dx.doi.org/10.6084/m9.figshare.644738
30. Timoshenko OV. Simulation technology achievement of students in physical education classes. *Physical Education of Students*, 2010;3:102 - 105.
31. Uskov SV. Formation of stress students in the process of notions of martial arts in high school. *Physical Education of Students*, 2013;5:88-92. http://dx.doi.org/10.6084/m9.figshare.771216
32. Fomenko EV. Practical recommendations for the implementation of health technologies to enhance physical fitness of students in extracurricular classes during non-traditional gymnastics. *Pedagogics, psychology, medical-biological problems of physical training and sports*, 2014;7:31-36. http://dx.doi.org/10.6084/m9.figshare.1015385
33. Furman YM, Salnikova SV. Improvement of aerobic energy supply processes in 37-49 yrs old women by means of complex aqua-fitness trainings' and methodic of endogenous - hypoxic breathing's application. *Pedagogics, psychology, medical-biological problems of physical training and sports*, 2015;7:59-63. http://dx.doi.org/10.15561/18189172.2015.0708
34. Shkola OM. *Teoriia ta metodika navchannia* [Theory and methodic of training]. Kharkov: FOP Brovin O.V., 2014. (in Ukrainian)
35. Adashevskiy VM, Iermakov SS, Firsova IuIu. Physical mathematical modelling of difficult elements of acrobatic rock-and-roll. Physical Education of Students, 2013, vol.3, pp. 3-10. http://dx.doi.org/10.6084/m9.figshare.662463
36.Buultjens M, Robinson P. Enhancing aspects of the higher education student experience. *Journal of Higher Education Policy and Management.* 2011;33(4):337–346. http://dx.doi.org/10.1080/1360080X.2011.585708.
37. Highstreet VD. Aerobics for All Ages: A Broadband Approach to a Diverse University Population. *Journal of American College Health.* 1983;32(3):125–127. http://dx.doi.org/10.1080/07448481.1983.9936156.
38. Iermakov SS. Bio-mechanical models of strike movements in context of perfection of sportsmen technical fitness. *Teoria ta metodika fizicnogo vihovanna,* 2010;4:11–18. (in Ukrainian)
39. Iermakov SS, Kriventsova IV, Minenok AA. Peculiarities of physical training of special health group students in pedagogic HEE. *Visnik Chernigivs'kogo derzhavnogo pedagogichnogo universitetu*, 2013;107(2):193-197. (in Russian)

40. Ivashchenko OV, Khudolii OM, Yermakova TS, Pilewska W, Muszkieta R, Stankiewicz B. Simulation as method of classification of 7-9th form boy pupils' motor fitness. *Journal of Physical Education and Sport (JPES),* 2015;15(1):142–147. http://dx.doi.org/10.7752/jpes.2015.01023
41. Ivashchenko OV, Yermakova TS, Cieslicka M, Zukowska H. Discriminant analysis in classification of motor fitness of 9-11 forms' juniors. *Journal of Physical Education and Sport (JPES)*. 2015;15(2):238–244. http://dx.doi.org/10.7752/jpes.2015.02037
42. Khudolii OM, Iermakov SS, Prusik K. Classification of motor fitness of 7-9 years old boys. *Journal of Physical Education and Sport (JPES),* 2015;15(2):245-253. http://dx.doi.org/10.7752/jpes.2015.02038
43. Klimenchenko VG, Kriventsova IV, Gorban' IIu, Makhonin IM. Features of the procedure of joint exercises for physical education with students of basic and special medical groups. *Pedagogics, psychology, medical-biological problems of physical training and sports,* 2014;4:18-21. http://dx.doi.org/10.6084/m9.figshare.950951
44. Prusik Krzysztof, Prusik Katarzyna, Kozina ZhL, Iermakov SS. Features of physical development, physical preparedness and functional state of boys and girls – students of Polish higher educational establishments. Physical Education of Students, 2013;1:54-61. http://dx.doi.org/10.6084/m9.figshare.96415
45. Zaycev VP, Iermakov SS, Manycharyan SV, Fedyay IA. Recreation as a scientific discipline and its historical aspects. *Pedagogics, psychology, medical-biological problems of physical training and sports,* 2012;12:46-52. http://dx.doi.org/10.6084/m9.figshare.105444

STRUCTURAL EQUATION MODELING (SEM) OF PERFORMANCE EVALUATION INDICES IN GENERAL DIRECTORATE OF YOUTH AND SPORT OF GUILAN PROVINCE WITH PARTIAL LEAST SQUARES (PLS)

Hamidreza Goharrostami[1], Mustafa Mollaei Nejad*[1],Rahim Ramezani Nejad[3] , Azam Abdollahi[4]
[1]Assistant Professor, Faculty of Physical Education, University of Guilan, Iran.
[2]M.A. Strategic Management of Sport Organizations at the University of Guilan, Iran.
[3]Professor, Faculty of Physical Education, University of Guilan, Iran.
[4]M.A. Strategic Management of Sport Organizations at the University of Guilan, Iran

Abstract. *Purpose*: to evaluate the performance evaluation the indexes of general directorate of youth and sport of Guilan province by using the BSC approach. *Material*: This was a descriptive and field -based survey. The population included managers and experts from the general directorate of youth and sport of Guilan province. The purposive sampling was used. A questionnaire was used to collect data. Content validity and reliability were approved by experts Cronbach's alpha test (0.89) respectively. For data analyzing and model fitting the structural equation modeling (SEM) with PLS software was used. *Results*: performance evaluation model of general directorate of youth and sport of Guilan province has four factors, 12 dimensions and 55 indicators. So that learning and development factor has 4 dimensions and 13 indicators, internal processes have 4 dimensions and 23 indicators, financial factor has 2 dimensions and 7 indicators and customer and sport results have 2 dimensions 12 indicators. Internal processes, customer and sporting results, learning and development and financial factors had coefficients of factor loading of 0.91, 0.83, 0.81 and 0.80 respectively. *Conclusion*: We concluded that, in evaluating the performance of the organization, special attention should be paid on four studied terms and their confirmed dimensions and indicators. Based on the factor loading priority of activities and evaluation should be allocated to internal processes, customer and sporting results, learning and development and financial factors. So this index can be used to design a model to evaluate the performance of the general directorate of youth and sport of Guilan province.

Keywords: balanced, scorecard, index, performance, evaluation.

Introduction

The function of continuous monitoring, identifying items and affecting factors on the function of organizational performance in manufacturing and servicing industries for a few decades has clearly shown its significance and owners of various industries are well aware about the key role of continuous oversight on the key points of performance [1].

Monitoring and evaluation of performance can make the service intelligent and can be considered as the main section of the development and organizational implementation of policy and can be very helpful in pushing the system toward the optimum use of resources [5]. All public and private organizations, for the development, growth and sustainability in today's competitive arena are in need of performance evaluation systems, through which be able to measure the efficiency and effectiveness of the programs of organizations, process and human resources. Efficient organizations do not suffice to simply gather and analyze data, they also use this data to improve their organization and achieve the mission and strategies. In other words, instead of evaluating the appraisal performance they consider the performance of management [4].

Performance evaluation is a process that seems to be essential in all organizations and this evaluation is in fact a form of hedging against pests ahead [18]. On the other hand, in evaluating the performance of sport organizations, there are always problems that make the accurate and reliable assessment almost impossible. There are a lot of criteria and indicators and many hidden cases which have made assessment as a complex issue in a way that even mathematical algorithms fail to provide an appropriate solution to build an efficient evaluation model [7]. Kaplan and Norton (2006) in the late twentieth century presented a tool to evaluate the performance of the organizations known as the Balanced Scorecard (BSC). These tools then evolved beyond an assessment tool and provided a framework for the implementation of the overall goals and strategies of organization [16]. Nowadays in the sport organizations of the country different models are used to evaluate the performance that each of them has a different approach to the context. One of these strategic models is the Balanced Scorecard where all aspects of an organization are checked equally [13]. In this study in order to evaluate the performance among the various presented models Balanced Scorecard was selected. This model, with a focus on four key aspects of development and learning, internal processes, customer and financial factors provided the needed criteria and indicators to evaluate the performance of the organization [4]. In order to perform the duties of the ministry of sport and youth in the provinces, the provincial departments of youth and sport is formed on the basis of the statute of the ministry of sport and youth. General department of youth and sport is an organization that is created in order to provide a favorable context for the development of professional sport, sport and community, cultural, education and research, organizing youth affairs, legal, parliamentary and provincial coordination, resource development and support and related public relations and motivating and attracting people to the sport and discover talents and raising the level of skills sport on the basis of the predicted principles and objectives of the federation and physical education organization.

This general department works under the organizational chart of the ministry of youth and sport and indeed is the representative and vicar of the ministry of youth and sport in the province that monitors the related activities in the province in coordination with the ministry of sport and with full respect of the relevant laws and regulations [2]. In this regard some researches have been done, e.g. Hosseini (2011) , in his study indicated that the financial and economic indicators had the greatest effect on performance of clubs and clubs to improve the performance, need to manage costs and create ways to increase their income, in addition, the stability of the players, management and club coaches had special significance in this study [8]. Saadatpour (2011), in a study evaluated the performance of staff in physical education offices of Khorasan Razavi province based on the Balanced Scorecard (BSC) and indicated that the importance of customer and financial areas is desirable but is not desirable in the case of internal processes, learning and development. His study also revealed that four aspects of balanced scorecard will not be equally important [19]. Mir Fakhredini et al (2012), in their study revealed that the department of physical education in Yazd province in both internal processes and learning and development had optimal performance and in both customer and financial factors (BSC) did not [14]. Alian (2013), in his study showed that the performance of the internal infrastructures of general directorate of youth and sport within Isfahan province based on the Balanced Scorecard (BSC) and its performance in terms of the effect of financial system, customers, internal processes, learning and continuous learning in the establishment of evaluation based on the Balanced Scorecard method was significantly lower than the average [2]. Mosaffa (2014), in his research found that in the sport model designed for the sport boards of Guilan Province internal processes have the highest importance and financial factor has the least importance [15]. ZhengMin et al (2005) in their study entitled the Balanced Scorecard performance management found that four (BSC) factors were not the main source of supplying strategic plan but as a method of performance management can be used for different purposes by different stakeholders. Therefore, any changes required at (BSC) can be achieved based on the proposed assumptions and follows the long-term strategic success of organization. Delaney (2008) during his study concluded that when university conducted the performance evaluation system in the sport section of university by the use of Balanced Scorecard it had 3 goals in operating financial, customer and learning and development factors and 4 goals at the internal processes through which the profitability of this segment and the tendency of students toward sportive activities, particularly competitive ones increased [6]. Alonso and Fernandez (2009) in a study investigated the effect of Balanced Scorecard on public investment in the field of sport and concluded that the performance indicators are the reason for the appropriateness, effectiveness, efficiency and durability [3]. O'Boyle (2015) in a study stated that organizational performance is an essential management function in the field of non-profit sport to increase the pressure on these organizations to provide high-quality services to stakeholders in an accountable and transparent manner [17]. So given that the performance evaluation of the departments of youth and sport is one of the first and most basic part of strategic planning, the researcher attempts to analyze the performance evaluation indicators of general directorate of youth and sport in Guilan province by the use of Balanced Scorecard so that by using these indicators and designed models can evaluate the organization's performance.

Methodology

This study was a descriptive-survey that was conducted within a field study and to explain the theoretical foundations of performance evaluation criteria of general directorate of youth and sport of guilan province, the available resources (reports, websites and documents) were used. In this regard, in order to clarify and enrich the study provided information used to identify the criteria and options to evaluate the performance of the general directorate of youth and sport, interviews were organized with some managers and experts from the general directorate of youth and sport, faculty members and professors and inaddtion to reviewing criteria and identified options, collecting and summarizing the results, four aspects of the balanced scorecard, 12 dimensions and 60 indexes were determined for the design of performance evaluation system in general directorate of youth and sport of Guilan province.

The studied population consisted of all managers and deputy director of the general directorate of youth and sport of Guilan province(n=80) who through purposeful or qualitative sampling were chosen as statestical sample. So a total of 80 questionnaires were distributed and 64 questionnaires were usable and 16 questionnaires were flawed. To collect the data a research made questionnaire (significance criterion) was used to determine the importance of each indicators in the evaluation of performance. To determine the validity and resolve possible ambiguities, questionnaire was studied by a group of professors and faculty members of sport management group in Guilan University and after making the necessary corrections, the questionnaires were distributed among the samples. The (AVE) criterion for desirableness is equal to or higher than 5.0 which in this study, the amount for all structures is above 0.5. In order to determine the reliability of the questionnaire Cronbach Alpha was used (α = 0.89). In this study, structural equation modeling (SEM) and partial least squares method using Smart PLS software for data analysis and model fitting and in descriptive statistics SPSS23was used.

Findings

The findings were divided into two parts. The first part by the use of data obtained from the questionnaire and second part through descriptive statistical techniques tried to analyze the quantitative data. Results indicated that the questionnaire respondents in terms of gender were 68% men and 32% female. In terms of educational level 42% of respondents had B.A., 36% had M.A., 14% had associate's degree 14%, 6% had Ph.D. and 2% had diploma. Work experience of respondents also included 15 years and older (42%), 10.6 years (27%), 15-11 years (19%) and less than 5 years (12%), respectively.

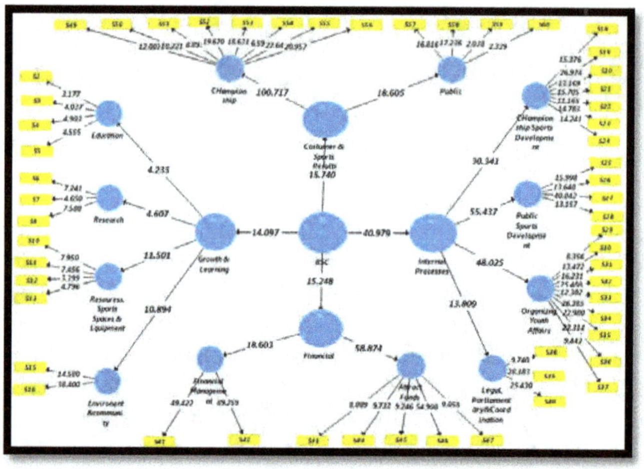

Figure1. The pattern of significant coefficients (z)

The second part included the analysis of the data using PLS model by the use of three measurements (validity, convergent reliability, divergent validity), structural model (correlation coefficient, determining coefficient and prediction coefficient) and general model (GOF criterion); that all these factors, approved and properly reported. After data analysis software output was given in Figures (1) and (2). To assess the significance of causal relationships between variables partial index of t value was used. Based on the significance level of 0.05 t value must be greater than 1.9 for less than this amount, the parameters of the model is not considered important. After determining the significance of relationships between variables standardized coefficients of related hypotheses investigated, Figure (2) shows the model with factor loadings; and at the end for overall fit of the research model GOF criterion was used that its output is given in the next section.

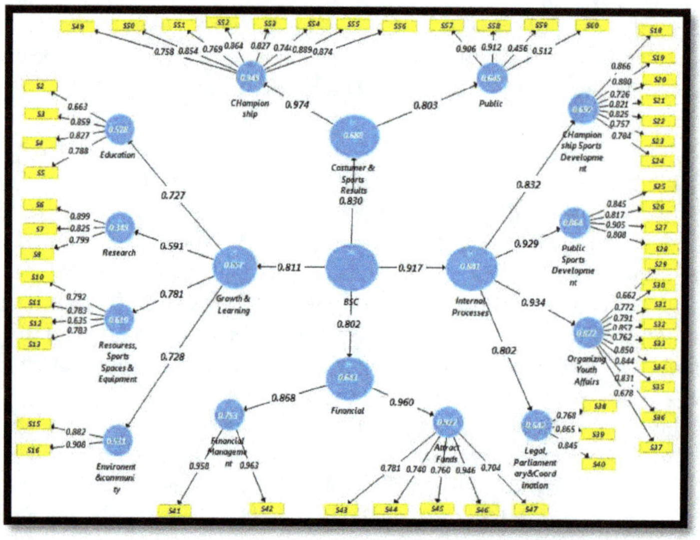

Figure2. The pattern of the values of factor loadings coefficients

Following the GOF criterion was used for overall fit of the model that calculated by the following formula:

$$GOF= \sqrt{\overline{communalities} \times \bar{R}^2}$$

$$GOF= \sqrt{\overline{communalities} \times \bar{R}^2} = \sqrt{0.56 \times 0.70} = 0/65$$

$$\overline{communalities} = \frac{0.63+0.60+0.52+0.50}{4} = 0.56 \quad R^2= \frac{0.65+0.84+0.64+0.68}{4} = 0.70$$

Regarding the three values of 0.01, 0.25 and 0.36 as weak, medium and strong values for this criterion, the value of 0/65 indicates strong overall fit of the model.

Table 1 - coefficients of factor loadings

Factors	Factor Loadings	Dimensions	Indicators	Indicators	Load Factor
Balanced Scorecard Internal processes	0.91	Organizing Youth Affairs	0.93	The number of individual and team ranks gained in festivals, cultural fairs at regional and national level	0.85
				The number of individual and team ranks gained in Quranic races	0.85
				The number of sport- cultural programs (celebration meetings and...)	0.84
				The number of meetings of marriage donors	0.83
				The number of dispatches to conferences, festivals and cultural at regional and national level in the field of youth	0.79
				The number of hosting conferences, festivals and cultural at regional and national level in the field of youth	0.77
				The number of dispatches to Quranic competitions at national level	0.76
				The number of national approved projects and running NGOs	0.67
				The number of active non-governmental sport organizations in province	0.66
		Development of public and rural sport	0.92	The number of hosting of sport competitions and rural and public festivals at national level	0.90
				The number of conferences held regarding the public sport in province	0.84
				The number of rural sport houses	0.81
				The number of dispatches to rural and public competitions and festivals at national level	0.80
		Athletics and professional sport development	0.83	The number of teams in Asian tournaments	0.88
				The number of teams in international events	0.86
				The number of hosts in various sport competitions in the country	0.82
				The number of hosts in various sport competitions in global, international and Asian levels	0.82
				The number of dispatch (individual and team) to various sport competitions in the country	0.78
				The number of dispatch (individual and team) to official competitions in global, international and Asian levels	0.75
				The number of teams in domestic leagues club competitions at various levels	0.72

		Legal, parliamentary and coordination	0.80	The number of estates resolved with the use of non-budgetary priority	0.86
				The number of annual performance appraisal of the departments of Youth and Sport in province	0.84
				The number of establishment licenses and constructed sport clubs	0.76
Customer and sport results	0.83	Results of athletics and professional sport	0.97	The number of shares acquired in Olympics	0.88
				The number of individual and team ranks gained in festivals, cultural fairs at regional and national level	0.87
				The number of individual and team ranks gained in Quranic races	0.86
				The number of sport- cultural programs (celebration meetings and...)	0.85
				The number of meetings of marriage donors	0.82
				The number of dispatches to conferences, festivals and cultural at regional and national level in the field of youth	0.76
				The number of hosting conferences, festivals and cultural at regional and national level in the field of youth	0.75
				The number of dispatches to Quranic competitions at national level	0.74

Table 1 - coefficients of factor loadings

	Factors	Load Factor	Dimension	Indicators	Load factor	Load Factor
Balanced Scorecard	Customer and Results		Results of public and rural sport	0.80	The number of individual and team ranks gained in competitions and festivals, rural and public sport at the country level	0.91
					The number of individual and team ranks gained in competitions and festivals, rural and public sport at international level	0.90
					The committee of women's organized sport insurance	0.51
					The committee of men's organized sport insurance	0.45
			Resources, sport spaces and equipments	0.78	Indoor sport space per capita (ratio of area to population)	0.79
					Outdoor space per capita (ratio of area to population)	0.78
					The number of active male and female referees	0.78
					The number of active male and female coaches	0.63
	Development and learning	0.81	Environment and Community	0.72	The number of agreements with other organizations in the field of championship, professional, public and educational sports	0.90
					The number of provincial experts in charge of general department in federations and national organizations	0.88
			Education	0.72	The number of arbitration courses held at national and international level in the province	0.85
					The number of people assigned to coaching courses at national and international level	0.82
					The number of people dispatched to arbitration enhancement courses at the country and international levels	0.78

		Research	0.59	The number of coaching courses held in national and international level in the province	0.66
				The number of executive- scientific meetings (such as academic meetings and the general department)	0.89
				Number of research - sport projects taking place in the province in the form of Master and Ph.D. thesis	0.82
				The number of scientific papers in seminars and congresses in interior and exterior levels	0.79
Financial	0.80	Absorption of financial resources	0.96	The provincial absorption of credit from other sources (cost, capital)	0.94
				The absorption of financial resources through donors	0.78
				The revenue from the ads and...	0.76
				The amount of income from the rent of properties	0.74
				The amount of income from the sale of properties	0.70
		Financial Management	0.86	Cost budget of the department of sport and youth	0.96
				Constructional budget of the department of sport and youth	0.95

Discussion and Conclusion

One of the managerial problems in the world is that the value creation of organizations has been changed but their performance evaluation tools have not been changed. This is why determining the appropriate model for assessing organizational performance is considered as one of the basic principles of the organization to develop and progress [11]. To this end the purpose of this study is to provide a structural equation modeling (SEM) for the performance evaluation indexes in general directorate of youth and sport of Guilan province through balanced scorecard approach which was done by reviewing the opinions of elected members of the general directorate of youth and sport of Guilan and the results showed that the factor of internal processes in the department of sport and the youth of Guilan indicates the most of the variations of scorecard balanced in the general directorate of youth and sport which has a loading factor of 0.91 that is consistent with the results of Mosaffa (2014).This factor has four dimensions the regarding their importance are namely the youth organization, process of public and rural sport development, process of the development of legal, professional and athletic sports, parliament and coordination of affairs (%93) (%92) (%83) and (%80) of all changes related to the Balanced Scorecard. Although the coefficients of factor loading of all four dimensions were high, two dimensions of organizing youth affairs and process of public and rural sport development with very few differences were more important than other two dimensions. The most important dimension is the organization of youth affairs, which indicates the importance of this dimension. The dimension of organizing youth affairs can be an important challenge for the country that some part of it is investigated at general directorate of youth and sport and executive activities in this area is important for young people. According to Table (1) in the factor of internal processes the public sport development is more important than the development of athletic sport that indicates the importance of this dimension and much attention has been paid by general directorate of youth and sport to public sport than athletic sport in the internal processes regarding the answers of respondents. Also the factor of customer and sportive results in the general directorate of youth and sport of Guilan province has a factor loading of 0.83. This factor has two dimensions that regarding their importance are namely the results of the athletics and professional sports (97%) and the results of public and rural sport (80%) can explain all changes that are related to the Balanced Scorecard. Given that the dimension of professional and athletic results is of the utmost importance, or indicates the amount of attention paid on professional and athletic results by managers and experts of general directorate of youth and sport, therefore sport organizations through professional sport can better indicate their position and its positive image in the country. Also in terms of sports results and customer according to the responses of respondents respectively indices of acquired shares in the Olympics, the quota acquired in the Paralympics, earned individual and team ranks in official international events (Olympic and world), invited male and female athletes in different sport fields to national teams, the number of ranks acquired in the individual and team events in Asian, the number of elite athletes in different sports (male and female), the number of different sport fields and the number of gained individual and team ranks in national events had the highest importance. In the third part of development and learning in the general directorate of youth and sport of Guilan province has a coefficient factor of 0.81. This factor has four dimensions that based on their importance, resources, spaces for sports and equipments, environment and communication, education and research explain (78%), (72%), (72%) and (59%) of all changes related to learning and development. Given that the dimensions of resources and sports spaces and equipments are of the utmost importance, this indicates the importance of this dimension. It means that in order to form an organization first of all human resources, sports spaces and equipment are needed within an organization. Therefore, lack of skilled human resources in organization can lead to the inefficient usage of sports equipments. According to Table (1) in the learning and development factor other indoor and outdoor space per capita regarding the factor of resources, increasing the agreements with other organizations in the field of professional, athletic, championship, educational and public sports regarding the factor of environment and communication, holding coaching and refereeing courses in the country and international level in the province regarding the factor of training and increasing scientific meetings; increasing support for sports research projects in province in the form of master and PhD thesis are the most important factor regarding the factor of study. Finally, the financial factor of general directorate of youth and sport in Guilan province has factor loading of 0.80. This factor has two dimensions that regarding to their importance, attracting financial resources and financial management respectively explain the (96%) and (86%) of the total changes that are related to financial factor. Given that this factor has upmost importance after absorption of financial resources this indicates that general directorate of youth and sport in Guilan province pays much attention to the attraction of financial resources more than financial management. In financial factors and its strategic indicators based on the responses of respondents, indicators of financial credits of sport and youth department, constructional budget of sport and youth department, the provincial attraction of credit from other sources (cost- capital), the absorption of funds by donors and the amount of income through renting is more than other indices. That indicates the attention of the general directorate of youth and sport of Guilan province to the importance of attracting financial resources and financial management and spending it on relevant topics. Thus, building a budget and codified financial resource in the form of income-generating projects and absorbing governmental and non-governmental financial resources seems necessary for the department of sport and youth. Thus, according to the survey results, it is suggested that in evaluating the performance of the department of sport and youth, more attention should be paid on four above mentioned factors and their dimensions and approved indicators. That based on factor loading the priority of activity and evaluation is dedicated to internal processes, especially two important issues that are related to organizing the youth affairs and rural and public development of sport, regarding the customer perspective and sport results especially on the results of the athletics and professional sports, regarding the factor of development and learning the special attention is on the dimension of resources, regarding sports spaces and the development of sports facilities and finally in the financial factor the special attention is on the financial resources.

Conflict of interests

The authors declare that there is no conflict of interests.

References:

1. Adams A, Armitage S, Mutuality for football clubs, lessons from the financial sector. *Studies in Economics and Finance,* 2002;22(1):26-41.
2. Alian Nafisa. *Exploring the possibility of implementing balanced scorecard approach for evaluating the performance of general directorate of youth and sport.* [PhD thesis]. Isfahan: University of Guilan; 2013.
3. Alonso Angle B, Fernandez Patricio S. The Balanced Scorecard of Investment in Sport: Proposal for Change. *Rivista di Diritto ed Economia dello Sport*, 2009;1: 1-10.
4. Amiri F. Performance evaluation of organizations through Kanji's Business Excellence Model. *Journal of Tadbir.* 2006;168:100-110.
5. Asmild M, Paradi JC, Pastor JT. Centralized resource allocation BCC models. *Omega*. 2009;37: 40-49.
6. Delaney D Daniel. *Accounting for Athletics: A Balanced Scorecard Approach. Thesis. University of Connecticut - Storrs.* Drive Performance. Harvard Business Review on Measuring Corporate Performance; 2008.
7. Delurgio SA. *Forecasting principles and applications*. McGrow Hill edition; 1998.
8. Hosseini Misagh. *Designing the performance evaluation of football premier league clubs in Iran using the Balanced Scorecard* [PhD thesis]. University of Guilan; 2011
9. Kaplan Robert S, David P Norton. *Translating Strategy in to Action.* Tehran: Published by Irans Commercial Studies and Research Institute; 2006.
10. Kaplan Robert S, Norton David P. *Strategy Oriented Organization.* Tehran: Publication of Industrial Management Institute. 2007
11. Kaplan RS, Norton DP. Putting the balance scorecard to work. *Harvard Business Review*. 1993;10:134-147.
12. Kaplan RS, Norton DP. *Using the Balanced Scorecard as a strategic*. 1996.

13. Mehrghan MR, Dehghan Mahmoud. Strategic model for the assessment of higher education institutions. *Journal of Research and Planning in Higher Education*, 2009;52:55-72.
14. Mir Fakhredini Heydar, Peymanfar MH, Khatibi Aghda Abd al-Nabi, Ali-Mohammadi H. *Evaluating the performance of sport organizations using an integrated model TOPSIS*. BSC (Case Study of Physical Education in Yazd province); 2013.
15. Mosaffa P. Designing a model for evaluating the performance of sport commissions in Guilan Province through balanced scorecard approach [PhD thesis]. Islamic Azad University of Karaj; 2014.
16. Nion Paul R. *Balanced Scorecard- step by step guide to design and implementation*. Tehran: Publication of Industrial Management Institute; 2007.
17. O'Boyle I. Developing a performance management framework for a national sport organisation. *Sport Management Review*. 2015;18(2):308316.
18. Parker C. Performance management. *Work study*, 2000;49(2):63-66.
19. Saadatpour Reza. *Evaluating the performance evaluation of employees in Physical education offices in Khorasan Razavi province based on the Balanced Scorecard (BSC)*. [M.A. thesis]. University of Guilan; 2011.

25

INFLUENCE OF INFORMATION TECHNOLOGIES ON TECHNICAL FITNESS OF STUDENTS IN SPORT-ORIENTED PHYSICAL EDUCATION

Kozina Zh. L.[1], Ol'khovyj O. M.[2], Temchenko V. A.[2]
[1]H.S. Skovoroda Kharkiv National Pedagogical University
[2]Kharkov National University

Abstract. _Purpose:_ to determine influence of information technologies in sport-oriented physical education on technical fitness of students, practicing football indoors. _Material:_ in the researches students (boys - n=40) of 18-20 years' age participated. Standard tests on physical condition were used. For determination of motor skills and abilities we used: juggling with ball; kick in pre-set sector of goal; shuttle run 4 x 10 meters with dribbling; kick for distance. _Results:_ structural model of sport-oriented students' physical education with application of information technologies has been formed. In the model all students are trained in sport-oriented academic groups by chosen kinds of sports (motor functioning). Such approach envisages holistic form of program material construction and unified algorithm of students' progress assessment. _Conclusions:_ the wholeness of sport-oriented physical education's functioning is ensured at the account of application of information technologies. It permits to optimize motor skills' training process. In this case single form of building of program material is created.
Key words: students, sport, physical education, information technologies, football indoors.

Introduction

Intensification of educational process in higher educational establishments resulted in tendency to weakening of students' motor functioning. The researchers note that reduction of motor functioning negatively influence on students' physical condition, physical fitness and functional state [21, 22]. In this connection importance of students' health protection and strengthening is increasing [28, 31, 32, 33, 35].

Scientific-technical progress facilitated computerization of all spheres of life [14, 24, 26]. Such shifts have two sides of changes in life. Increase of communication opportunities owing to computer informational technologies is accompanied by rapid growth of quantity and quality of information in all spheres of life. Increase of time for motor functioning results in weakening of functional potentials and physical fitness of students [2, 6, 8, 10]. Some authors think that usage of computer informational technologies permits to individualize physical education process and increase students' activity [6]. Useful and final result of it is increase of effectiveness of students' physical education.

At present a number of methodic on creation of complex image of structure and specificities of technical-tactic elements and exercises' fulfillment has been developed [7, 8, 9, 10]. However, in sport-oriented physical education application of informational technologies shall differ from analogous technologies for qualified sportsmen [1, 3, 4, 5, 15]. It is connected with peculiarities and level of students' physical and special fitness. Application of informational technologies shall also comply with tasks of healthy life style formation and consider students' perception of presented information [4, 5, 18, 20].

In system of students' progress in discipline "Physical education" assessment it is purposeful to consider quality, expressed in presence of skills and abilities to fulfill physical exercises; ability to work independently at lessons and in extra-curriculum time [11-13]. In this connection it would be logical to assume that active mastering of informational technologies and their implementation in sport-oriented physical education shall facilitate effectiveness of educational process.

Purpose, tasks of the work, material and methods

The purpose of the works is to determine influence of information technologies in sport-oriented physical education on technical fitness of students, practicing football indoors.

Material and methods: experimental group was composed of 19 students, practicing football indoors; control – 21 students. At the beginning and at the end of academic year we conducted pedagogic testing for determination of physical and technical fitness. As tests we used standard tests for physical and technical fitness [16, 17, 19, 23, 25, 27, 29, 30]. For determination of physical fitness we conducted pedagogic testing: forward bending from sitting position; shuttle run 4×9 meters; long jump from the spot; 100 meters' run; rising in sitting position from lying on back position; chin ups. For determination of motor skills and abilities we used: juggling with ball; kick in pre-set sector of goal; shuttle run 4 × 10 meters with dribbling; kick for distance.

In experimental group we used informational technologies for training of motor skills and abilities in football indoors. Control group was trained without informational technologies' application. Total duration of forming experiment was 9 months (2013-2014 academic year). All tested were informed about research and gave written consent for participation in the research. All researches were conducted in compliance with standards of Helsinki declaration, 2008.

The received data were processed with the help of program Microsoft Excel "Data analysis", SPSS. By each indicator we found mean arithmetic X, mean square deviation σ (standard deviation), assessment of confidence of differences between initial and final parameters.

Results of the researches

On the base of systemic analysis of educational process organization we formed structural model of students' sport-oriented physical education with application of informational technologies. In the model all students are trained in sport-oriented academic groups by chosen kinds of sports (motor functioning). Such approach envisages holistic form of program material construction and unified algorithm of students' progress assessment.

Formation of academic groups by kinds of sports is a specific feature of sport-oriented physical education. Wholeness of sport-oriented physical education functioning is ensured by application of informational technologies. It permits to optimize training of motor skills. In this case single form of program material construction is created.

Usage of university's informational-communicative technologies is one of forms of informational technologies: university's, physical education department's, sport club's sites; organs of students' self-governing. The created by us Internet-site of physical education department plays key role in the research. The site contains the following information: scientific-pedagogic staff of the department; schedule of trainings with annotations of kinds of sports and references. The site is an informational technology of open type and is accessible for all students.

In experimental groups we used "closed" informational technologies for motor skills' training: animation video-programs with accentuated visualization of separate technical and tactic elements; films on principles of theory and methodic of the chosen kind of sports. Besides, we used printed manual with detail illustrations of techniques' video-grams. In experimental groups we used video-technologies for understanding of organism's work under physical load. It permitted to realize students' conscious approach to physical education classes. Thus, in the research we widely used methods of activation of conscious perception of motor actions. Demonstration of learning material was realized directly at practical classes.

In experimental group we observed confident increase of technical fitness results (see table 1):

- "Juggling with ball" from 25.47 times to 32.47 c ($t=6.13, p<0.001$);
- "Kick to goal for distance" – from 28.26 m to 33.11 m ($t=7.23, p<0.001$);
- "Kick to pre-set sector of goal" – from 3.95 times to 6.95 times ($t=8.02, p<0.001$);
- "Shuttle run 4 × 10 meters with ball" – from 12.22 sec. to 11.69 sec. ($t=6.88, p<0.001$).

In control group there were also confident changes in indicators of tests "Juggling with ball" ($p<0.01$) and "Shuttle run 4×10 meters with ball" ($p<0.001$). Dynamic of the rest of indicators was statistically not confident ($p>0.05$). In experimental group we noticed improvement of results in tests: "Kick in pre-set sector of goal" (by 76%, $t=8.02, p<0.001$); "Juggling with ball" (by 27.48%, $t=6.13, p<0.001$); "Kick to goal for distance" (by 17.13%, $t=7.23, p<0.001$). Minimal change of results was registered in test "Shuttle run 4 × 10 meters with ball" (by 4.31%, $t=6.88, p<0.001$).

Table 1. Indicators of technical fitness of control group students (n=21) and experimental group students (n=19) before and after experiment

Testing indicators	Period of testing	Group	$\overline{X}$	S	m	Changes %	t BE-AE	p BE-AE	t CG-EG BE	p CG-EG BE	t CG-EG AE	p CG-EG AE
Juggling with ball, times	BE*	EG*	25.47	3.92	0.90	27.48	6.13	0.001	0.63	0.54	5.67	0.00
	AE		32.47	3.06	0.70							
	BE	CG	26.10	2.21	0.48	6.93	2.80	0.01				
	AF		27.90	1.97	0.43							
Kick to goal for distance, m	BE	EG	28.26	2.23	0.51	17.13	7.23	0.001	0.68	0.50	5.35	0.00
	AF		33.11	1.88	0.43							
	BE	CG	27.76	2.39	0.52	5.15	1.84	0.07				
	AF		29.19	2.64	0.58							
Kick to pre-set sector of goal from 10 meters' distance (10 attempts), quantity of hits	BE	EG	3.95	1.18	0.27	76.00	8.02	0.001	0.37	0.72	7.39	0.00
	BE		6.95	1.13	0.26							
	AF	CG	3.81	1.21	0.26	16.25	1.79	0.08				
	BE		4.43	1.03	0.22							
Shuttle run 4 × 10m with ball, sec.	AF	EG	12.22	0.25	0.06	4.31	6.88	0.001	1.57	0.13	5.36	0.00
	BE		11.69	0.22	0.05							
	AF	CG	12.36	0.31	0.07	2.16	3.07	0.01				
	AE		12.10	0.25	0.05							

*Notes: BE- before experiment; AF – after experiment; CG – control group; EG – experimental group.

Experiment showed confident change of technical indicators in control group in tests "Shuttle run 4x9 meters with ball" (by 2.16%, p<0.001) and "Juggling with ball" (by 6.93%, p<0.01). Maximal change of technical fitness indicators in control and experimental groups was registered in test "Kick to pre-set sector of goal" (16.25%). In test "Kick to gal for distance we registered change of indicators by 5.15%. However, in control group these changes were not confident (p>0.05).

Discussion

In works by L.N. Barybina [1; 2] researches in higher educational establishments with sport-oriented physical education are described. The author offers algorithm of training process's individualization. Wide usage of these recommendations is possible exclusively in conditions of sport-oriented physical education. From this point of view our research confirms these data. From the point of view of informational technologies' application, in researches by Zh.L. Kozina et al. [7; 10] computer programs, permitting to quickly and effectively determine students' psycho-physiological characteristics are offered. In this aspect our research is a continuation and expansion of the offered results.

Our research also expands results of Zh.L. Kozina [8, 10] and S.S. Iermakov [4]. The authors substantiated effectiveness of development and application of informational technologies for ensuring of visibility in technical tactic training. In works of Zh.L. Kozina [8, 10] informational multi-media for application in sport functioning are studied. Our research is devoted to working out methodic of informational technologies' application in sphere of students' sport-oriented physical education.

Program provisioning can successfully be applied on all stages of students' perfection in chosen kind of sports (motor functioning). By it, results of our researches expands and supplements results of Zh.L. Kozina, L.N. Barybina [7]. Researches of these authors have been expanded and supplemented by the data of our work. Our work points at influence of informational technologies on students' physical and technical fitness.

A number of authors [11; 14] points that young people have great quantity of diseases. Unfortunately, correct eating and taking vitamins do not solve this problem. People can not eat ecologically pure products and live in areas with pure air and water.

The data of our research confirm and supplement results of V.A. Kashuba et al. [6] in respect to approaches and peculiarities of formation of students' demand in healthy physically active life style. Strategic purpose of higher education shall be creation of optimal medium. Such medium shall facilitate students' physical and moral improvement; preservation of actual health; formation of healthy life style habits; education of health culture. Theoretical approaches to the set problems' studying permit to mark directions of health related technologies' realization in higher educational establishments. It permits to determine their essence, components, criteria and directions of development [5; 6; 12; 13].

In works of Kozina Zh.L. et al. [5] innovative technology of game-oriented aqua-fitness for integral influence on girl students' functional and psycho-physiological potentials is offered. Such technology includes: regulated rules of basketball in water with the help of technical equipment; methodic of training of movements in water for basketball in water; methodic of aqua-fitness exercises in combination with training of basketball [5].

It should be noted that application of progressive innovative technologies can be effectively realized in system of students' sport-oriented physical education. In this connection our research is a scientific-methodic basis for practical realization of modern progressive innovative technologies. In the same way our research is a scientific-methodic basis for realization of body-flex and Pilates methodic, presented in works of A.S. Ilnitskaya [18].

Comparison of the received data with results of other scientists' researches permits to formulate scientific novelty of our work in the following way.

In the work we supplemented and specified results of researches of S.S. Iermakov [4], Zh.L. Kozina et al. [15] in respect to advantage of sport-oriented form of physical education classes, comparing with traditional. It is expressed in students' higher interest in physical culture as well as in students' provisioning with the newest modern information about health perfection and physical fitness. In our research, for the first time we found positive influence of informational on students' physical fitness and on development of motor skills and abilities in chosen kinds of sports (on example of game kinds of sports).

The prospects of further researches imply determination of informational technologies' influence on HEE students' physical and technical fitness in chosen kinds of sports with sport-oriented physical education.

Conclusions

We have been substantiated ways of application of information technologies in sport-oriented physical education in higher educational establishments. Such approach envisages the following: working out and usage of physical education department's site and sites of sport clubs; application of printed editions, video and multi-media technologies.

Application of informational technologies confidently improves students' physical and technical fitness. Indicators in test "Juggling with ball", in test for distance of kick, for quantity of hits in pre-set sectors of goal and for speed of movements with ball confidently increased. In control group changes of these indicators was less expressed and in a number of cases they were not confident.

The received results confirm and prove purposefulness of information technologies' application in organization of sport-oriented physical education of higher educational establishments' students.

Acknowledgements

The research has been conducted in compliance with the following:

- "Combined plan of scientific-research works in sphere of physical culture and sports for 2011-2015" by topic 2.4 "Theoretical-methodic principles of individualization in physical education and sports" (state registration № 0112U002001);
- Scientific research work of Ministry of education and science of Ukraine for 2013-2014 "Theoretical-methodic principles of application of informational, pedagogic and medical-biological technologies for formation of healthy life style" (State registration № 0113U002003)
- Scientific-research work of Ministry of education and science of Ukraine for 2015-2016 "Theoretical-methodic principles of application of means of informational, pedagogic and medical-biological

orientation for motor and mental development and formation of healthy life style" (State registration № 0115U004036).

Conflict of interests

The authors declare that there is no conflict of interests.

References:

1. Barybina LN. Vliianie primeneniia sistemy individualizacii fizicheskogo vospitaniia v vysshem uchebnom zavedenii na funkcional'noe sostoianie studentok [Influence of application of physical education individualization system in higher educational establishment on girl students' functional state]. *Pedagogics, psychology, medical-biological problems of physical training and sports,* 2012;10:10–15. (in Russian)
2. Barybina LN, Kozina ZhL, Grin' LV. Psikhofiziologicheskie vozmozhnosti i ob"em vospriiatiia studentov raznykh sportivnykh specializacij [Psychological potentials and volume of perception of different sport specializations students]. *Zdorov'esberegaiushchie tekhnologii, fizicheskaia reabilitaciia i rekreaciia v vysshikh uchebnykh zavedeniiakh*, 2010;1:19–21. (in Russian)
3. Borisov VV, Olejnik ON, Timoshenko VV. Motivacionnoe obespechenie uchebno-vospitatel'nogo processa s ispol'zovaniem tekhnologii sportivno-orientirovannogo fizicheskogo vospitaniia v vuze [Motivational provisioning of educational process with application of technology of sport-oriented physical education in HEE]. *Molodoj uchenyj,* 2014;17:459–461. (in Russian)
4. Iermakov SS, Ivashchenko SN, Guzov VV. Osobennosti motivacii studentov s primeneniem individual'nykh programm fizicheskoj samopodgotovki [Specificities of students' motivation with application of individual physical education self-training programs]. *Physical education of students*, 2012;4:59–61. (in Russian)
5. Kozina ZhL, Iermakov SS, Bazyliuk TA, Voloshina EV Innovacionnye tekhnologii akvafitnesa igrovoj napravlennosti s primeneniem tekhnicheskikh ustrojstv v fizicheskom vospitanii studentok [Innovative technologies of game-oriented aqua-fitness with application of technical means in girl students' physical education]. *Physical education of students*, 2012;1:42–47. (in Russian)
6. Kashuba VA, Futornyj SM, Golovanova NL. K voprosu ispol'zovaniia informacionnykh tekhnologij v processe fizicheskogo vospitaniia studencheskoj molodezhi [On the problem of informational technologies' application in process of students' physical education]. *Slobozhans'kij naukovo-sportivnij visnik*, 2011;4:157–163. (in Russian)
7. Kozina ZhL, Barybina LN. Kharakteristika psikhofiziologicheskikh pokazatelej studentov razlichnykh sportivnykh specializacij [Characteristic of different sport specialties students' psycho-physiological indicators]. *Physical education of students*, 2010;4:38–47. (in Russian)
8. Kozina ZhL. Avtorskie informacionnye, pedagogicheskie i mediko-biologicheskie tekhnologii dlia formirovaniia zdorovogo obraza zhizni [The author's informational, pedagogic and medical-biological technologies for formation of healthy life style]. *Visnik Chernigivs'kogo derzhavnogo pedagogichnogo universitetu*, 2013;3:44–48. (in Russian)
9. Kozina ZhL. Faktorni modeli fizichnoi pidgotovlenosti volejbolistok visokogo klasu riznogo igrovogo amplua [Factorial models of different game roles elite female volleyball players' physical fitness]. *Pedagogics, psychology, medical-biological problems of physical training and sport*, 2007;9:80–85. (in Ukrainian)
10. Kozina ZhL, Cerkovna OV, Vorobjova VO. Viznachennia efektivnosti zmagal'noi diial'nosti v basketboli za dopomogoiu zastosuvannia informacijnikh tekhnologij [Determination of competition functioning effectiveness in basketball with the help of information technologies' application]. *Slobozhans'kij naukovo-sportivnij visnik*, 2008;1–2:151–158. (in Ukrainian)
11. Ol'khovij OM. Dinamika fizichnogo stanu iunakiv 17–22 rokiv u procesi profesijno-prikladnoi fizichnoi pidgotovki [Dynamic of 17–22 years' age boys' physical condition in process of professional-applied physical training]. *Sportivnij visnik Pridniprov'ia*, 2014;1:219 – 224. (in Ukrainian)
12. Temchenko VA, Sirenko RR. Sekcionnaia forma organizacii fizicheskogo vospitaniia studentov [Sport-circle form of organization of students' physical education]. Physical education of students, 2010;3:99–101. (in Russian)
13. Temchenko VA, Petrenko IuM, Makhonin IN. Ocenivanie uspevaemosti studentov, zanimaiushchikhsia futzalom [Assessment of progress of students, who practice football indoors]. IX *mezhdunarodnaia nauchnaia*

konferenciia, 8–9 fevralia 2013 goda "Problemy i perspektivy razvitiia sportivnykh igr i edinoborstv v vysshikh uchebnykh zavedeniiakh" [9th international scientific conference, February 8–9, 2013 "Problems and prospects of sports games and martial arts development in higher educational establishments"], 2013; P. 341–345. (in Russian)

14. Futornyj CM, Kashuba VA. Rol' fizicheskogo vospitaniia i sporta v orientacii studentov na zdorovyj obraz zhizni [Role of physical education and sports in orientation of students for healthy life style]. *Physical education of students*, 2011;3:94–98. (in Russian)
15. Kozina ZhL, Barybina LN, Lugina IV, Kozin AV. Eksperimental'noe obosnovanie sistemy individualizacii v fizicheskom vospitanii studentov [Experimental substantiation of individualization system in students' physical education]. *Physical education of students,* 2012;4:77–86. (in Russian)
16. Toke S. Aidt, Bernard Leong, William C. Saslaw, Daniel Sgroi. A power-law distribution for tenure lengths of sports managers. *Physica A: Statistical Mechanics and its Applications*, 2006;370(2,15):697–703.
17. Roberto da Silva, Mendeli H Vainstein, Luis C Lamb, Sandra D Prado. A simple non-Markovian computational model of the statistics of soccer leagues: Emergence and scaling effects. *Computer Physics Communications*, 2013;184(3):661–670.
18. Ilnitskaya AS, Kozina ZL, Barybina LN, Kolomiez NA, Cieślicka Mirosława, Stankiewicz Błażej, Pilewska Wiesława. Author's internet blog as information and communication technologies in the educational space within the physical education students. *Physical education of students*, 2014;1:22–26. http://dx.doi.org/10.6084/m9.fgshare.903689
19. Burrows L, McCormack J. School culture meets sport: A case study in New Zealand. *European Physical Education Review*, 2011;17:301–312.
20. Connolly J, Dolan P. Sport, media and the Gaelic Athletic Association: the quest for the «youth» of Ireland. *Media Culture Society*, 2012;34:407–423.
21. Peker K, Bermek G. Predictors of Health-Promoting Behaviors Among Freshman Dental Students at Istanbul University. *J Dent Educ.*, 2011;75:413–420.
22. Dzikus L, Hardin R, Waller SN. Case Studies of Collegiate Sport Chaplains. *Journal of Sport and Social Issues*, 2012;36:268–294.
23. Goumas C. Modelling home advantage in sport: a new approach. *Int J Perf Anal Sport*, 2013;13:428–439.
24. Kaufman P, Wolff EA. Playing and Protesting: Sport as a Vehicle for Social Change. *Journal of Sport and Social Issues*, 2010;34:154–175.
25. Kerr R. Integrating Scientists into the Sports Environment: A Case Study of Gymnastics in New Zealand. *Journal of Sport and Social Issues*, 2012;36:3–24.
26. Roseli AF Romero, Edson Prestes, Marco AP Idiart, Gedson Faria. Locally oriented potential field for controlling multi-robots. *Communications in Nonlinear Science and Numerical Simulation*, 2012;17(12):4664–4671.
27. Page L, Page K. The second leg home advantage: evidence from European football club competitions. *J Sports Sci*, 2007;25:1547–1556.
28. Murphy MH, Donnelly P, Shibli S, Foster C, Nevill AM. Physical activity, walking and leanness: An analysis of the Northern Ireland Sport and Physical Activity Survey (SAPAS). *Preventive Medicine*, 2012;54 (2):140–144.
29. Pollard R. Worldwide regional variations in home advantage in association football. *J. Sports Sci*, 2006;24:231–240.
30. Roberto da Silva, Silvio R. Dahmen Universality in the distance between two teams in a football tournament. *Physica A: Statistical Mechanics and its Applications*, 2014;398(15):56–64.
31. Stefanie P, Petra J. Different mental rotation performance in students of music, sport and education. *Learning and Individual Differences*, 2012;9(22,1):159–163.
32. Ilnitskaya AS, Kozina ZhL, Lakhno EG, Ilnitskaya LV, Cieślicka Mirosława, Stankiewicz Błażej, Pilewska Wiesława. Students' attitude to the possibility of applying modern information and communication

technologies in the educational process in physical education. *Physical education of students*, 2014;2:18–24. http://dx.doi.org/10.6084/m9.fgshare.906369

33. Tucker P, Irwin JD. University Students' Satisfaction With, Interest in Improving, and Receptivity to Attending Programs Aimed at Health and Well-Being. *Health Promot Pract*, 2011;12:388–395.

34. Wakefield CJ, Adie JW. Evaluating sport psychology teaching through action research. *Journal of Hospitality, Leisure, Sport & Tourism Education*, 2012;11(2):125–130.

35. Marchwant Przemysław, Cieślicka Mirosława, Muszkieta Radosław, Zukow Walery, Iermakov Sergii. The impact of training on the efficiency overall and special players Youth Sports Training Center in Bydgoszcz and MLKS Wlokniarz Okonek [Wpływ treningu na sprawność ogólną i specjalną piłkarzy Ośrodka Szkolenia Sportowego Młodzieży w Bydgoszczy i MLKS Włókniarza Okonek]. *Journal of Education, Health and Sport*, 2015; 5(5):463–486. http://dx.doi.org/10.5281/zenodo.18158 (in Polish)

26

CORRECTION OF PHYSICAL EDUCATION PROGRAM FOR TECHNICAL HIGHER EDUCATIONAL ESTABLISHMENT GIRL-STUDENTS ON THE BASE OF THEIR HEALTH INDICATORS

Kolumbet A.N., Dudorova L.Yu.
Kiev National University of Technology and Design

Abstract. _Purpose:_ to illustrate opportunities of physical education in health strengthening of technical HEE girl-students through correction of their biological age components. _Material:_ 127 girl-students participated in the research. _Results_: the authors' program of biological age correction permitted to increase breathing pauses, hand strength, time of static balance and reduce blood pressure. Knowledge of biological age and mechanisms of too early ageing facilitates practicing healthy life style and formation of body-motor conditions. We offered trainings of biological age correction' methodic, oriented on prophylaxis of organism's ageing, reduction of biological age and prolongation girl-students' active life. _Conclusions:_ specially determined biological age of an individual can be used as integral characteristic of his/her health condition.
Key words: physical, education, biological, age, health, girl-students.

Introduction

The problem of health protection and strengthening is one of main tasks of our society. Modern conditions of education in higher educational establishments set high requirements to students' health. Absence of healthy life style and low motor activity condition sharply accelerated ageing, characteristic for all age groups. It reflects general tendency to worsening life quality, health and physical fitness. Besides it determines the demand in prophylaxis of too early ageing and working out health related technologies.

To day actually every forth patient and fifth citizen of workable age have diseases of cardio-vascular system, [22, 41, 50]. Vegetovascular dystonia is one of the most frequent cardio-vascular diseases among young persons. With it among women it is 2-3 times more frequent than among men [1, 25, 43, 46].

Recent scientific researches witness that in health rehabilitation and strengthening active role is played by complexes of rehabilitation measures. Such complexes are directed at treatment of existing pathological; syndromes and improvement of students' health. Physical education means engage important place in these complexes that is proved by scientific works [10, 18, 26, 53]. Systemic physical exercises' practicing facilitates significant strengthening of students' organism's resistance and physical fitness [34, 42, 47, 51]. With it harmony of he whole organism is achieved.

Compliance of students' individual morphological functional level with mean statistic standard of this population reflects non-uniformity of development, maturity and ageing of different physiological systems. The temp of organism's adaptation potentials' age changes determines such model conception as biological age [11, 32, 44, 48]. Biological age is an indicator of wear out of structure and organism's definite structural element or group of elements and organism in the whole, expressed in units of time. It is found by correlating the measured individual bio-markers with reference mean population curves of these bio-markers' dependences on calendar age [5, 8, 11, 17].

It is known that mean biological age of Ukrainians is much higher than in their European peers. This age is nearly equal to Africans' age [6, 30, 37, 38]. Comparing with Europe, in Ukraine youth more frequent has diseases [4, 9, 35].

The problem of too early ageing is relevant due to its biological and economic consequences. It is known that early ageing significantly influences on period of working and creative activity. In Ukraine this indicator is 30 years (in the range of age from 20-25 – to 50-55 years). In poorer countries it lasts 45-50 years [2, 12, 31, 36].

If to analyze literature sources chronologically it is seen that interest to too early ageing was manifested by many authors. In modern literature the problem of students' biological and passport age correlation is regarded in the works of many authors [3, 13, 20, 23]. In these works it is pointed that students' biological age is, in average, from 40 to 46 years, Discrepancy between biological and passport age is from 10 to 40 years. Approximately 15-20 years ago this difference was 4-5 years [14, 27, 39, 45].

In scientific works significance of biological and passport age coincidence is noted. If biological age of heart is much higher than passport age there appears a risk of cardio-vascular system's disease and too early heart's ageing [16, 24, 40, 52].

From medical sources it is known that every person's organism ages hetero-chronically. In different life periods, ageing of people from different countries and continents is different [19, 29, 33, 49]. In respect to Ukrainians, there is no mentioning of "age strata" with higher ageing temps. Also it is unknown, if ageing temps are equal for men and women in Ukraine. In scientific journals there are very few works, devoted to biological ageing and its correction by physical education means, especially in respect to students.

Hypothesis: it was assumed that partial individualization of girl-students' physical education on the base of data about their health would permit to raise the level of their physical fitness.

The purpose of the research: is to illustrate opportunities of physical education in health strengthening of technical HEE girl-students through correction of their biological age components.

Material and methods

Participants: in the research 127 1-st – 2nd year girl-students of 17-21 years' age, from Kiev national university of technology and design participated. All girl students were practically healthy (I.e. did not have any health problems). The girl-students were divided into experimental and control groups.

Organization of the research: the research was conducted in 2015-2016. At the beginning of 2015 we registered girl-students' biological age, detected weak organism' systems, worked out individual program of physical education. At the end of 2016 we again registered biological age of the same girl-students. The experiment implied working out means for biological age correction and implementation of the authors' program and methodic in educational process.

For determination of personal biological age we used some modified methods [25]. For biological age assessment we used indicators of separate organism systems' maturity. The assessment was fulfilled by comparing girl-students' appropriate indicators with standards, characteristic for this age group. For correct assessment of biological age it is desirable to use several indicators in heir combination. However, in practice, when doing mass examinations, one has to consider separate indicators, which reflect human state rather satisfactory. Biological age assessment shall reflect clear age changes, which can be measured or described. The method of such changes' assessment shall not be harmful for the health and shall not cause unpleasant feelings. It shall be suitable for screening of great number of girl-students. We used abbreviated method of biological age determination [25]: determination of obesity degree (weight-height indicator); hand power (hand dynamometry); testing of cardio-vascular system (heart beats rate –HBR after 20 squats); state of nervous system (Romberg's test); state of respiratory system (vital capacity of lungs – VCL); determination of blood vessels' elasticity (blood pressure); functional state of respiratory and blood circulation systems (Genchi's test).

Statistical analysis:

For processing of the research's results we used mathematical statistic methods. For every indicator we calculated mean values and mean square deviation. Confidence of results was assessed with Student's t-criterion at 1% and 5% significance levels.

In conduct of complex pedagogic and biologic testing of girl-students we observed health protection laws of Ukraine and Helsinki declaration 2000; directive №86/609 of European community on human participation in medical-biological researches.

Results

Results of preliminary research (2015) showed that girl-students' average biological age (27.9 years) does not correspond to passport age (18.6 years) exceeding it. Accelerated temps of ageing are observed in 99% girl-students. Distribution by biological age is not uniform and the rage of variations is 27.0 years. In 17% girl-students biological age is within from 23 to 26 years; in 10% from 27 to 30 years; in 31% - from 31 to 34 years; in 21% - from 35 to 38 years; in 14% it is from 39 to 50 years; 4% have biological age from 51 to 60 years; 1% - from 61 to 70 years. Thus, biological age of most of girl-students is in the range form 30 to 40 years. The quantity of girl –students with low biological age (18-20 and 20-22) is insignificant and is not obligate (1% and 1% accordingly).

By results of preliminary testing in 83 girl-students we registered low health level; in 29 – below average and in 15 girl-students – average level. Thus, the girl-students' health can not be assessed as above average. Therefore, no one of them is in "safe zone". It is connected with deficiency of physical functioning and absence of systemic sports practicing.

Other mean-statistic data of our research are given in table 1.

The youngest biological age was 19.7 years. It exceeds passport age by 1.7 years. It should be noted that it is the best indicator. In all other cases biological age indicators are much worse.

The methodic of biological age assessment did not envisage study of volume and content of motor functioning. That is why we could not analyze influence of the latter on biological age.

Pedagogic experiment implied initial testing of control and experimental groups' girl-students. During academic year experimental group was trained by the authors' program of biological age correction. After finishing pedagogic experiment we received results of finalizing testing of these groups' biological age (see table 1).

Table 1. Girls-students' biological age indicators before and after application the authors' program

№№	Indicators	Before experiment	After experiment	Confidence
1	Weight-height indicator, conv.un.	21.9	22.2	P≥0.05
2	Static balance (Romberg's test), sec.	51.4	45.6	P≤0.05
3	Blood pressure, mm.merc.col.	34.9	29.2	P≤0.05
4	Breath pause (Genchi's test), sec.	33.5	30.3	P≤0.05
5	Hand dynamometry, kg	38.5	31.7	P≤0.05
6	VCL, liters	18.1	18.2	P≥0.05
7	HBR restoration after 20 squats, beats per sec.	17.8	18.2	P≥0.05
8	Mean passport age, years	17.6	18.6	P≥0.05
9	Mean biological age, years	27.9	23.3	P≤0.05

It is undoubted that influence of physical education means on student's organism is extremely necessary. However, to influence on biological age it is required to determine the most significant indicators. With Pearson's method of pair correlation we determined correlation coefficients. The highest rating belonged to indicator of pause after exhale (r=0.91); the second place is taken by static balancing on one leg with closed eyes (r=0.59); third place belonged to blood pressure (r=0.43). All these were considered in selection of the authors' program means.

The worked out authors' program included theoretical part. This part is a cycle of lectures targeted to open main principles and sense of the studies conceptions. The second part included content of practical, methodic and independent trainings. In the process of trainings we practically familiarized girl-students with complex of targeted means, oriented on human biological age correction and on application of the received knowledge in practice. As a result of this part's realization girl-students mastered therapeutic physical culture exercises, vestibular and fine motor exercises, breathing methodic, psycho-correction techniques. Besides, the girl-students knew methods of determination of human biological age and learnt to independently find it by calculations.

Independent trainings by the authors' methodic were directed at better mastering of material. Practical classes were conducted in the process of compulsory academic hours on discipline "Physical education". In our opinion group practical classes shall be conducted with application of individual approach to girl-students. It will permit for them to self-influence by correction and prophylaxis exercises. Means for biological age correction can include: therapeutic physical exercises, breathing exercises and exercises for psycho-correction relaxation [15, 16, 19].

The repeated testing of biological age showed that in 21% girl-students it is within from 23 to 26 years; in 16.0% - from 27 to 30 years; in 32.0% - from 31 to 34 years; in 17.0% - from 35 to 38 years; in 10.0% - from 39 to 50 years and in 1.0% -from 51 to 60 years. The quantity of girl=student with low biological age (18-20 and 20-22) remained insignificant (1% and 2% accordingly). The main is: period of breath pause, hand strength and period of static balance increases as well as blood pressure reduced (see table 1). With it the following indicators nearly did not change: weight-height indicator, VCL, HBR after 20 squats (restoration of pulse).

As it follows from the received data the authors' program of girl-students' biological age correction and its realization methodic showed their confident effectiveness by most of the tested indicators.

Discussion

The results of presented here work can be called deplorable: they witness about significant passport age exceeding by biological age. In the future this gap can only increase owing to accelerated ageing. If now biological age is about 28 years, then in the nearest 5 years it can raise up to 40 years. It is necessary to think about control over this process and improvement girl-students' health.

It should also be noted that ageing is a multi-factor process of biologically conditioned objective and subjective factors' influence, which depend on a person [19, 26, 33]. It can be assumed that correction of a number of physical defects is possible with the help of specially selected physical exercises. On the base of the present work we can conclude that one training a week is not enough for health strengthening and improvement. It is necessary to think about independent trainings (for example in sport circles). With it individual condition of girl-students shall be considered [15, 37, 40].

As a result of the authors' program application we registered that girl-students' heaviest problems appear in respiratory system. By Genchi's test 55.6% have low health level, 18.5% - health below average. For cardio vascular and respiratory systems aerobic kinds of sports can be proposed. For example: run or power walking, swimming bicycle racing, dances, skating (roller skating) or skiing, outdoor games with ball (basketball, football, volleyball and etc.) [15, 21, 28].

Besides, Romberg's test showed the presence of problems with nervous system in girls. Indeed, balancing, as one of coordination qualities, directly influences on professional qualities of technologists and designers [26, 40].

We compared the received data with the data of other authors, who studied this problem earlier. Results of biological age study in the whole coincide with the data of other authors, living in Ukraine.

Conclusions

1. Specially determined girl-students' biological age can be used as an integral characteristic of their health.

2. As far as human biological age is conditioned by physiological, functional and adaptation organism's potentials, physical education means can be considered to be the most rational mean for ensuring longevity and prevention from too early ageing. They permit to mobilize adaptation mechanisms of young people, who are bent to pathologies of different organism's organs and systems.

3. Knowledge of biological age essence and mechanisms of too early ageing can facilitate the tasks of girl-students' self-perfection, healthy life style and formation of body-motor conditions; self-correction of organism's systems and functions.

4. Within the frames of "Physical education" discipline in university it is purposeful to realize the course by choice. This course is based on mastering biological age correction methodic; reduction of biological age and prolongation of girl-students' active life.

5. It is purposeful to introduce lectures, methodic and practical classes in the process of physical education in university. Such classes will be mainly directed at future technologists (designers, engineers) preparation for ageing prophylaxis through biological age reduction and active life prolongation.

The prospects of future studies imply development and implementation of too early ageing prophylaxis program for students.

Conflict of interests

The authors declare that there is no conflict of interests.

References:

1. Abbakumov SA, Makolkin VI, Sapozhnikova AA. *Nejrocirkuliatornaia distoniia* [Neuro-circulatory dystonia], Cheboksary: Chuvashia; 1995. (in Russian)
2. Amosov NM., Bendett MA. *Fizicheskaia aktivnost' i serdce* [Physical functioning and heart], Kiev: Health; 1989. (in Russian)
3. Anan'ev VA. *Psikhologiia zdorov'ia* [Psychology of health], Sankt Petersburg: Speech; 2006. (in Russian)
4. Apanasenko GL. *Izbrannye stat'i o zdorov'e* [Selected papers about health], Kiev; 2005. (in Russian)
5. Akhaladze MG. *Ocinka tempu starinnia, stanu zdorov'ia i zhittiezdatnosti liudini na osnovi viznachennia biologichnogo viku. Dokt. Diss.* [Assessment of ageing temp, health state and person's vitality on the base of biological age. Dokt. Diss.], Kiev; 2007. (in Ukrainian)
6. Bazhal A. Ukrains'ki khroniki: smertnist' [Ukrainian chronicles: mortality]. *Dzerkalo tizhnia*, 2010;46:8. (in Ukrainian)
7. Belozerova LM. *Metody opredeleniia biologicheskogo vozrasta i umstvennoj i fizicheskoj rabotosposobnosti* [Methods of determination of biological age and mental and physical workability], Perm: PGMA; 2000. (in Russian)
8. Bulich EG. *Sovremennye dostizheniia nauki o zdorov'e* [Modern achievements of science of health]. Teoriia i praktika fizicheskoj kul'tury, 2004;1:62-63. (in Russian)
9. Bushuiev IuV. *Riven' fizichnogo zdorov'ia studentiv iak kliniko-fiziologichna osnova fizichnogo vikhovannia u vuzi. Kand. Diss.* [Students' physical health level as clinic-physiological base of physical education in HEE. Cand. Diss.], Dnepropetrovsk; 2007. (in Ukrainian)
10. Vojtenko VP. *Biologicheskij vozrast* [Biological age]. Leningrad: Science; 1982. (in Russian)
11. Vojtenko VP, Tokar AV, Rudaia ES. Metodika opredeleniia biologicheskogo vozrasta [Methodic of biological age determination]. *Voprosy gerontologii*, 1989;11:9-16. (in Russian)
12. Griban VG. *Valeologiia* [Valueology], Kiev: Center educational literature; 2005. (in Ukrainian)
13. Zakharina E. The analysis of Classic Private University student's physical health. *Pedagogics, psychology, medical-biological problems of physical training and sports,* 2009;7:61-63.
14. Zeleniuk OV. Fizicheskoe vospitanie v upravlenii sostoianiem zdorov'ia studencheskoj molodezhi [Physical education in control of students' health]. *Fizicheskoe vospitanie studentov tvorcheskikh special'nostej*, 2002;2:75-82. (in Russian)
15. Kalinkina OM. Doslidzhennia mozhlivosti vikoristannia pokaznika biologichnogo viku dlia viznachennia vplivu stanu navkolishn'ogo seredovishcha na zdorov'ia liudej [Study of possibility of biological age indicator's usage for determination of environmental conditions' influence on people's health]. *VI Mizhnarodna naukova konferenciia "Okhorona navkolishn'ogo seredovishcha ta racional'ne vikoristannia prirodnikh resursiv"* [6th International scientific conference "Protection of environment and rational usage of natural resources", Donets'k], Donets'k; 2007. P.134-135. (in Ukrainian)
16. Kishkun AA. *Biologicheskij vozrast i starenie* [Biological age and ageing], Moscow: GEOTAR Media; 2008. (in Russian)
17. Klapchuk VV, Samoshkin VV. *Kil'kisna ocinka rivnia fizichnogo zdorov'ia ta rekreacijno-ozdorovchi rezhimi* [Quantitative assessment of physical health level and health related recreational regimes], Dnepropetrovsk: DDIFKIS; 2009. (in Ukrainian)
18. Kopko IIe, Fil' VM. Biologichnij vik iak biomarker diagnostiki rivnia zdorov'ia students'koi molodi [Biological age as bio-marker of students' health]. *Naukovo-pedagogichni problemi fizichnoi kul'turi*, 2011;13:249-254. (in Ukrainian)
19. Korol SA. Assessment of physical health and physical fitness of students of technical specialties of I course. *Pedagogics, psychology, medical-biological problems of physical training and sports,* 2014;11:23-29. doi:10.15561/18189172.2014.1105
20. Loshits'ka TI. Biological age and rates of senescence of organism of students. *Pedagogics, psychology, medical-biological problems of physical training and sports,* 2010;7:50-53.
21. Lugaj MI, Dorogij AP. Zakhvoriuvanist' i smertnist' vid khvorob sistemi krovoobigu v Ukraini [Morbidity and mortality, resulted from blood circulation system's diseases in Ukraine]. Nova medicina, 2002;3:18-21. (in Ukrainian)
22. Mandrikov VB, Salaznikova LV, Miculina MP. O problemakh ocenki funkcional'nogo sostoianiia studentov special'nogo uchebnogo otdeleniia [On problems of assessment of special department students' functional state]. *Sovremennye nauchno-metodicheskie razrabotki v fizicheskom vospitanii studentov, imeiushchikh otklonenie v sostoianii zdorov'ia*, 2001;1:36-38. (in Russian)
23. Martiniuk O, Pechena V, Kravchenko K. Analiz riznomanitnikh metodik ocinki rivnia fizichnogo zdorov'ia students'koi molodi [Analysis of different assessment methodic for students' physical health]. *Fizichna kul'tura, sport ta zdorov'ia nacii*, 2014;18(1):183-189. (in Ukrainian)

24. Pokalev GM. *Nejrocirkuliatornaia distoniia* [Neuro-circulatory dystonia], N. Novgorod: NSPU; 1994. (in Russian)
25. Prisiazhniuk SI. *Biologichnij vik ta zdorov'ia students'koi molodi* [Biological age and students' health], Kiev: Center educational literature; 2010. (in Ukrainian)
26. Raevskij RT, Kanishevskij SM. *Zdorov'e, zdorovyj obraz zhizni i ozdorovitel'nyj obraz zhizni studentov* [Health, healthy life style and health related life style of students], Moscow: Science and Technology; 2008. (in Russian)
27. Romanchishin ON, Sidorko OJ, Dyka MV. Somatic health, adaptable potential, physical condition and biological age of students of pedagogical college. *Pedagogics, psychology, medical-biological problems of physical training and sports,* 2010;11:98-102.
28. Solov'ev VN. Fizicheskoe zdorov'e kak integral'nyj pokazatel' urovnia adaptacii organizma studentov k uchebnomu processu [Physical health as integral indicator of students' organism adaptation to educational process]. *Fundamental'nye issledovaniia*, 2005;6:61-66. (in Russian)
29. Timkiv K. Biologichnij vik ukrainciv [Biological age of Ukrainians]. *Korespondent*, 2011;46:85. (in Ukrainian)
30. Tserkovna OV, Nefedova AL, Osipov VN, Mirgorod OA. Biological age and rates of ageing at students with different level of impellent activity. *Physical Education of Students*, 2011;1:130-133.
31. Abar B. Promoting tobacco cessation utilizing pre-health professional students as research associates in the emergency department. *Addictive Behaviors*, 2015;40(3):73-76.
32. Al-Hariri MT, Al-Hattami AA. Utilization of internet by health colleges students at the University of Dammam. *Journal of Taibah University Medical Sciences,* 2015;10(1):66-73.
33. Berger H. Mental health of students and its development between 1994 and 2012. *Mental Health & Prevention,* 2015;3(1-2):48-56.
34. Dolan E, Hancock E, Wareing A. An evaluation of online learning to teach practical competencies in undergraduate health science students. *The Internet and Higher Education,* 2015;24(6):21-25.
35. Feuerman VV. Influence of socio-philosophical and spiritual values on the formation of social orientation and physical health specialists the sphere of physical culture and sports. *Physical Education of Students,* 2014;2:41-45. doi:10.6084/m9.figshare.906859
36. Goginava SE, Rumba OG. On improving effect combining aerobic and anaerobic loads of character in the classroom for physical training in universities. *Physical Education of Students,* 2014;3:18-29. doi:10.6084/m9.figshare.974492
37. Golod NR. Principles of developing a well-rounded program of physical rehabilitation for female students in the special medical group with consideration of physical activity impairment. *Pedagogics, psychology, medical-biological problems of physical training and sports,* 2015;5:9-15. doi:10.15561/18189172.2015.0502
38. Hadden KB. Health literacy training for health professions students. *Patient Education and Counseling,* 2015;98(7):918-920.
39. Holm-Hadulla RM, Koutsoukou-Argyraki A. Mental health of students in a globalized world: Prevalence of complaints and disorders, methods and effectivity of counseling, structure of mental health services for students. *Mental Health & Prevention,* 2015;3(1-2):1-4.
40. Iermakova TS. Development of the idea of forming health culture of a person in the world educational thought. *Pedagogics, psychology, medical-biological problems of physical training and sports,* 2014;4:8-12. doi:10.6084/m9.figshare.950949
41. Iermakova TS. Education of children in Polish family in a context of forming health culture. *Pedagogics, psychology, medical-biological problems of physical training and sports,* 2014;11:17-22. doi:10.15561/18189172.2014.1104
42. Iermakova TS. Forming a health culture of future teachers in Polish educational establishments. *Physical Education of Students*, 2014;5:14-19. doi:10.15561/20755279.2014.0503
43. Iermakova TS. Peculiarities of forming health culture of pupils in Poland: historical aspect. *Pedagogics, psychology, medical-biological problems of physical training and sports,* 2014;6:16-20. doi:10.6084/m9.figshare.1004090
44. Kozina ZhL, Kozhuhar LV, Sobko IN, Vaksler MA, Tihonova AA. Workability's recreation methodic with application of cupping massage and autogenic training of women student teams' basketball players. *Pedagogics, psychology, medical-biological problems of physical training and sports,* 2015;5:16-21. doi:10.15561/18189172.2015.0503
45. Lapkin ST, Levett-Jones C. Gilligan Using the Theory of Planned Behaviour to examine health professional students' behavioural intentions in relation to medication safety and collaborative practice. *Nurse Education Today* 2015;35(8):935-940.
46. Malenyuk TV, Kosivska AV. Training at sport circle as priority form of organization of students physical

education (on example of shaping). *Pedagogics, psychology, medical-biological problems of physical training and sports,* 2015;4:38-42. doi:10.15561/18189172.2015.0407

47. Petrenko NV, Loza TA. Model of recreational and training sessions based on the use of funds aqua professionally applied in the preparation of students of economics. *Physical Education of Students,* 2014;4:32-36. doi:10.6084/m9.figshare.974481
48. Pichurin VV. Psychological and psycho-physical training as a factor of personal anxiety at students. *Pedagogics, psychology, medical-biological problems of physical training and sports,* 2015;3:46-51. doi:10.15561/18189172.2015.0307
49. Prosvirina LN, Kolokoltsev MM, Kolchanova MA, Cieslicka Miroslawa, Stankiewicz Blazej. The characteristic of the engine qualities of the students of technical institute of III functional health group (special medical group). *Physical Education of Students,* 2015;1:43-49. doi:10.15561/20755279. 2015.0107
50. Siri A, Rui M. Distance Education for Health Professions' Students. *Procedia-Social and Behavioral Sciences,* 2015;174;9:730-738.
51. Stanishevska TI, Gorna OI, Berezhniak AS, Horban DD. Daily dynamic of indicators of girl-students' blood micro-circulation. *Pedagogics, psychology, medical-biological problems of physical training and sports,* 2015;6:23-29. doi:10.15561/ 18189172.2015.0604
52. Usher K et al. Australian health professions student use of social media. *Collegian,* 2014;21(2):95-101.
53. Yermakova TS. Individualization of forming health culture in schoolchildren of Polish schools. *Pedagogics, psychology, medical-biological problems of physical training and sports,* 2015;1:29-33. doi:10.15561/18189172.2015.0106

27

METHODIC OF PERFECTION OF HIGHER PEDAGOGICAL EDUCATIONAL ESTABLISHMENTS GIRL STUDENTS' RHYTHM

Kolumbet A.N., Dudorova L.Yu.
Kiev National University of Technology and Design

Abstract. *Purpose:* to study influence of methodic of rhythm perfection on girl students' coordination abilities. *Material:* in the research 264 girl students participated. We assessed individual and collective rhythm, internal and external motor rhythm; rhythm in exercises with musical accompaniment. *Results:* we have determined that creative motor tasks require variable conditions for their realization. We have proved demand in appropriate criteria for their assessment. It is noted that there is a demand in development of rhythm, considering its main kinds and manifestations, which are formed with some peculiarities. Individual rhythm is determined by activation of attention and its level. It is perfected more successfully rather with stimulated development than with natural. It was found that with age the character of natural progressing of rhythm preserves. *Conclusions:* it is recommended to develop rhythm in compliance with its kinds and manifestations. Progressing and perfection of rhythm is a long lasted process and shall be realized during all period of girl students' studying. Such approach forms girl students' demand in finding of purposeful motor rhythm in all their new motor actions. It ensures optimality of their fulfillment.
Key words: physical education, coordination abilities, rhythm, girl students.

Introduction

Rhythm is the basis of live systems' functioning. Self regulation of processes, adaptation to environmental changes; preservation of homeostasis are impossible without it, as well as synchronization of physiological processes under influence of physical loads. Motor actions also have certain rhythm: natural alteration of different efforts [2, 16, and 18].

When training physical exercises it is necessary to build theoretical model of rhythmic movements, which would be the content of them. Their visible simplicity, high orderliness in space and time can create an image of excess easiness and simplicity. Actually, for achievement of high results in moving much more time and efforts are spent. Free motor rhythms completely depend on human will and are the highest degree of motor acts' organization.

One of important tasks of physical education is development of strive for beauty and perfectness; search of new ways of effectiveness increase. For this purpose, it is necessary to strive for variable content of trainings; cultivate girl students' demand in everyday physical exercises; teach them to strive for purposeful motor actions and their variability [4, 24, 28, 30-34].

Significance of rhythm (as coordination ability) is determined by the fact that with its help optimal correlation of motor act's different parts is achieved; its continuity and joining are ensured as well as rational distribution of efforts in space and time. This coordination quality requires more attention to its development and perfection.

The problems of coordination qualities' development have always been paid great attention. Researches of a number of authors are devoted to perfection of coordination qualities in youth [7, 9, 14, 15, 18, 25, and 35]. Alongside with it, the authors did not manage to completely elucidate the problem of rhythm development in pedagogic HEEs' girl students.

Hypothesis: we assumed that our research (in the process of long lasted experiment) of rhythm's kinds will permit to mark out its main components, determine its assessment criteria. It will permit to offer renewed methodic of rhythm stimulated perfection in HEEs' girl students.

The purpose of the research is analysis of influence of rhythm stimulated perfection methodic on pedagogic HEEs' girl students' coordination abilities.

Material and methods

Participants: in the research 264 1st – 3rd year girl students (17-21 years' age) of Chernigov national pedagogic university, named after T.G. Shevchenko and Kiev university, named after Boris Grinchenko, participated. All girl students belonged to main health group.

Procedure: the research was fulfilled during 2008-2010. Rhythm indicators were determined by every kind at the beginning, in the middle and at the end of academic year. We used five tests, offered by the authors earlier **[13; 19].**

Individual rhythm was assessed with test 1. When walking by lunges foot drops on the floor with certain accent from toe to full foot. The sound of foot's contact with floor shall be equal by strength and uniform by duration. The assessment of motor rhythm was as follows: 5 points – leg drops on toe without sound and with accent – from toe on all foot, through equal periods of time. Amplitude of movements shall be equal, carriage – good, actions shall be free and expressive. 4 points: there is certain tension and stiffness, but movements are uniform and accented. 3 points – movements are accented with good amplitude with one or two disorders in steps' uniformity.

Collective rhythm was assessed with the help of test 2. Girl student stood facing group of 3-5 persons, who fulfilled general exercises. Then, synchronously with other girl students she reproduced the same movements. We assessed degree of coincidence by direction, temp, amplitude, expressiveness. 5 points meant complete coincidence by all main parameters; actions are expressive and accurate; 4 points – actions coincide by direction, temp and amplitude, but are stiff and not expressive; 3 points – movements coincide in general by main parameters with two-three failures in temps and direction.

External rhythm of movements was assessed with the help of test 3. The tested copied the showed by teacher exercise: walking with forward rising of straight leg (up to horizontal level), moving hands aside (at shoulder level). It is necessary to keep the picture of movement, its form, amplitude, dynamic. We assessed the coincidence of the fulfilled exercise with the task. 5 points mean complete coincidence: leg is straight, risen up to horizontal level with stretched toe, arms are straight, moved accurately aside, making straight line, head is up, back is straightened; 4 points – leg is in horizontal position but toe is not sufficiently stretched; hands are moved exactly aside but head is a little dropped; 3 points mean leg positioned lower than horizontal position, hands are moved aside not accurately, movements are stiffed.

Internal rhythm was assessed with test 4. The tested girl students fulfilled the showed by teacher dance movement: forward waltz step with forward and aside hands' moving, radiating gay and merry mood. We assessed coincidence of movement's external form with radiated mood: 5 points – movements are correct by form and smooth, eyes follows hands' movement, expression of face is happy; 4 points – movements are correct by form and character of fulfillment, smile is stiffed; 3 points – movements are correct by direction and amplitude, but there are no emotions.

Rhythm in exercises with musical accompaniment was assessed with test 5. Having listened to musical fragment, the tested girl students fulfilled exercise in compliance with its character. We assessed compliance of character of movement with content of musical fragment: 5 points meant complete coincidence of movements with character of musical accompaniment (march sounds – the tested fulfills drill step; waltz sounds - wide steps' walking or lunges; polka sounds – jumps by both legs and etc.); 4 points – insignificant coincidence of movements with character of musical accompaniment; movements are chosen correctly but do not coincide sufficiently by amplitude and temp. 3 points were given for one or two incomplete coincidence with character of melody: jumps under march music; run under waltz melody.

Statistical analysis: for processing of the research's results we used commonly accepted methods of mathematical statistic. For each of the tested indicators we calculated mean values and mean square deviation. Assessment of differences' confidence was fulfilled by Student's t-criterion at 1% and 5% significance levels. We calculated increment of the studied indicators. Increment temps was calculated by formula of S. Broudy:

$$W = V_2 - V_1 / 0,5 \text{ x } (V_2+V_1) \text{ x } 100 \%$$

where: V1 and V2 – accordingly, initial and final results in control testing.

In fulfillment of complex pedagogic and biological examinations, in which girl students participated, we observed legislation of Ukraine about health protection, the Declaration of Helsinki 2000, Directive №86/609 of European community on participation of people in medical – biological researches.

Results

Methodic of stimulated rhythm's development implied introduction of motor tasks in every training by all rhythm's kinds: *activation of attention, training of motor memory, distribution and applying of efforts, orientation in space and time and ability to general actions.* Depending on type of training (its tasks, purpose), special exercises were given to girl students in warming up (main and finalizing) parts, in different sequence and scope. These exercises were of different complexity. For example light athletics training had subject: run in various directions and with different speed, throwing of small ball for distance. The task was to familiarize with peculiarities of runs with changing of direction and speed; to perfect technique of small ball throwing for distance from the spot. Warming up part included exercises for activation of attention as necessary condition of rhythm's perfection: in walking first and third steps were to be marked with claps; after every third step – right hand rising with left on the waist; after five steps – turn by 360°; determination and memorizing of distance between steps in run and walking; memorizing of efforts in walking, calm run and with acceleration, Moving in column the tested shall fulfill general and warming up exercises synchronously with leading girl student.

In main part of training girl students were offered warming up and special exercises for main rhythm's kinds development: in run by right side of the gym every fifth step was fulfilled with turn to the right and every tenth step – with turn to the left by 180°; in run by left side of gym left leg was put with accent. Steps should have been equal by amplitude with uniform speed; in diagonal running – double acceleration at the beginning (10-12 m) and in the middle of distance. The offered run tasks had clear rhythm and required certain fitness. That is why girl students were permitted to fulfill these exercises independently in free time.

For mastering of *throw rhythm* of small ball throwing for distance we used motor actions for activation of attention: visual inspection of place for ball throw, noting of some guide points; compare different by value efforts for preparatory movements (dropping of hand with ball, moving hand backward - upward) and main motor action (throw); concentration of attention on difference in applied efforts for fulfillment of main part of ball throw.

Development of *motor memory* was realized with the help of the following tasks: count and remember quantity of run steps in right and left sides of gym with accented putting of right and left legs. Determine the quantity of run steps in first and second accelerations in diagonal run and all additional steps before and after acceleration; remember the value of efforts in run with changing of direction and speed and in period of acceleration.

For training of *rhythm of applying and distribution of efforts* the following exercises were envisaged: run with turns to the right and to the left by 360°, run with back forward, prolongation of run step up to maximal amplitude, run with shortened steps and many other.

For perfection of small ball *throwing* girl students also fulfilled a number of movements: throw behind marked line from stance "on one knee", from sitting position with straightened legs, with closed eyes, with quarter of strength, with half of strength and so on.

For better orientation in space girl students fulfill run by the right and left sides of gym within definite corridors (width 1-1.5 m), marked with chalk or paper strips. Having remembered the width of corridor and steps' amplitude, they were to repeat the task without additional guide points. Having determined speed of 10 meters' segment run by diagonal they were to keep it at longer (20 meters') segment.

When throwing small bal for distance the girl students were offered: a) remember ball's trajectory in the best attempt and repeat it several times; b) determine amplitude of additional and main movements, when throwing, compare throw distance with different arm's amplitude and additional step forward; c) compare different feelings, when throwing ball in gym and outdoors.

Training and perfection of *collective rhythm* (ability to collective actions) was realized in the process of sports game at the end of main part of training. Besides, girl students mastered Greek folk dance "Sirtaki" with accented rhythmic movements, which are fulfilled first slowly and then - with gradual acceleration. For better feeling of mutual actions girl students positioned their hands on shoulders of each other. In finalizing part of training there were exercises for attention, fixing of motor memory and other: a) walking with accented foot putting on toe ("acute" step), with arms' movement (rising on tip toes – hands up, when dropping on full feet – hands down), hands behind head with keeping straight carriage; b) walk, rolling from heel to toes with accent on vertical position in upper point (position - on toes), arms aside with palms upward and other.

By the end of first year training for rhythm's development and perfection some results became obvious (see table 1). Girl students became able to fulfill exercises with higher amplitude, correctly find required accents. Culture of movements improved. Materials of the research point at demand in development of rhythm, considering its main kinds and manifestations, which are formed with some peculiarities. For example, *individual rhythm* was determined by degree of attention's development and activation. It is perfected more successfully in stimulated development than in natural.

Analysis of rhythm increment by level of *motor memory* permitted to find that with age the character of rhythm's natural development is preserved. Indicators are gradually improved. In stimulated formation of this rhythm's kind it was registered that experimental trainings favorably influenced on increment temps. Girl students reproduce by form a lot of motor actions with rather high accuracy. In their age, for mastering of motor action's character application of visible patterns is quite sufficient. Systemic fulfillment of different game exercises by girl students with their gradual complication facilitates development of motor memory.

Some peculiarities of rhythm increment were observed when fulfilling collective actions (*collective rhythm*). This kind of rhythm is connected with some specific requirements. They include ability to distribute very accurately muscular efforts, orienting on movements of team members. The pre-set amplitude requires accuracy of exercise's fulfillment by space characteristics. Targeted perfection facilitated better increment of indicators; the offered motor tasks did not require significant strength. With game or competition methods they facilitated more successful transformation of motor actions' individual rhythm into collective.

Analysis of data on formation of *rhythm in exercises with musical accompaniment* showed that natural increment of indicators has tendency to improvement with age. Application of stimulated development methodic for this rhythm kind showed the highest increment temps of experimental girl students' indicators.

Table 1. Increment of indicators (%) of different kinds of rhythm

№	Tests	Period of research	Control group		Experimental group		p
			M	±m	M	±m	
1	2	3	4	5	6	7	8
1	Individual rhythm	1st year	2.28	0.18	8.14	0.26	<0.05
		2nd year	4.62	0.20	10.22	0.36	<0.05
		3rd year	3.78	0.30	11.53	0.46	<0.05
2	Collective rhythm	1st year	2.60	0.15	9.17	0.42	<0.05
		2nd year	3.05	0.15	8.95	0.40	<0.05
		3rd year	3.31	0.26	10.56	0.45	<0.05
3	Internal and external rhythm of movements	1st year	3.40	0.14	4.00	0.26	>0.05
		2nd year	4.00	0.31	4.78	0.27	>0.05
		3rd year	3.74	0.28	5.15	0.27	>0.05
4	Rhythm in exercises with musical accompaniment	1st year	2.63	0.09	4.57	0.27	>0.05
		2nd year	4.12	0.18	5.77	0.38	>0.05
		3rd year	3.99	0.29	4.27	0.25	>0.05

Discussion

Man is able to control free motor act, in the base of which there is definite rhythm. In this case we speak about higher level of muscular functioning's organization. In the process of active muscular functioning motor rhythm is generated by motor system itself. With impulses' entering nervous system their transformation occurs. As a result new algorithms of motor actions appear. Main elements of muscular functioning (neuron connections of central nervous system, nervous-muscular apparatus) switch in organized movement of all motor system with definite clear rhythm [1, 10, and 21].

Functional system ensures reverse afferentation – connection from working organ to regulating nervous centers [11, 20, and 24]. Receptor signal circulates by closed ring from muscular, ligament and tactile receptors in the form of neuron impulses. Simultaneously it fulfills a role of timer and program, determining rhythm.

Information about space-time and space-power characteristics of motor action is conditioned by appearing of certain rhythm. The emerged impulses transform in mechanical movement. Depending on external conditions (age of a trainee, physical fitness, character of motor task and etc.) there happens constant modification of motor program. As a result rational motor team, amplitude, distribution of efforts and optimal rhythm take place [2, 17].

Rhythm conditions required correlation of motor act's separate phases, continuity of muscular functioning during pre-set time, coincidence and amplitude of movements. Physical exercise has certain speed (temp) and regulated distribution of efforts (dynamic). The temp and dynamic of motor act are closely interconnected and influence on each other. It is not possible to voluntarily change temp of run or distribution of efforts. The higher is temp of run for long jump the more efforts are required for their rational distribution in order to create optimal conditions for fulfillment of main motor act [3, 19, 28]. With too high temp of run fulfillment of preparatory actions for push off becomes more difficult. That is why at the last step and the step before last speed is reduced. It permits to more completely realize motor potential. Temp, dynamic and harmony are the main components of rhythm.

Temp is speed of fulfillment of motor act's separate elements. Physiological functions to large extent are determined by speed. The higher it is the stronger muscular load's influence on organism. With insufficient speed training influence is absent as well as positive effects *[2, 4, 18]*.

Dynamic (distribution of efforts in fulfillment of physical exercises) is one more component of rhythm. Motor act consists of several components, which require different muscular efforts. For example, long jump from the sport with push by two legs and arms' waving includes the following preparatory actions: squatting, moving arms backward, re-distribution of muscular-skeletal apparatus's links; then – push forward by two legs with quick arms' waving (main phase is accompanied by maximal muscular efforts), landing and keeping body balance (final phase, in which efforts sharply reduce).

If temp of movements coincides with dynamic of muscular efforts' distribution, then change of many nervous centers and inter-centers relations' functional state take place; conditional reflex activity improves, coincidence of motor and vegetative functions' activity increases. As a result *harmony* of movements is achieved [1, 9, 14, 15].

Harmony is manifested as more perfect control over body with fulfillment of physical exercises. With coincidence of temp and dynamic less time and efforts are required for motor act with higher movements' amplitude. In this connection in practicing of physical exercises it is necessary to work out individual rhythm. Feeling of lightness of movements, "muscular joy", satisfaction of trainings are important signs of individual rhythm's formation. Without it, it is impossible to cultivate demand in motor functioning, strive for achievement its optimal scope, ensuring required level of health.

The character of rhythm depends on specificity of motor actions. Physical exercises are fulfilled individually and collectively. In cyclic and non cyclic exercises rhythm is different. Rhythm is greatly influenced by musical accompaniment. We can mark out the following main kinds of rhythm, characteristic for motor functioning: individual rhythm; collective rhythm, external rhythm; internal rhythm; rhythm in cyclic physical exercises; rhythm in non cyclic physical exercises and rhythm in exercises with musical accompaniment [6, 15, 16, 22].

Different kinds and manifestations of rhythm determine content of methodic of definite motor functioning training. For mastering new physical exercise it is necessary to determine its rhythm; to find principle moment of efforts' application (to make program of actions) [2, 5, 8, 12, 23]. With it, rhythm's manifestation depends on a number of factors and is assessed with the help of special criteria [7, 19, 20, 27].

It would not be correct to speak about development and perfection of rhythm in general. It is known that at one or several trainings it is possible to form one or another kind of motor coordination, depending on tasks of training.

Conclusions

1. Rhythm is a kind of coordination qualities, which has its own kinds and manifestations. With it, its perfection implies usage of various exercises.
2. Creative motor tasks imply different conditions for their realization. For their assessment appropriate criteria are required.
3. Rhythm training shall be in compliance with its kinds and manifestation. It requires appropriate approach to content of the methodic and its perfection.
4. Targeted development of rhythm, considering its kinds and manifestations results in improvement of its indicators with different temps of increment. It positively reflects on girl students' physical fitness.
5. Development and perfection of rhythm is of long term character and shall be realized during all period of girl students' studying at HEE. Such approach forms girl students' demand in finding of purposeful motor rhythm in all new motor actions that ensures optimality of their fulfillment.

Acknowledgements

The researches have been fulfilled in compliance with scientific program of Chernigov national pedagogic university, named after T.G. Shevchenko physical education faculty by topic "Didactic principles of motor function's formation in persons, who practice physical education and sports" (state registration number 0108U000854).

Conflict of interests

The authors declare that there is no conflict of interests.

References:

1. Anokhin PK. *Uzlovye voprosy teorii funkcional'noj sistemy* [Key problems of functional system theory], Moscow: Science; 1980. (in Russian)
2. Bernshtejn NA. *O lovkosti i ee razvitii* [On dexterity and its training], Moscow: Physical Culture and Sport; 1991. (in Russian)
3. Bojchenko SD, Karseko EN, Leonov VV, Smotrickij AL. Problemy koncepcii koordinacii i koordinacionnykh sposobnostej v fizicheskom vospitanii [Problems of coordination and coordination conception in physical education]. *Pedagogics, psychology, medical-biological problems of physical training and sports*, 2002;2:53-55. (in Russian)
4. Bojchenko SD, Karseko EN, Leonov VV, Smotrickij AL. O nekotorykh aspektakh izucheniia koordinacionnykh sposobnostej v teorii fizicheskogo vospitaniia i teorii sporta [On some aspects of coordination abilities study in theory of physical education and theory of sports]. *Teoriia i praktika fizicheskoj kul'tury*, 2003;8:19-22. (in Russian)
5. Bojchenko SD, Ejder E, Iashanina N, Leonov V, Iashanin Ia, Bojchenko T. Koordinacionnye sposobnosti kak veshchestvennye korreliaty effektivnosti obucheniia dvigatel'nym dejstviiam [Coordination abilities as substantial correlates of effectiveness of motor actions' training]. *Pedagogics, psychology, medical-biological problems of physical training and sports*, 2003;11:39-43. (in Russian)
6. Bryukhanova NA, Bulgakova OV, Mokrova TI, Bogashchenko YA. Determination of possibilities of the use of high-intensive trainings facilities on lessons health aerobics. *Physical Education of Students*, 2013, vol.2, pp. 25-29. doi:10.6084/m9.figshare.156376
7. Vlasiuk OO. Vikoristannia elementiv suchasnikh tanciv i khoreografii na zaniattiakh z fizichnogo vikhovannia studentok 17-18 rokiv [Application of modern dances and choreography elements in physical education classes of 17-18 years' age girl students]. *Visnik Chernigivs'kogo nacional'nogo pedagogichnogo universitetu*. 2012;98(1):93-97. (in Ukrainian)
8. Volkov VL. *Rozvitok fizichnikh zdibnostej studentiv u sistemi fizichnoi pidgotovki* [Development of students' physical abilities in system of physical training], Kiev: Education Ukraine; 2011. (in Ukrainian)

9. Gibaeva NN, Liulina NV, Zakharova NV. Osobennosti ispol'zovaniia fitnes programm po fizicheskoj kul'tury studentov [Specific features of fitness programs on students' physical culture application]. *Physical Education of Students*, 2010;6:16-19. (in Russian)
10. Donskoj DD. Psikhomotornoe edinstvo upravleniia fizicheskimi uprazhneniiami kak dvigatel'nymi dejstviiami (ot «mekhaniki zhivogo» k psikhobiomekhanike dejstvij [Psycho-motor unity of physical exercises control as motor actions (from mechanic of "alive" to psycho-bio-mechanic of actions)]. *Teoriia i praktika fizicheskoj kul'tury*, 1994;5-6:23-26. (in Russian)
11. Zhidenko AA. Psikhofiziologicheskie osnovy upravleniia dvizheniem [Psycho-physiological principles of motor control]. *Visnik Chernigivs'kogo nacional'nogo pedagogichnogo universitetu*. 2012;102(1):168-173. (in Russian)
12. Zaporozhanov VA, Borchinski T. Sovershenstvovanie ocenki koordinacionnykh sposobnostej zanimaiushchikhsia fizicheskimi uprazhneniiami [Perfection of coordination abilities' assessment of physical exercises' trainees]. *Pedagogics, psychology, medical-biological problems of physical training and sports*, 2009;9:52-55. (in Russian)
13. Kolumbet OM. *Rozvitok koordinacijnikh zdibnostej molodi* [Development of youth's coordination abilities], Kiev: Education Ukraine; 2014. (in Ukrainian)
14. Kozhevnikova LK. Vospitanie koordinacionnykh sposobnostej na zaniatiiakh po fizicheskomu vospitaniiu [Training of coordination abilities at physical education classes]. *Physical Education of Students*, 2012;1:38-41. (in Russian)
15. Kurganskij AV. O vozniknovenii i koordinacii ritmicheskikh dvizhenij [On appearing and coordination of rhythmic movements]. *Teoriia i praktika fizicheskoj kul'tury*, 1996;11:44-49. (in Russian)
16. Litvinova OP. Vliianie ozdorovitel'noj aerobiki na razvitie dvigatel'nykh kachestv devushek 18-20 let [Influence of health related aerobics on development of motor qualities of 18-20 years' age girls]. *Pedagogics, psychology, medical-biological problems of physical training and sports*, 2009;10:118-122. (in Russian)
17. Liakh VI. *Dvigatel'nye sposobnosti shkol'nikov* [Motor abilities of schoolchildren], Moscow: Terra-Sport; 2000. (in Russian)
18. Maliar IeI, Lebid' RM. Pedagogichni umovi realizacii programi rozvitku koordinacijnikh zdibnostej [Pedagogic conditions of realization of coordination abilities' development program]. *Pedagogics, psychology, medical-biological problems of physical training and sports*, 2010;4:87-90. (in Ukrainian)
19. Nazarenko LD, Ignat'eva ZhA. Teoreticheskoe obosnovanie i metodika razvitiia ritmichnosti [Theoretical substantiation and methodic of rhythm's development]. *Fizicheskaia kul'tura*, 2000;1:45-50. (in Russian)
20. Sinajskij MM. *Fiziologicheskie proiavleniia koordinacionnykh sposobnostej u sportsmenov* [Physiological manifestations of sportsmen's coordination abilities]. Moscow; 2007. (in Russian)
21. Farfel' BC. *Upravlenie dvizheniiami v sporte* [Control over movements in sports], Moscow: Physical Culture and Sport; 1975. (in Russian)
22. Fizner LN. *Upravlenie koordinaciej dvizhenij* [Control over motor coordination], Moscow: Science; 1971. (in Russian)
23. Chernovsky SM, Kolumbet AN. Determination of future designers' professionally important coordination qualities. *Physical education of students,* 2016;2:38–44. doi:10.15561/20755279.2016.0206
24. Hirtz P. *Koordinative Fahigkeiten im Schulsport* [Coordinative abilities in school sports], Berlin: Volk und Wissen, Volksseigener Verlag; 1985.
25. Iermakov SS, Apanasenko GL, Bondarenko TV, Prasol SD. Physical culture is a basic instrument of culture of health. *Pedagogics, psychology, medical-biological problems of physical training and sports*, 2010;11:31-33.
26. Iermakov SS, Ivashchenko PI, Guzov VV. Features of motivation of students to application of individual programs of physical self-preparation. *Physical Education of Students*, 2012;4:59-61.
27. Kolumbet AN. Influence of stimulated plasticity training method on coordination indicators of high pedagogic educational estableshments' girl students. *Physical Education of Students*, 2015;6:31-37. doi:10.15561/20755279.2015.0604
28. Kolumbet AN. Dynamic of girl students' psycho-physiological indicators in process of their study at

pedagogical higher educational establishment. *Physical Education of Students*, 2016;1:29-36. doi:10.15561/20755279.2016.0104

29. Kopylov YuA, Jackowska LN, Kudryavtsev MD, Kuzmin VA, Tolstopyatov IA, Iermakov SS. The concept of structure and content of health related trainings for higher educational establishments' students. *Physical Education of Students,* 2015;5:23–30. doi:10.15561/20755279.2015.0504
30. Lopatenko GO. Optimization of training process in pre-start fencing training on the base of out-of-training means' of mobilization orientation application. *Pedagogics, psychology, medical-biological problems of physical training and sports*, 2016;20(2):34-39. doi:10.15561/18189172.2016.0205
31. Marc R Lochbaum, Javan Jean-Noel, Zişan Kazak Çetinkalp, Felipe Andrés Vallejo-Reyes, Jose Mena-Campbell. 2 x 2 achievement goals profiles in chilean Competitive and recreational athletes: a first look. *Pedagogics, psychology, medical-biological problems of physical training and sports*, 2016;1:41-46. doi:10.15561/18189172.2016.0106
32. Michael Chia, Marcus Lee. Body weight satisfaction and disordered eating among youth who are active in sport in Singapore. *Pedagogics, psychology, medical-biological problems of physical training and sports*, 2015, vol.4, pp. 51-58. doi:10.15561/18189172.2015.0409
33. Nishan Singh Deol, Davinder Singh. A comparative analysis of flow state in basketball performance: a psychological probe. *Pedagogics, psychology, medical-biological problems of physical training and sports*, 2016;1:47-51. doi:10.15561/18189172.2016.0107
34. Podrigalo LV, Iermakov SS, Alekseev AF, Rovnaya OA. Studying of interconnections of morphological functional indicators of students, who practice martial arts. *Physical Education of Students*, 2016;1:64-70. doi:10.15561/20755279.2016.0109
35. Skurikhina NV, Kudryavtsev MD, Kuzmin VA, Iermakov SS. Fitness yoga as modern technology of special health groups' girl students' psycho-physical condition and psycho-social health strengthening. *Physical Education of Students*, 2016;20(2):24-31. doi:10.15561/20755279.2016.0204

28

INTEGRATIVE ASSESSMENT OF KICK BOXERS' BRAIN BLOOD CIRCULATION AND BIO-ELECTRICAL ACTIVITY IN CONDITIONS OF CORRECTION TECHNOLOGIES' APPLICATION

Romanov Y.N.[1], Isaev A.P.[1], Shevtsov A.V.[2], Romanova L.A.[1], Cieslicka M.[3], Muszkieta R.[3]
[1]South Ural State University Institute of Sport, Tourism and Service, Chelyabinsk, Russia
[2]Lesgaft National State University of Physical Education, Sport and Health, St.-Petersburg, Russia
[3]Kazimierz Wielki University in Bydgoszcz, Poland.

Abstract. *Purpose:* to scientifically substantiate the role of para-vertebral impacts on blood circulation and bio-electrical activity of kick boxers' cortex. *Material:* in the research participated kick boxers (main group, n=62) and university students (control group, n=25) of 18-23 years' age. Assessment of para-vertebral impacts with device "Armos" and classic massage was fulfilled with the help of the following methodic: trans-cranial dopplerography of head main arteries and cortex EEG of the tested. *Results:* it was found that with the help of para-vertebral impacts by device "Armos" linear velocity of cerebral blood flow reduces to normal limits and in- and inter-hemispheres' interaction strength increases. *Conclusions:* para-vertebral impacts by device "Armos" activate integrative processes and inter-hemispheres' interactions of different cortex areas of kick boxers. It can witness about better formation of functional systems, ensuring sports efficiency.
Key words: kickboxing, device "Armos", cerebral dopplerography, electroencephalography, linear velocity of blood flow, coherence.

Introduction

Kickboxing is characterized by high physical, psycho-physiological and emotional tension, in connection with kick/punch impacts; by rather high temp of duels and actions of high static-kinetic level. That is why, in our work modern approaches to training technologies is presented. In basic period technology includes training of local-regional muscular endurance, accurate actions and formation of resistance to hypoxia. It requires assessment of blood flow borders (cerebral inclusive and bio-electrical activity of brain). It is connected with the fact that kick-boxers' sports functioning often is accompanied by brain micro-traumas and disorders in sportsmen's body segments. Kick-boxers endure muscular-fascial imbalance and disorder of static-kinetic stability. Comparative analysis of correction technologies' influence showed high effectiveness of some of them in influence on cerebral blood circulation and brain's bio-electrical activity. We showed some priorities of the applied technologies, comparing our data with control data received in fitness technologies' practicing. We also found specific mechanisms of functional changes, characteristic for this kind of sports.

Kickboxing requires from sportsman comprehensive fitness and adaptive ability to fulfill intensive motor actions in short periods of time. In connection with the above said, kick-boxers can endure muscular-fascial imbalance, resulting in fatigue and risk of traumas [8, 16, and 20]. It should be also noted that kick/punch impacts in head area can cause micro-traumas [17, 18, 19, and 25] and other deeper disorders of organs [21, 23, and 24]. Application of brain bio-electric activity and dopplerography methodic in trainings permits to open sports potentials of the tested [6, 10].

In materials of sports physiology and kinesiology there is quite a number of works on rehabilitation of sportsmen with nervous-muscular disorders [2, 3, and 9]. In these works weak links are revealed and technologies of manual-muscular testing, functional eating are offered; creation of artificial training-correction medium system, reflex moving to sports influences are described [1] (including overloads and disorders of adaptation).

The researches of N.A. Volynkina [4] showed that compensated compression of peripheral tissue was a factor, reducing sportsmen's adaptation reserve. Correction influences permit to increase the reserves, spent on adaptation-compensatory processes in conditions of average degree traumas. O.G. Sukhorukova [12] offered technique of dura mater restoration during 2-5 minutes, in conditions of competitions. In works of Shitikov T.A. [15] potentials of manual therapy and applied kinesiology in correction of athletes with post traumatic vascular disorders are shown. Such correction causes reduction of increased excitability of brain's segmental structures, which ensure tonic reactions of cranial and cervical muscles, normalization of muscle tonus under metabolic-trophic disorders. These integrative processes facilitate strengthening of connections between neuron chains and mobilization of organism's reserves for sports efficiency. Klimesch W. [22] found that organism's integrative functioning is based on cortical/sub-cortical connections and mobilization of neuron circuits with frequency of external rhythm. It happens against the background of increase of nervous organization's plasticity, which regulates processes in conditions of unexpected factors.

Hypothesis: It is assumed that the conducted rehabilitation measures permitted for complex scientific group and coach to timely eliminate appearing dysfunctions and, at the same time, use organism's reserves for increasing of its functioning. Sportsmen's relaxation increase resistance of brain structures to synchronization and activation at inter-neuron level. Integrative processes and inter-hemisphere interactions of different areas of kick-boxers' brains are activated. It can witness about better formation of functional systems, ensuring sports efficiency.

The purpose of the research is to scientifically substantiate the role of manual-correction influence with devise "Armos" and classis massage impacts on blood flow and bio-electrical activity of kick boxers' cortex and comparison of these data with the data of fitness practices.

Material and methods

Participants: in the research participated kick-boxers from first spots grade to masters of sports (main group, n=62 and students of ФГБОУ ВПО "South-Ural State university". The students practiced fitness technologies 2 times a week (control group, n=25). All participants were of 18-23 years' age. Kick-boxers were the main group (2nd group, n=62), which was divide into two sub-groups: 3rd (n=40) and 4th (n=22).

Procedure (organization of the research): By standard methodic all tested kick-boxers and control group students (n=87) twice (before and after corrections) endured two diagnostic procedures. The first was supersonic trans-cranial dopplerography («Digi-lite» of «Rimed» Co, Israel) for study of blood flow in frontal, middle, vertebral (4th segment) brain arteries of both hemispheres; main (basilar) artery (MA), basal vein of Rosenthal. Then we registered electroencephalogram (EEG) from symmetric outlets of occipital (O1, O2), parietal (P3, P4), central (C3, C4), forehead (Fp1, Fp2, F3, F4, F7, F8), temple (T3, T4, T5, T6) with separate ear indifferent electrodes. In the range from 1 to 35 Hz we calculated spectrums of coherence with resolution by frequency of 0.2 Hz for segments 2 from monopole EEG. Average coherence level is calculated automatically for all EEG frequency band in the whole and for separate physiological rhythms. On the base of mean coherence level we assessed coherence spectrums. Besides, we studied statistical linear connections of electric processes of two brain areas. They were assessed by value of connection by every separate frequency of oscillations independent on their amplitude [5].

After preliminary testing by two above mentioned methodic, 2nd main group of kick-boxers was divided into two sub-groups. With device "Armos" we conducted 10 days' course of influencing on para-vertebral areas in sub-group 3 (n=40) and 10 days' course of classis massage (back and neck) in sub-group 4 (n=22).

Device "Armos" is a rigid structure with special protrusions. Lying on back, sportsman puts this device turn-by-turn under cervical, thoracic and lumbar spines. After dozed pressing by weight of own body on the mentioned backbone segments unloading is achieved. It reduces possible pain and increases backbone mobility. This method is based on deep penetration of "Armos" device protrusions in muscular fascial tissues of backbone system. It stretches shortened muscles and opens bootastic joints that restore their mobility [14]. Technology and methodic of apparatus-manual correction "Armos" implied stimulation of nervous-muscular and fascial segments of backbone, ensuring keeping of dynamic postures, support and defense of organism from shocks. Fascias have cell memory and form myo-fascial chains. Fascias ensure regulation of neighboring muscles and other organs' tonus. In case of patho-bio-mechanical dysfunctions there happens disordering of impulses' passing from muscles to organs, ensuring static-kinetic balance. EEG and brain blood stream registration permits to find left- or right hemisphere motor- cerebellum thalamo basilar conductivity for diagnosis of main and compensatory sides of affection.

Statistical analysis: statistical processing of the research material was fulfilled with the help of programs Statistica 10.0, SPSS 17 on the basis of key methods. Confidence of differences between groups was determined with Mann-Whitney test.

Results of the research

Results of testing of kick-boxers' and control group blood flow are given in table 1. Comparison of kick-boxers' and control group indicators before and after correction influences with apparatus-manual method showed confident differences by all spectrum of brain arteries ($p \leq 0.05$-0.01). Exclusion was left front brain artery, right brain artery and main artery. It can be assumed that higher diameter of left carotid and left backbone arteries (as well as asymmetry of kick-boxers' dynamic positions in duel) results just in such re-distribution of blood stream. In most of arteries, under impact of apparatus-manual complex "Armos" excess of brain blood flow substantially decreased. Vein blood flow in basal vein of Rosenthal was studied with method of trans-cranial dopplerography. Parameter of blood flow systolic velocity (LVBF – linear velocity of blood flow with norm of not more than 19 cm/sec) and indicator of artery-vein balance (correlation of final diastolic velocity in carotid artery with maximal systolic velocity in internal jugular vein) are the main indicators of brain vein blood circulation. In control group these indicators were in reference limits.

Table 1. Characteristics of brain blood flow in the tested groups before and after corrections

Parameters of cerebral blood stream		1st control group (n=25)	2nd group before correction (n=62)	I3rd subgroup after "Armos" (n=40)	IV subgroup after massage (n=22)
Linear velocity of blood flow in middle brain artery (cm/sec.)	right	93.9±18.8	136.3±18.1*	95.48±16.11**	128.95±17.93
	left	96.3±19.7	124.85±18.9*	95.5±16.0**	121.38±19.09
Resistivity index in middle brain artery	right	0.56±0.07	0.64±0.04*	0.55±0.05**	0.62±0.07
	left	0.55±0.21	0.73±0.17*	0.54±0.02**	0.68±0.77
Linear velocity of blood flow in frontal brain artery (cm/sec.)	right	77.1±13.20	87.15±15.82*	87.03±11.94**	91.05±13.27
	left	77.3±18.1	83.76±17.31*	81.88±13.28**	84.92±16.08
Resistivity index in frontal brain artery	right	0.58±0.03	0.69±0.05*	0.55±0.07**	0.64±0.06
	left	0.54±0.05	0.66±0.11*	0.55±0.34**	0.60±0.24
Linear velocity of blood flow in back brain artery (cm/sec.)	right	54.7±17.1	78.95±13.2*	54.39±8.11**	68.60±10.13
	left	56.9±16.3	64.34±10.25*	58.01±9.35**	60.65±10.53
Resistivity index in back brain artery	right	0.56±0.19	0.75±0.25*	0.54±0.12**	0.59±0.09
	left	0.56±0.08	0.75±0.09*	0.53±0.07**	0.68±0.09
Linear velocity of blood flow in 4th segment of backbone artery (cm/sec.)	right	57.2±8.1	31.97±12.45*	58.10±7.11**	43.91±9.21
	left	56.1±4.1	37.22±13.17*	56.95±7.89**	41.56±12.24
	right	0.53±0.06	0.60±0.06	0,52±0,04	0.59±0.72

Parameters of cerebral blood stream	1st control group (n=25)	2nd group before correction (n=62)	I3rd subgroup after "Armos" (n=40)	IV subgroup after massage (n=22)
Resistivity index in 4th segment of left backbone artery	0.54±0.05	0.66±0.07*	0.51±7.21**	0.62±0.08
Linear velocity of blood flow in main brain artery (cm/sec.)	59.1±12.3	74.43±14.14	67.55±13.78	72.09±13.33
Resistivity index in main brain artery	0.51±0.05	0.64±0.07*	0.54±0.05**	0.60±0.25
Inter-hemisphere asymmetry by middle brain artery, (%)	4.2±1.5	10.99±11.2*	0.98±1.5**	8.03±11.87
Inter-hemisphere asymmetry by frontal brain artery, (%)	2.5±1.5	4.6±0.7*	0.8±0.05**	6.99±13.83
Parameters of cerebral blood flow	1st control group (n=25)	2nd group before correction (n=62)	I3rd subgroup after "Armos" (n=40)	IV subgroup after massage (n=22)
Inter-hemisphere asymmetry by back brain artery (%)	3.9±2.8	16.9±16.1*	4.9±2.9**	16.05±19.02
Inter-hemisphere asymmetry by backbone arteries, (%)	1.3±12.0	13.5±8.9*	4.8±2.8**	12.15±11.10

Notes: * - confident differences between indicators of 1st and 2nd groups ($p < 0.05$); ** - confident differences between indicators of 2nd group and 3rd subgroup ($p < 0.05$); *** - confident differences between indicators of 2nd group and 4th subgroup ($p < 0.05$).

In group of kick boxers indicator of artery-vein balance before correction was less than 1 and velocity of blood stream in basal vein of Rosenthal was by 43% higher than normal. In the whole it worsened blood circulation because of complicated vein outflow of dystonic character. After fulfilled corrections in subgroups 3 and 4 we registered physiological orientation of both parameters – statistically significant in "Armos" group. In conditions of ischemic progressing of brain substance it is important to realize self-regulation of brain circulation. We found parameters of blood circulation regulation reserves (anatomic, myogenic and metabolic) when making compressing test, tests with breathing pauses and hyper-ventilation with calculation of cerebral vascular reactivity index. The results of these tests are presented in table 2.

With computer electroencephalograph "Neuron-Spectr – 4" ("Neuro-Soft", Russia) we registered EEG from symmetric occipital (O1, O2), parietal (P3, P4), central (C3, C4), forehead (Fp1, Fp2, F3, F4, F7, F8), temple (T3, T4, T5, T6) outlets with separated ear indifferent electrodes. In frequency band from 1 to 35 Hz we calculated coherence spectrums with resolution by frequency 0.2 Hz for segments 2 of monopole EEG. On the base of mean coherence level (calculated automatically for all frequency band of EEG in the whole and for separate physiological rhythms) we assessed coherence spectrums. Besides, we studied statistical linear connections of electric processes of both brain areas. They were assessed by value of connection by every separate frequency of oscillation, independent on their amplitude.

Table 2. Characteristic of vein outflow in tested contingent before and after corrections, (M±m)

Indicator	1st control group (n=25)	2nd group before correction (n=62)	I3rd subgroup after "Armos" (n=40)	IV subgroup after massage (n=22)
Linear velocity of blood flow in basal vein of Rosenthal (cm/sec.)	19.00±3.15	27.22±4.92*	18.89±4.15**	22.78±5.75
Artery-vein balance	1.00±0.65	0.78±0.45*	0.97±0.15*	0.83±0.37
Circle of Willis (%of separation)	55.35	35.15	39.58	34.76
Auto-regulatory response (myogenic reserve), %	75.18±2.46	66.39±16.35*	83.68±10.45**	72.69±17.54***
Metabolic reserve (index of cerebral vascular reactivity), %	52.41±2.95	29.66±12.98*	59.89±18.01	41.15±21.22

Notes: * - confident differences between indicators of 1st and 2nd groups ($p < 0.05$); ** - confident differences between indicators of 2nd group and 3rd subgroup ($p < 0.05$); *** - confident differences between indicators of 2nd group and 4th subgroup ($p < 0.05$).

In table 3 we present in-hemisphere coherences of different cortex areas of three groups' kick boxers. We found high coherence in frontal lobe, significant coherence in other areas, in left- right side correlations in conditions of apparatus-manual influence "Armos". According to the found coherences kick boxers have rather good functions of prediction, formation of movement's idea, pre-motor programming of movement and its realization. A little less coherence was noticed when influencing on analyzers' systems as well as with visual perception of movements, in which frontal brain artery (FBA), middle brain artery (MBA) and back brain artery (BBA) are engaged. Concerning regulation of movements, in the order of significance frontal lobe, central, parietal and occipital areas are engaged.

Table 3. Indicators of in-hemisphere coherences of alpha rhythm in tested groups

Cortex zones	Background electroencephalogram			Electroencephalogram with hyper-ventilation		
	II, n=62	III, n=40	IV, n=22	II, n=62	III, n=40	IV, n=22
Fp1-Fp2	0.62±0.004	0.66±0.005	0.61±0.007	0.62±0.004	0.68±0.005	0.63±0.006
F3-F4	0.65±0.003	0.69±0.006	0.64±0.007	0.63±0.004	0.67±0.004	0.62±0.006
C3-C4	0.63±0.003	0.70±0.005	0.61±0.008	0.63±0.005	0.64±0.006	0.61±0.007
P3-P4	0.60±0.004	0.67±0.006	0.60±0.007	0.59±0.005	0.62±0.005	0.61±0.006
O1-O2	0.53±0.005	0.61±0.007	0.56±0.008	0.49±0.005	0.54±0.006	0.53±0.007
F7-F8	0.44±0.004	0.52±0.007	0.47±0.008	0.39±0.004	0.42±0.006	0.41±0.007
T3-T4	0.40±0.005	0.46±0.007	0.39±0.008	0.35±0.004	0.36±0.006	0.33±0.007
T5-T6	0.35±0.005	0.39±0.007	0.31±0.008	0.27±0.005	0.25±0.007	0.21±0.008

Notes: Fp1-Fp2 – pole of frontal lobe; F3-F4 – frontal lobe (pre-motor cortex); C3-C4 – central area (motor cortex); P3-P4 –parietal area; O1-O2 –occipital area; F7-F8 – back forehead area (additional motor area); T3-T4 – frontal temple area; T5-T6 – back temple area; * – confidence of differences $p \leq 0.05$.

In 3rd subgroup of kick boxers we registered confident distinction of in-hemisphere coherence from group 2 by central, back forehead, parietal-occipital and temple areas of analyzers' fields. We also found prevailing (by 8-15%) development of 3rd subgroup sportsmen's two motor regulation components: involuntary, caused by sensor stimuli and arbitrary, caused by internal motive.

By alpha frequencies range of kick boxers we studied compatibility degree in short and longs pairs of in-hemisphere coherences (see table 4)

Table 4. Indicators of in-hemispheres' coherences of alpha rhythm in tested groups

Cortex zones	Background EEG			EEG with hyper-ventilation (HV)		
	II, n=62	III, n=40	IV, n=22	II, n=62	III, n=40	IV, n=22
Fp1F3	0.74±0.004	0.75±0.005	0.74±0.006	0.72±0.004	0.74±0.005	0.74±0.006
F3C3	0.71±0.004*	0.76±0.005	0.70±0.007	0.68±0.004	0.72±0.005	0.68±0.006
C3P3	0.67±0.005*	0.73±0.005	0.66±0.006	0.63±0.004	0.69±0.006	0.68±0.006
P3O1	0.65±0.004	0.67±0.006	0.68±0.007	0.65±0.005	0.65±0.006	0.67±0.006
Fp2F4	0.73±0.004*	0.81±0.006	0.79±0.007	0.75±0.004	0.82±0.005	0.79±0.006
F4C4	0.72±0.005	0.72±0.006	0.68±0.008	0.70±0.004	0.71±0.007	0.68±0.007
C4P4	0.65±0.005	0.66±0.007	0.60±0.008	0.63±0.004	0.61±0.006	0.60±0.006
P4O2	0.76±0.005	0.72±0.007	0.65±0.008	0.75±0.004	0.65±0.006	0.61±0.007
F7T3	0.72±0.005	0.75±0.006	0.73±0.008	0.69±0.004	0.71±0.007	0.67±0.007
T3T5	0.60±0.005	0.64±0.006	0.53±0.006	0.55±0.005	0.59±0.007	0.52±0.008
F8T4	0.71±0.005	0.73±0.007	0.69±0.006	0.66±0.005	0.64±0.007	0.66±0.006
T4T6	0.57±0.005	0.61±0.006	0.57±0.007	0.53±0.005	0.54±0.007	0.51±0.007

Notes: * – confident differences form indicator of control group, ** – in groups of sportsmen, $p<0.05$. FpF3 – pre-frontal cortex of frontal lobe from the left; F3C3 – pre-motor cortex of frontal lobe from the left; C3P3 –motor cortex of frontal lobe from the left; P3O1 –parietal-occipital area from the left; Fp2F4 – pre-frontal cortex of frontal lobe from the right; F4C4 – pre-motor cortex of frontal lobe from the right; C4P4 – motor cortex of frontal lobe from the right; P4O2 – parietal-occipital area from the right; F7T3 – forehead-temple area from the left; T3T5 – temple area from the left; F8T4 – forehead-temple area from the right; T4T6 – temple area from the right.

Discussion

In the course of writing the article there appeared some discussible moments. In opinion of M.V. Koroliova [7], increased brain blood circulation is an adequate functional reaction to muscular impacts. They require increased oxygen supply to motor cortex neurons. However, in opinion of Shevtsov A.V. [14] increased brain blood circulation shall be regarded as a state of system's tension, which can result in pre-morbid status and even in pathology of brain blood vessels. It should be added that excessive blood flow trail in rest state requires additional energy supply. Probably, myocardium shall work more intensively. Results of our mutual researches permitted to specify mechanisms of the processes, which take place and take neutral position in this duel of opinions. Actually, Koroliova M.V. is right, thinking that the found in our researches (see table 1) increased blood flow in kick boxers can be regarded as a symptom of working hyperemia. It witnesses about increasing of functional demand of motor neurons depending on the following: the higher neurons' demand in oxygen and glucose are the higher is blood flow. But Shevtsov A.V. is also right to some extent because owing to continuous increase of competition and training functioning's tension in muscular-skeletal apparatus of practically healthy sportsmen different physiological-bio-mechanical disorders are diagnosed. It can become a factor, provoking a number of borderline states of different organs and systems, for example myo-fascial pain syndrome with "trigger" zones, initiating pain, local muscular hyper-tonuses and etc. [11, 26, and 27]. Technique of many kick attacks, especially in kickboxing disciplines "low-kick" and "K1", results in twisting of backbone, when attacking legs, because of torso inertia, one-side overload and over tension of muscular skeletal apparatus. It causes tissues' lesion [6]. In parallel with it trophic dysfunctions of metabolic, autogenic and vascular-vegetative character appear. It results in imbalance of central, periphery and cerebral blood circulation [13]. There appears a question if increase of cerebral haemo-dynamic parameters occurs only as a result of increase of motor neurons' functional demands. The answer was received after rick boxers' recreational correction with device "Armos". Such correction influence on reflex areas in muscular-ligament apparatus of disordered segments, recovers static dynamic disorders of backbone and blocked joints' functions. These manipulations permit to eliminate blockages in joints and muscles with normalization of cerebral blood circulation and improvement of vein outflow. Our experiment showed confident reduction of brain blood circulation velocity parameters. Though, we observed increase of control data. It witnessed in favor of Koroliova's M.V. opinion about working hyperemia in perfusion-metabolic coupling. To the above said it should be added that we had not found referent borders of cerebral blood flow in different areas of localization velocity parameters. Now information material is accumulated, which will permit to analyze differentially localization of linear blood flow velocities. It is the task of next researches.

Conclusions

1. Analysis of indicators of kick boxers' brain cortex bio-electrical activity, fulfilled with technology "Armos", permitted to determine bran resistance to stress impacts and better stability of functional state, comparing with group of kick boxers, who endured classic massage and control group.

2. In hyper-ventilation test we registered increase of inter-hemisphere interaction strength in pre-frontal cortex in group 3. We found confident distinctions from control group in increase of in-hemisphere coherence in forehead pre-frontal cortex from the right by 12% in group 3 and decrease by 15% in right parietal-occipital region in groups 3 and 4.

3. Application of device-manual procedure "Armos" reduced brain blood flow and increased reserves of 3rd group kick boxers' functional system (decrease in right and left middle brain arteries, in right and left back brain arteries, $p \leq 0.001$). Besides, we found increase of blood flow linear velocity (earlier reduced) up to referent borders in right and left backbone arteries ($p \leq 0.001$).

4. We also observed inter-hemisphere asymmetry in middle, front and back brain arteries ($p \leq 0.01$). In resistive indices confident shifts were registered in right and left middle brain arteries, in right and middle back brain arteries; in right and left backbone arteries and main basilar artery.

Conflict of interests

The authors declare that there is no conflict of interests.

References:

1. Bershtejn NA. *Fiziologiia dvizhenij i aktivnost'* [Physiology of movements and activity], Moscow: Science; 1990. (in Russian)
2. Vasil'eva LF. Vozmozhnosti prikladnoj kineziologii v sporte vysshikh dostizhenij [Possibility of applied kinesiology in elite sports]. *Vserossijskaia nauchno-prakticheskaia konferenciia s mezhdunarodnym uchastiem "Prikladnaia kineziologiia v sporte vysshikh dostizhenij"* [All-Russian scientific-practical conference with international participation "Applied kinesiology in elite sports"], Moscow; 2016. P. 10-16. (in Russian)
3. Vasil'eva LF. *Manual'noe myshechnoe testirovanie* [Manual muscular testing], Moscow; 2008. (in Russian)
4. Volynkina NA. Kompensirovannaia kompressiia nervnoj tkani kak prichina snizheniia adaptacionnykh rezervov u sportsmenov [Compensated compression of nervous tissue as the reason of reduction of sportsmen's adaptation reserves]. *Vserossijskaia nauchno-prakticheskaia konferenciia s mezhdunarodnym uchastiem "Prikladnaia kineziologiia v sporte vysshikh dostizhenij"* [All-Russian scientific-practical conference with international participation "Applied kinesiology in elite sports"], Moscow; 2016. P. 54-57. (in Russian)
5. Zhirmunskaia EA. *V poiskakh ob"iasneniia fenomenov EEG* [On explanation of EEG phenomena], Moscow: Biola; 1997. (in Russian)
6. Isaev AP, Lichagina SA, Gatgarov RU. Osobennosti sokratitel'nykh i relaksacionnykh kharakteristik myshc u sportsmenov vysokikh kvalifikacij razlichnykh vidov sporta [Characteristics of contraction and relaxation characteristics of elite sportsmen's muscles of different kinds of sports]. *Teoriia i praktika fizicheskoj kul'tury,* 2006;1:28-33. (in Russian)
7. Koroleva MV, Koroleva VV, Isaev AP, Nenasheva AV. Osobennosti mozgovogo krovoobrashcheniia zhenshchin, vedushchikh aktivnyj obraz zhizni [Brain blood circulation in women, practicing active way of life], *Vestnik IuUrGU*, 2009;27(20):10-15. (in Russian)
8. Kuznecov OV. Vozmozhnosti prikladnoj kineziologii dlia povysheniia effektivnosti rezul'tatov u legkoatletov [Possibilities of applied kinesiology in increase of light athletes' effectiveness]. *Vserossijskaia nauchno-prakticheskaia konferenciia s mezhdunarodnym uchastiem "Prikladnaia kineziologiia v sporte vysshikh dostizhenij"* [All-Russian scientific-practical conference with international participation "Applied kinesiology in elite sports"], Moscow; 2016. P. 17-24. (in Russian)
9. Liv D. *Prikladnaia kineziologiia v sportivnoj medicine* [Applied kinesiology in sports medicine].]. 5-j

mezhdunarodnyj seminar [5th international seminar], Moscow; 2011. P. 80-85. (in Russian)

10. Romanov IuN, Kasymova MF, Redchina OA. Modulirovanie fiziologicheskogo sostoianiia kikbokserov posredstvom vozdejstviia na sensornye, sosudistye i motornye sistemy golovnogo mozga v sisteme integral'noj podgotovki, vliiaiushchej na sportivnuiu rezul'tativnost' [Simulation of kick boxers' physiological state by impact on sensor, vascular and motor systems of brain in system of integral training, influencing on sports efficiency]. *Vestnik IuUrGU*, 2014;14(2):42-51. (in Russian)
11. Sabir'ianov AR, Sabir'ianova ES, Epishev VV. Dinamika variabel'nosti central'nogo krovoobrashcheniia u zdorovykh pod vozdejstviem massazha vorotnikovoj zony [Dynamic of central blood circulation variability of healthy people under influence of collar area massage]. *Voprosy kurortologii, fizioterapii i lechebnoj fizicheskoj kul'tury*, 2004;6:13-15.
12. Sukhorukov OG. Rasshirenie kompensatornykh vozmozhnostej organizma sportsmena pri pomoshchi ustraneniia torzii tverdoj mozgovoj obolochki [Expansion of sportsman organism's compensatory potentials by elimination of dura mater tarsia]. *Vserossijskaia nauchno-prakticheskaia konferenciia s mezhdunarodnym uchastiem "Prikladnaia kineziologiia v sporte vysshikh dostizhenij"* [All-Russian scientific-practical conference with international participation "Applied kinesiology in elite sports"], Moscow; 2016. P. 58-61. (in Russian)
13. Terekhina EN. *Osobennosti funkcional'nogo sostoianiia central'noj nervnoj sistemy i oporno-dvigatel'nogo apparata sportsmenov-bokserov v usloviiakh optimizacii trenirovochnogo processa. Cand. Diss.* [Specific features of boxers' central nervous system and muscular-skeletal apparatus functional state in conditions of optimization of training process. Cand. Diss.], Chelyabinsk; 2007. (in Russian)
14. Shevcov AV, Lichagina SA, Iumaguen VR. Fiziologicheskoe obosnovanie sistemnoj mobilizacii kikbokserov vysshej kvalifikacii v period podgotovki k social'no-znachimym sorevnovaniiam [Physiological substantiation of systemic mobilization of elite kick boxers in period of preparation for solially important competitions], *Vestnik IuUrGU,* 2005;4:33-38. (in Russian)
15. Shitikov TA. Voprosy diagnostiki, korrekcii, reabilitacii posttravmaticheskikh cerebrovaskuliarnykh narushenij u sportsmenov s poziciej prikladnoj kineziologii [Problems of diagnostic, correction and rehabilitation of sportsmen's post traumatic cerebral vascular disorders from positions of applied kinesiology]. *Vserossijskaia nauchno-prakticheskaia konferenciia s mezhdunarodnym uchastiem "Prikladnaia kineziologiia v sporte vysshikh dostizhenij"* [All-Russian scientific-practical conference with international participation "Applied kinesiology in elite sports"], Moscow; 2016. P. 63-67. (in Russian)
16. Chao S, Pacella MJ, Torg JS. The pathomechanics, pathophysiology and prevention of cervical spinal cord and brachial plexus injuries in athletics. *Sports Med.* 2010;40(1): 59–75.
17. Dunn RN, van der Spuy DS. Rugby and cervical spine injuries - has anything changed? A 5-year review in the Western Cape. *Afr Med J.* 2010;100(4):235–238.
18. Engebretsen L, Steffen K, Alonso JM. Sports injuries and illnesses during the Winter Olympic Games 2010. *Br. J. Sports Med.* 2010;44(11):772–780.
19. Gavett BE, Stern RA, McKee AC. Chronic traumatic encephalopathy: a potential late effect of sport-related concussive and subconcussive head trauma. *Clin Sports Med.* 2011;30(1):179–188.
20. Graham MR, Myers T, Evans P. Direct hits to the head during amateur boxing is associated with a rise in serum biomarkers for brain injury. *Int J Immunopathol Pharmacol.* 2011;24(1):119–125.
21. Hasiloglu ZI, Albayram S, Selcuk H, Ceyhan E, Delil S, Arkan B, Baskoy L. Cerebral microhemorrhages detected by susceptibility-weighted imaging in amateur boxers. *AJNR Am J Neuroradiol.* 2011;32(1):99–102.
22. Klimesch W, Sauseng P, Hanslmayr S. EEG alpha oscillation: The inhibition – timing hypothesis. *Brain Res. Rev.* 2007;53:63-88.
23. Rainey CE. Determining the prevalence and assessing the severity of injuries in mixed martial arts athletes. *N Am J Sports Phys Ther.* 2009;4(4):190–199.
24. Rihn JA, Anderson DT, Lamb K. Cervical spine injuries in American football. *Sports Med.* 2009;39(9):697–708.
25. Stern RA, Riley DO, Daneshvar DH, Nowinsk CJ, Cantu RC, McKee AC. Long-term consequences of repetitive brain trauma: chronic traumatic encephalopathy. *PM R.* 2011;3(10):460–467.

PHYSICAL CONDITION OF PEDAGOGIC COLLEGE GIRL STUDENTS UNDER INFLUENCE OF CHEERLEADING EXERCISES

Masliak I.P., Krivoruchko N.V.
Kharkov State Academy of Physical Culture

Abstract. *Purpose:* to determine degree of cheer-leading exercises' influence of physical condition of pedagogic college girl students. *Material:* in the research 385 1st-3rd years girl students participated. Physical condition level of girl students was determined by indicators of body composition harmony (index of Kettle 2), functional potentials of respiratory system, organism's resistance against hypoxia factors (Skibinsky's index), regulation of cardio-vascular system (Robinson's index). Body length and mass, chest, hip and waist circumferential sizes, vital capacity of lungs, breathing pause after inhale (Stanger's test), systolic and diastolic blood pressure, heart beats rate in rest were measured. *Results:* As a result of initial testing "low" level of girl students' physical condition was registered. Age distinctions in the tested indicators were regarded. Positive influence of cheerleading exercises on functional potentials of respiratory system and organism's resistance against hypoxia factors; on regulation of cardio-vascular, system was found. *Conclusions:* Application of cheerleading exercises' in physical education positively influenced on physical condition level of pedagogic college girl students.
Key words: physical condition, physical education, girl students, cheerleading.

Introduction

Recent time the problem of pupils and students' health has been becoming still more important. The data of scientific literature witness that there is steady tendency to worsening of students' health [5, 29], which, to large extent, is determined by physical condition [6]. Physical education takes one of priority places in control over physical condition, in formation of health culture, full and comprehensive development of personality; in cultivation of physical qualities [15, 19]. Traditional knowledge in physical education still less attracts pupils and students. It results in significant reduction of their motor functioning and worsening of health [14, 21, 32]. In this connection, seeking of innovative methods of physical education's optimization in different educational establishments is rather an urgent problem [15, 30].

Analysis of scientific methodic literature showed presence of large quantity of works, devoted to application of non-traditional forms of pupils and students' physical education. In pupils' physical education rugby-5 trainings [37], hiking [35], cheerleading [1], shaping [7] are practiced; in students' physical education [24] – aerobics [20], Pilates and body flex [31], Pranayama Bhastrica [28]. In our opinion, cheerleading is an innovative mean of physical education. Cheer-leading positively influence on physical condition of pre-school age children and physical health and motor functioning of secondary forms' pupils [1-3, 23, 26, 27]; on physical condition and physical workability of girl students [22]; formation of wide motor skills' arsenal in students [9]; on level of physical fitness and functional state of pedagogic educational establishments girl students [36]. Other authors found the following: high interest of pedagogic college girl students to cheer-leading trainings [14]; positive influence of cheer-leading on definite parameters of physical condition [11] and motor abilities [12, 13, 32, and 34].

With it, the question about cheerleading exercises' influence on general physical condition of pedagogic college girl students of 15-17 years' age has been studied insufficiently.

Purpose, tasks of the work, material and methods

The purpose of the work is to determine degree of cheerleading exercises' influence of physical condition of pedagogic college girl students.

The methods of the research are theoretical analysis and generalization of scientific-methodic literature data, medical-biological methods, pedagogic experiment, and methods of mathematical statistic.

Physical condition level of 15-17 years' age girl students was determined by indicators of body composition harmony (index of Kettle 2), functional potentials of respiratory system, organism's resistance against hypoxia factors (Skibinsky's index), regulation of cardio-vascular system (Robinson's index). Body length and mass, chest, hip and waist circumferential sizes, vital capacity of lungs, breathing pause after inhale (Stanger's test), systolic and diastolic blood pressure, heart beats rate in rest were measured.

The research was conducted on base of pedagogic college of Kharkov humanitarian pedagogic institute. In the research 385 1st-3rd years girl students of not physical culture profile participated. They were organized in 3 control and 3 experimental groups: 1st group – 1st year girl students; 2nd group – 2nd year girl students and 3rd group – 3rd year girl students. All girl students related to main and preparatory health groups. In the course of experiment, girl students of control groups were trained as per state program of physical education. In program of experimental groups, cheerleading elements (basic movements, jumps and so on) were included.

Results of the research

Analysis of anthropometrical measurements results showed absence of confident differences between indicators of control and experimental groups' girl students ($p > 0.05$). (See table 1).

Table 1. Anthropometrical indicators of experimental and control groups' girl students before and after experiment

Groups	I		II		III	
	Before experiment	**After experiment**	**Before experiment**	**After experiment**	**Before experiment**	**After experiment**
	Indicators $\overline{X}$ ± m					
	Body length (cm)					
n	*75*		*108*		*95*	
Experimental	163.4± 0.66	164.1± 0.65	163,9± 0.50	164.1± 0.50	164.4± 0.52	164.5± 0.51
n	*23*			*34*		*50*
Control	163.0± 1.41	164.1± 1.32	164.3± 1.14	165.5± 1.11	162.9± 0.68	163.0± 0.68
t	0.27	0.03	1.12	1.15	1.77	1.74
p	>0.05	>0.05	>0.05	>0.05	>0.05	>0.05
	Body mass (kg)					
Experimental	54.49± 0.39	55.03± 0.34	56.95± 0.69	56.53± 0.62	58.48± 0.63	58.03± 0.58
Control	54.00± 1.76	54.87± 1.64	55.41± 1.13	55.71± 1.03	59.55± 0.88	59.47± 0.80
t	0.62	0.09	1.16	0.68	0.98	1.45
p	>0.05	>0.05	>0.05	>0.05	>0.05	>0.05
	Circumference of chest (cm)					
Experimental	85.43± 0.48	85.59± 0.47	86.21± 0.49	86.50± 0.50	87.33± 0.57	87.71± 0.55
Control	84.87± 1.08	85.13± 1.01	86.10± 1.01	86.62± 0.93	87.24± 0.83	87.52± 0.83
t	0.47	0.41	0.09	0.11	0.09	0.19
p	>0.05	>0.05	>0.05	>0.05	>0.05	>0.05
	Circumference of waist (cm)					
Experimental	68.46± 0.48	68.56± 0,47	69.32± 0.60	68.94± 0.53	69.78± 0.54	69.18± 0.55
Control	67.28± 1.38	67.61± 1.30	69.15± 0.99	69.57± 0.91	68.55± 0.84	69.04± 0.80
t	0.81	0.69	0.15	0.60	1.24	0.14
p	>0.05	>0.05	>0.05	>0.05	>0.05	>0.05
	Circumference of hip (cm)					
Experimental	53.75± 0.40	53.83± 0.40	53.70± 0.38	53.71± 0.42	54.72± 0.45	54.57± 0.45

Control	52.98± 0.88	53.13± 0.83	53.99± 0.76	54.37± 0.68	54.93± 0.66	55.01± 0.61
t	0.79	0.76	0.33	0.82	0.27	0.59
p	>0.05	>0.05	>0.05	>0.05	>0.05	>0.05

Analysis of the received indicators in age aspect showed that with age they increase (though not always confidently, p>0.05). Confident differences were observed between indicators of body mass of 1st and 3rd experimental groups' girl students, 1st and 2nd experimental groups and 2nd and 3rd control groups. The same concerns chest circumference in 1st and 3rd experimental groups (differences were confident, p <0.01 – 0.001).

As per indicators of body composition's harmony (index of Kettle 2) and assessment scale [17] girl students of all tested groups correspond to mark 1 point ("corpulent body composition"). After application of cheerleading exercises at physical culture lessons (see table 1) anthropometrical indicators did not change substantially in experimental and control groups (p>0.05). Repeated calculation of Kettle 2 index also did not result in significant changes. Thus, application of specially selected cheerleading exercises in pedagogic college 1st -3rd year girl students' physical education did not influence noticeable on harmony of body composition.

Analysis of indicators of respiratory system functional state (see table 2) showed absence of confident differences between control and experimental groups' girl students (p> 0.05).

Table 2. Indicators of respiratory system's functional state of experimental and control groups' girl students before and after experiment

Groups	**I**		**II**		**III**	
	Before experiment	**After experiment**	**Before experiment**	**After experiment**	**Before experiment**	**After experiment**
	Indicators $\overline{X}$ ± m					
	Vital capacity of lungs (l)					
n	*75*		*108*		*95*	
Experimental	2,61± 0.05	2.78± 0.04	2.70± 0.04	2.86± 0.03	2.76± 0.05	2.95± 0.05
n		*23*		*34*		*50*
Control	2.67± 0.07	2.78± 0.07	2.72± 0.07	2.81± 0.07	2.76± 0.06	2.83± 0.06
t	0.65	0.02	0.26	0.56	0.03	1.58
p	>0.05	>0.05	>0.05	>0.05	>0.05	>0.05
	Stanger's test (sec)					
Experimental	29.40± 0.59	32.05± 0.54	30.32± 0.75	32.51± 0.70	27.92± 0.65	30.96± 0.55
Control	29.48± 1.17	31.96± 1.14	30.71± 0.97	32.03± 0.84	28.70± 0.79	30.36± 0.74
t	0.06	0.08	0.31	0.44	0.77	0.65
p	>0.05	>0.05	>0.05	>0.05	>0.05	>0.05

Analysis of the mentioned data in age aspect showed that with age vital capacity of lungs improves (differences are not confident. p>0.05). Exclusions are results of 1st and 3rd experimental groups (differences are confident, p<0.05). Analysis of Stanger' test showed wave and not confident character (p> 0.05). Exclusion were indicators of 2nd and 3rd experimental groups' girl students, where differences were confident, p<0.05).

Comparing received results by Skibinsky's index with assessment scale [17] we found that indicators of girl students of all tested groups corresponded to 2 points (level "below average"). After application of specially selected cheerleading exercises at physical culture lessons (see table 2) it was found that all indicators of respiratory system of experimental groups' girl students significantly improved (changes were confident, p<0.05–0.001). The most expressed improvement was in 17 years' girls.

The same analysis of control groups' results showed that they also improved a little. However, these changes were not confident, p>0.05. Analysis of secondary indicators in age aspect showed absence of significant changes in comparison with initial data. Exclusions were indicators of Stanger's test in 2nd and 3rd experimental groups (though differences were not confident, p>0.05). Comparing of results of Skibinsly's index calculation with assessment scale [17] showed improvement of experimental groups' results by 1 point ("average" level). In control groups there were no changes by assessment criteria.

Thus, application of specially selected cheerleading exercises positively influenced on functioning of respiratory system of pedagogic college girl students. The most noticeable improvements were in 17 years' girl students. Analysis of cardio-vascular system's indicators (see table 3) permitted to determine absence of confident differences between experimental and control groups girl students (p> 0.05).

Table 3. Indicators of cardio-vascular system's functional state of experimental and control groups' girl students before and after experiment

Groups	I		II		III	
	Before experiment	After experiment	Before experiment	After experiment	Before experiment	After experiment
	Indicators $\overline{X} \pm m$					
n	*75*		*108*		*95*	
	Systolic blood pressure (mm of merc.col.)					
Experimental	111.2± 0.94	110.5± 0.88	112.1± 0.95	112.4± 0.72	114.3± 0.90	114.5± 0.69
Control	11.,2± 1.42	119.8± 1.80	113.4± 1.15	11.,2± 1.03	115.7± 1.08	115.3± 0.87
t	0.58	0.37	0,87	0.66	0.99	0.74
p	>0.05	>0.05	>0.05	>0.05	>0.05	>0.05
	Diastolic blood pressure (mm of merc.col.)					
Experimental	66.93± 0.58	66.53± 0.49	70.46± 0.71	70.42± 0.53	72.00± 0.76	71.42± 0.54
Control	65.22± 1.22	65.00± 0.96	69.41± 1.31	69.85± 1.04	73.50± 0.85	74.90± 0.61
t	1.27	1.42	0.70	0.48	1.32	4.24
p	>0.05	>0.05	>0.05	>0.05	>0.05	<0.001
	Heart beats rate (b.p.m. $^{-1}$)					
Experimental	80.28± 1.21	77.27± 1.01	82.06± 0.94	77.72± 0.80	79.43± 0.99	75.11± 1.08
Control	81.57± 2.03	79.35± 1.66	83.26± 1.70	81.68± 1.45	77.50± 1.51	75.48± 1.32
t	0.54	1.07	0.62	2.39	1.07	0.22
p	>0.05	>0.05	>0.05	<0.01	>0.05	>0.05

Analysis of indicators of cardio-vascular system in experimental and control groups in age aspect permitted to find that blood pressure indicators increase with age. With it, differences between systolic pressure indicators are not confident ($p > 0.05$). Results of diastolic pressure were confident ($p<0.05$–0.001). Analysis of heartbeats rate data showed that there were no age distinctions ($p>0.05$). Exclusions were only results of 2nd and 3rd groups' girl students, differences between which were confident ($p<0.05$). Analysis of cardio-vascular system's regulation by Robinson's index [17] permitted to determine that indicators of girl students of all tested groups corresponded to 3 points ("average" level).

Application of specially selected cheerleading (see table 3) exercises positively influenced on functional state of cardio-vascular system of experimental groups' girl students (though changes were mainly not confident, $p>0.05$). Confident changes were observed only in heartbeats rate indicators of 2nd and 3rd age groups ($p<0.05$ – 0.001). Analysis of repeated data in age aspect did not show substantial distinctions, comparing with initial data.

Comparing of secondary results of Robinson's index calculation with assessment scale [17] showed increase of experimental groups' indicators by 1 point and mark became 4 points (level "above average"). In control groups, no changes by assessment criteria were observed.

Thus, application of specially selected cheerleading exercises in physical education of pedagogic college 1st-3rd year girl students positively influenced on functional state of cardio-vascular system of girl students.

Analysis of girl students' initial physical condition (body composition harmony, functional state of respiratory and cardio-vascular systems) showed that it corresponded to 2 points (level "below average") in all tested groups. The same comparison of data after experiment showed increase of physical condition in experimental groups. It became equal to 3 points ("average" level). In control groups there were no changes as per assessment scale. Thus, implementation of cheerleading exercises in physical education process influenced positively on experimental groups' girl students physical condition.

Discussion

Analysis of scientific-methodic literature showed that there was insignificant quantity of works, devoted to influence of cheerleading on girl students' functional state. Some works study cheer-leading influence on physical condition of pre-school age children [23], on girl students of technical university [22] and humanitarian pedagogic academy [36]; on physical health of secondary forms' pupils [1, 2, 27].

Basing on analysis and generalization of our research's results we found that implementation of cheer-leading exercises in physical education of 1st-3rd year girl students did not influence noticeably on anthropometrical indicators ($p>0.05$). It coincides with the data, presented in works of number of authors [8, 10, and 25]. The authors note that the tested age period is characterized by completion of growth and organism's formation processes. Most of body dimensions reach final value. That is why in this age rational physical load does not noticeably influence on them.

Analysis of respiratory system's indicators after application of cheerleading exercises permitted to state that in experimental groups they significantly and confidently improved ($p<0.05$–0.001). In the tested control groups parameters of functional state of respiratory system also improved to some extent, but not expressively and not confidently, ($p>0.05$). The received results are consistent with other authors' researches [1, 2, 27, and 36]. We found positive influence of different kinds of cheerleading on respiratory system functioning in secondary forms' pupils and in students of higher educational establishments. It is explained by the fact that with systemic practicing of physical exercises oxygen consumption increases significantly, blood circulation improves, metabolism is activated and functional potentials of respiratory system are indirectly strengthened.

Analysis of cardio-vascular system's indicators after experiment showed that in experimental groups they improved (though, mainly, not confidently, $p>0.05$). Confident character of changes was observed only in 2nd and 3rd age groups ($p<0.05$ – 0.001). In this case we observed general tendency to reduction of heart beats rate. In control groups results also improved a little (they were not confident ($p>0.05$). The received data are consistent with the data of other authors [1, 2, and 27]. These authors found that cheerleading exercises did not confidently influenced on functioning of cardio-vascular system of secondary school age children. Besides, they noted a general tendency to reduction of heart beats rate. The above said is confirmed by the data of I.I. Zemtsova [8]. The author says that systemic practicing of physical exercises for endurance reduces heartbeats rate. These changes witness about economic character of heart functioning, strengthening of its reserves and are consistent with main laws of age development.

As a result of our researches, it was found that implementation of cheerleading exercises in physical education process of pedagogic college girl students positively influenced on general physical condition level of the tested experimental groups. This level increased from "below average" to "average" level. In the tested control groups, no changes in physical condition were registered. The received results are consistent with the data of other authors. These authors affirm that such changes are observed in secondary forms' pupils [1, 2, and 27] and in higher educational establishment's students [22, 36].

Thus, on the base of analysis and generalization of our research's results we supplemented the data of T.M. Bala, I.P. Masliak [3, 26], I.A. Zinchenko [9], N.V. Krivoruchko, I.P. Masliak, I.N. Zhuravliova [11-13, 32, 34] about influence of cheerleading on different spheres of trainees' life activity. Besides, we confirmed the data of T.M> Bala, I.P. Masliak [1, 2, 27], V. Piatnitskaya [36], O.V. Timopheyeva. [22] about positive impact of cheer-leading on parameters of trainees' physical condition. For the first time we determined influence of cheerleading exercises on general level of physical condition of pedagogic college girl students. Besides, we found the most sensitive to cheerleading organism's systems and the most favorable age periods for improvement of physical condition by means of cheerleading.

Conclusions

1. As a result of initial testing, we registered "low" level of 15-17 years' age girl students' physical condition.
2. Application of cheerleading exercises in physical education process positively influenced on physical condition level of pedagogic college girl students.

The further researches in this direction can be realized by determination of cheerleading exercises' influence on girl students' physical fitness.

Acknowledgement

The researches were conducted in compliance with topical plan of scientific and research works of Kharkov state academy of physical culture for 2013-2015, by topic 3.5.29. "Theoretical and applied principles of building of physical condition and physical fitness monitoring in different population strata".

Conflict of interests

The authors declare that there is no conflict of interests.

References:

1. Bala TM, Masliak IP. Zmina rivnia fizichnogo zdorov'ia shkoliariv 5-6-kh klasiv pid vplivom vprav cherlidinga [Change of physical health level of 5-6 forms' pupils under influence of cheer-leading exercises]. *Moloda sportivna nauka Ukraini*, 2011; 15: 10-15. (in Ukrainian)
2. Bala TM, Masliak IP. Zmina rivnia fizichnogo zdorov'ia shkoliariv 7-9-kh klasiv pid vplivom vprav cherlidinga [Change of physical health level of 7-9 forms' pupils under influence of cheer-leading exercises]. *Sportivnij visnik Pridniprov'ia*, 2011; 2: 21-23. (in Ukrainian)
3. Bala TM, Masliak IP. *Chirliding u fizichnomu vikhovanni shkoliariv* [Cheer-leading in physical educationof pupils], Kharkov; 2014 (in Ukrainian)
4. Bezverkhnia GV, Maievs'kij MI. Motivaciia do zaniat' fizichnim vikhovanniam studentok pedagogichnikh special'nostej [Motivation of pedagogic specialties' girl students for physical education]. *Slobozhans'kij naukovo-sportivnij visnik,* 2015; 2: 28-33. (in Ukrainian)
5. Budag'ianc GM. Zdorov'ia starshoklasnikiv i jogo zalezhnist' vid zovnishn'ogo otochuiuchogo seredovishcha [Health of senior pupils and its dependence on surrounding medium]. *Pedagogics, psychology, medical-biological problems of physical training and sports,* 2010; 8: 15-17. (in Ukrainian)
6. Ermakov SS, Apanasenko GL, Bondarenko TV, Prasol SD. Fizicheskaia kul'tura – osnovnoj instrument kul'tury zdorov'ia [Physical culture as main tool of health culture]. *Pedagogics, psychology, medical-biological problems of physical training and sports,* 2010; 11: 31-33. (in Ukrainian)
7. Zhdanova OM, Chekhovs'ka LIa, Shevciv US. Zmini antropometrichnikh pokaznikiv divchat-starshoklasnic' pid vplivom urokiv shejpingu [Change of anthropometrical indicators of senior schoolgirls

under influence of shaping trainings]. *Slobozhans'kij naukovo-sportivnij visnik*, 2008; 3: 11-13. (in Ukrainian)

8. Zemcova II. *Sportivna fiziologiia* [Sports physiology], Kiev, Olympic literature; 2008 (in Ukrainian)
9. Zinchenko IA. *Pobudova trenuval'nogo procesu sportsmeniv u cherlidingu na etapi specializovanoi bazovoi pidgotovki. Cand. Diss.* [Building of sportsmen's training process in cheer-leading on stage of specialized basic training. Cand. Diss.], Kharkov; 2013 (in Ukrainian)
10. Zilov VG, Smirnov VM. *Fiziologiia detej i podrostkov* [Physiology of children and adolescents], Moscow, Medical News Agency; 2008. (in Russian)
11. Krivoruchko NV. Vpliv vprav chirlidingu na pokazniki fizichnogo rozvitku studentok VNZ I-II rivnia akreditacii [Influence of cheer-leading exercises on physical condition indicators of girl students of 1st, 2nd accreditation levels' HEEs], *Moloda sportivna nauka Ukraini*, 2013; 19: 119–124. (in Ukrainian)
12. Krivoruchko N, Masliak I. Dinamika pokaznikiv rozvitku koordinacijnikh zdibnostej studentiv VNZ pid vplivom vprav chirlidingu [Dynamic of indicators of coordination abilities of HEE students under influence of cheer-leading exercises]. *Moloda sportivna nauka Ukraini*, 2013; 17: 87-91. (in Ukrainian)
13. Krivoruchko N, Masliak I. Dinamika pokazatelej urovnia razvitiia gibkosti pod vliianiem uprazhnenij chirlidinga [Dynamic of flexibility indicators under influence of cheer-leading exercises]. *Physical education and sport,* 2015;1:145-147. (in Russian)
14. Krivoruchko N. V. Doslidzhennia vidnoshennia studentok vishchogo navchal'nogo zakladu I-II rivnia akreditacii do zaniat' z fizichnogo vikhovannia [Study of 1st-2nd accreditation levels' HEEs girl students' attitude to physical education lessons]. *Slobozhans'kij naukovo-sportivnij visnik*, 2011; 2: 25-28. (in Ukrainian)
15. Masliak IP, Mameshina MA, Zhuk VO. Stan vikoristannia innovacijnikh pidkhodiv u fizichnomu vikhovanni oblasnikh zagal'noosvitnikh navchal'nikh zakladiv [Application of innovative approaches to physical education in regional comprehensive educational establishments]. *Slobozhans'kij naukovo-sportivnij visnik*, 2014; 6 (44): 69-72. (in Ukrainian)
16. Matveev L. P. *Teoriia i metodika fizicheskoj kul'tury* [Theory and methodic of physical culture]. Moscow; 2004 (in Russian)
17. Poliakov SD, Khrushchev SV., Korneeva IT. *Monitoring i korrekciia fizicheskogo zdorov'ia shkol'nikov* [Monitoring and correction of pupils' physical health], Moscow; 2006 (in Russian)
18. Sinicia S, Shesterova LIe. Dinamika morfo-funkcional'nikh pokaznikiv studentok pid vplivom zaniat' ozdorovchoiu aerobikoiu [Dynamic of morphological-functional indicators of girl students under influence of health related aerobic trainings]. *Teoriia ta metodika fizichnogo vikhovannia i sportu*, 2011; 3: 78-83. (in Ukrainian)
19. Solovej A, Rimar O. Viznachennia osoblivostej motivacii do zaniat' fizichnimi vpravami studentiv vishchikh navchal'nkh zakladiv III-IV rivniv akreditacii [Determination of 3rd-4th accreditation HEES' students' motivation for physical exercises practicing]. *Moloda sportivna nauka Ukraini*, 2012; 2: 194-198. (in Ukrainian)
20. Sichova T, Koriagina O. Zmicnennia zdorov'ia studentok zasobami tanciuval'noi aerobiki [Strengthening of girl students' health by means of dance aerobic]. *Sportivnij visnik Pridniprov'ia*, 2013; 2: 176-179. (in Ukrainian)
21. Sichova T. Stavlennia studentok do zaniat' fizichnogo vikhovannia u vishchomu navchal'nomu zakladi [Attitude of girl students to physical education classes in higher educational establishment]. *Moloda sportivna nauka Ukraini*, 2011; 2: 233-236. (in Ukrainian)
22. Timofeeva OV. Chirliding v sisteme fizicheskogo vospitaniia studentok [Cheer-leading in system of girl students' physical education]. *Teoriia i praktika fizicheskoj kul'tury*, 2008; 11: 36-38. (in Russian)
23. Timofeeva TN, Tatarinova OO, Vladimirovna SM. Cherliding dlia doshkol'nikov [Cheer-leading for pre-school age children]. *Detskij sad: teoriia i praktika*, 2011; 10: 68-75. (in Russian)
24. Usachov Iu. Osoblivosti morfofunkcional'nogo stanu divchat, iaki zajmaiut'sia ozdorovchim fitnesom [Characteristics of morphological functional state of girls, who practice health related fitness]. *Teoriia ta metodika fizichnogo vikhovannia i sportu,* 2007; 3: 86-89. (in Ukrainian)

25. Fomin NA. *Fiziologiia cheloveka* [Physiology of man], Moscow, Education; 1982 (in Russian)
26. Bala T. Change in the level of strength and endurance development of 5-6 grades pupils under cheerleading exercises influence. *Slobozhanskyi herald of science and sport*, 2015; 3: 14-18.
27. Bala TM. The influence of cheerleading exercises on the schoolchildren's physical health of 5-9th forms. *Pedagogics, psychology, medical-biological problems of physical training and sports,* 2012; 4: 12-16.
28. Baljinder Singh Bal. Effects of short term practice of bhastrika pranayama on metabolic fitness (metf) and bone integrity (BI). *Pedagogics, psychology, medical-biological problems of physical training and sports*, 2015;7:72-78. http://dx.doi.org/10.15561/18189172.2015.07100
29. Garkusha SV. Current trends in the health of children and young people in learning environments. *Pedagogics, psychology, medical-biological problems of physical training and sports*, 2013;10:7-11. http://dx.doi.org/10.6084/m9.figshare.775315
30. Gruzhevsky VA. Appropriateness of the use of innovative technologies in the formation of personality oriented motivation of students to physical education. *Pedagogics, psychology, medical-biological problems of physical training and sports*, 2014;3:19-24. http://dx.doi.org/10.6084/m9.figshare.936958
31. Kozina ZhL, Ilnizaya AS, Kolomiez NA, Barybina LN, Cieślicka Mirosława, Stankiewicz Błażej, Pilewska Wiesława. Effects of integrated improving technique pilates and bodyflex level of functionality on students. *Pedagogics, psychology, medical-biological problems of physical training and sports*, 2014;1:24-30. http://dx.doi.org/10.6084/m9.figshare.899192
32. Kryvoruchko NV, Masljak IP, Zhuravlyova IN. Impact on the display of power cheerleading ability of university students I-II levels of accreditation. *Pedagogics, psychology, medical-biological problems of physical training and sports*, 2013;9:38-42. http://dx.doi.org/10.6084/m9.figshare.749696
33. Lachno OG. Motivation for physical culture as factor of students' functional state optimization. *Physical Education of Students*, 2015;5:31-38. http://dx.doi.org/10.15561/20755279.2015.0505
34. Masliak IP. Quickness and endurance fitness of pedagogic college girl students under influence of cheerleading. *Physical Education of Students*, 2015;4:24-30. http://dx.doi.org/10.15561/20755279.2015.0404
35. Mulyk KV, Grynova TI. Influence of hiking trainings on 13 years old adolescents' health. *Pedagogics, psychology, medical-biological problems of physical training and sports*, 2015;8:40-44. http://dx.doi.org/10.15561/18189172.2015.0806
36. Pyatnickaya DV. Development of girl-students' physical qualities at extracurricular cheer-dance classes (cheer-dance show). *Physical Education of Students*, 2015;4:31-38. http://dx.doi.org/10.15561/20755279.2015.0405
37. Filenko LV, Filenko IU, Martirosyan AA. Research of indexes of physical development, physical preparedness and functional state of students aged 10-11 years under the influence of engagement in rugby-5. *Pedagogics, psychology, medical-biological problems of physical training and sports*, 2013;6:53-58. http://dx.doi.org/10.6084/m9.figshare.714940

30

PHYSICAL WORKABILITY AS THE BASE OF STUDENTS' FUNCTIONAL POTENTIALS

Samokih I.I.
Odessa National O. S. Popov Academy of Telecommunications

Abstract. *Purpose:* to assess the level of students' physical workability and find its connection with physical fitness. *Material:* we tested 150 students (86 girls and 64 boys) of 17-19 years' age. All students were in main health group. The students fulfilled test on stationary bicycle. The complex of tests for physical fitness was used. *Results:* it was found that boys' physical workability results were better than girls'. Analysis of correlation matrix showed that physical workability parameters had close correlations with physical workability. Exception was only some pedagogic tests for explosive power of arms and torso as well as flexibility. *Conclusions:* physical workability indicators were within age and gender standards. Analysis of correlations showed that physical workability parameters substantially influence on results of control tests for physical fitness.
Key words: physical, workability, fitness, functional, testing, students, correlation.

Introduction

It was found that physical workability indicators are the base of functional potentials. Physical workability is an integral indicator, which permits to determine coordinated work of organism's organs and systems, health state, physical condition and functional state of human organism [2, 5]. It is known that physical workability depends on a number of factors, which determine and limit it. Demand in determination of the so-called dynamic health is also paid attention to [1].

In pedagogic researches the main source of information about functional potentials is different test batteries for physical fitness. The same situation exists in physical education process in different educational establishments. In physical education control exercises for physical fitness are used as main criterion of students' functional potentials [11, 12]. When creating factorial structure of girl-students (17-18, 18-19, and 19-20 years' age) functional potentials it is necessary to consider the following indicators: physical condition, physical fitness, physical workability, energy level, cardio-vascular system's condition, effectiveness of cardio functioning regulation and central nervous system [4]. Cardio vascular system's functioning influences on general endurance, speed-power abilities and coordination [15].

In other works it was noted:

- Determination of dynamic of students' somatic health, physical condition, physical and mental workability changes under impact of comprehensive school load [29];
- Substantiation of basketball and volleyball health related influence on functional state of first year students' visual analyzer in period of their adaptation to learning loads. Application of visual trainings at physical education classes permits to improve visual analyzer's indicators [18];
- Control of physical functioning in out-of-class time and at curriculum lessons [24];
- Purposefulness of fitness-yoga for strengthening of psycho-physical and psycho-social state of special health group girl-students at physical culture recreational and training classes [31];
- Raising of schoolchildren's motor fitness through pedagogic control t physical culture lessons [21, 28];
- Weakening of harmful habits' influence on students' workability 25, 26];
- Increase of students' mental workability [20, 27];
- Consideration of perceived tension under game loads [23].

The authors note that:

- Physical workability dynamic depends on period of week and terms of students' studying at educational establishments [30];
- The most important factors in complex fitness of physical rehabilitation group students are power and functional potentials [32];
- Application of modified variant of Harvard step-test permits to completely assess functional potentials of

students with deviations in their health [22];

– Application of oriental gymnastics increase students' physical workability [19].

By completeness of information physical fitness indicators yield the data of physical workability. Especially it concerns the data, received with the help of modern functional tests. However, pedagogic control exercises inform about condition of certain physical qualities.

Physical fitness and physical workability complex study [5] permits to wider assess functioning of children and youth's organisms. In physical culture lessons at educational establishments the received data will permit for teacher and instructor to control educational process at higher quality as well as to have more exact information about pupils/students' physical condition.

For better understanding the structure and correlations of functional potentials' parameters it is necessary to fulfill comparative analysis. When realizing pair correlation it is possible to analyze inter-influence of separate components within certain structure.

The purpose of the work is to assess 17-19 years' age students' physical workability within physical education process and determine its interconnection with physical fitness.

Material and methods

Participants: we tested 150 students (86 girls and 64 boys) of 17-19 years' age. All students were in main health group.

Procedure: for determination of physical workability we used methodic by D.N. Davidenko et al [5]. The students fulfilled test on stationary bicycle (60 rpm $^{-1}$). Load intensity changed with permanent speed (200 kg.m.min $^{-1}$) by closed cycle: first – from zero to heart beats rate (HBR) 153-155 bpm^{-1} (the moment of reverse); then at the same speed it reduced to zero (see fig.1). For this methodic modern software was created [2], which permitted to quicker receive the required information.

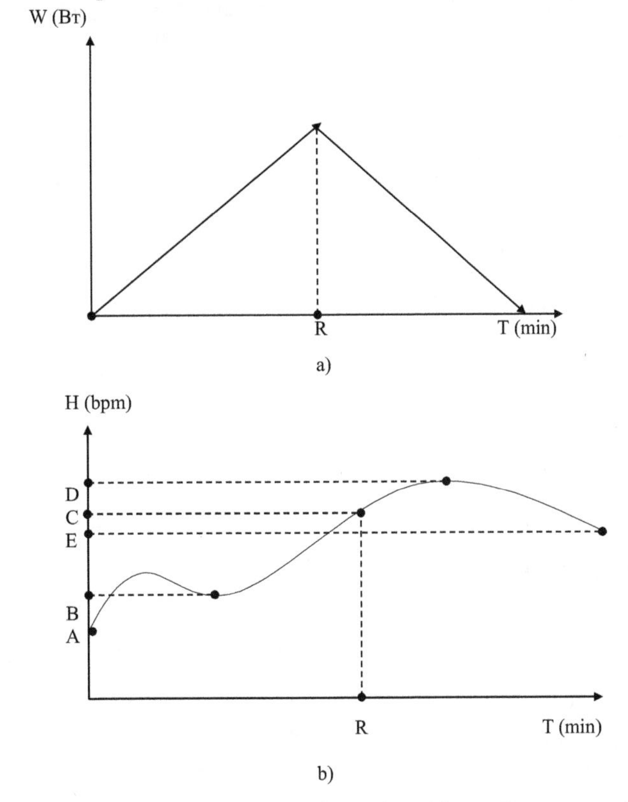

Fig.1. Dynamic of stationary bicycle load (upper part of figure) and heart beats rate changes during test (lower part of figure): W – power of load; R – power of load at reverse; T – time of testing; H – heart beats rate (HBR); A – initial HBR; B – threshold HBR; C – reverse HBR; D – maximal HBR; E – HBR of coming out of load.

The testing was conducted in the following way:

- Sensors of pulse were fixed on student's body;
- Student took seat on stationary bicycle and adapted to appropriate conditions during several minutes;
- Student started to fulfill test according to methodic;
- After test student was on stationary bicycle 1 minute more for recreation.

In the process of testing correlation of heart beats rate and physical load's power were registered in the form of hysteretic loop. Hysteretic loop reflects organism's systemic adaptation to physical load (see fig.2).

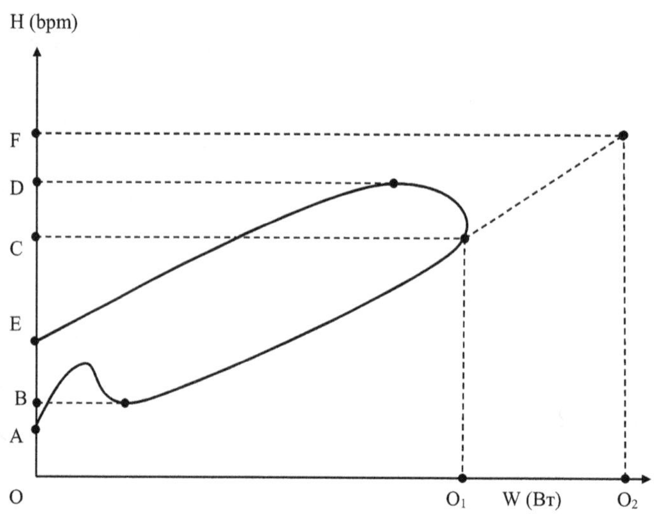

Fig.2. Dynamic of heart beats rate in functional testing: H – heart beats rate (HBR); W – power of load; A – initial HBR; B – threshold HBR; C – reverse HBR; D – maximal HBR; E – HBR of coming out of load. F –HBR=170 bpm^{-1}.

The methodic permits to assess the components of systemic organism's reaction: functions tension under load test; energy and regulatory components of systemic organism's reaction; general physical workability (see table 1).

Table 1. Indicators of physical workability

Indicators	**Description of indicators**
T_{tot}, sec.	Period of work during testing
W_{rev}, Watt	Physical workability at HBR = 153-155 bpm^{-1} (the moment of load reverse). To be determined by segment O-O_1 in fig.2.
A_{tot}, kJ	Scope of work during testing. To be determined by formula: $A_{tot} = W_{rev} \bullet T_{gen}/2$.
PWC_{170}, Watt	Level of physical workability at HBR = 170 bpm^{-1}. To be determined by segment O-O_1 in fig.2.

Test battery for functional fitness included the following control exercises: 30 meters' run; 60 meters' run; 1000 meters' run; shuttle run (4×9 m); long jump from the spot; high jump from the spot; triple jump from the spot; legs' raising during 30 sec. lying on back; throw of filled ball from sitting position (ball mass – 1 kg); pressing ups; torso bending from sitting position with feet apart.

Statistical analysis: experimental data were processed with statistical programs SPSS 16. For every studied parameter we determined mean arithmetic (M), error of mean arithmetic (m). In our work we used correlation (by Pearson) analysis. The confidence of the received results was checked by application of standard diagnostic methodic (Student's t-criterion).

Results of the research

In our research we received the following data (see table 2).

Total time of work fulfillment (T_{tot}) of girl students was 442±13.6 sec., of boy students – 535.05±14.1 sec. Average difference between them was 93.4 sec. Scope of fulfilled work (A_{tot}) in girls' group was within 18.4±0.4 kJ, and boys'– 27.9±0.5 kJ. The distinctions of the received results was confident at $p < 0.001$ and was within 9.5 kJ.

It should be noted that determination of PWC_{170} indicators by the offered methodic is the most accurate. When predicting this indicator, we used great number of points on graph. Other methods are less confident. For example, determination of PWC_{170} with the help of one-moment and two-moment functional tests [9].

Table 2. Indicators of 17-19 years' age students (M±m)

Indicators	Girls (n=86)	Boys (n=64)
T_{tot}, sec.	442.1±13.6	535.5±14.1**
A_{tot}, kJ	18.4±0.4	27.9±0.5**
PWC_{170}, W	109.2±4.4	152.1±4.9**
PWC_{170}/kg, BW•kg^{-1}	1.64±0.08	1.85±0.09
W_{rev}, W	82.4±2.5	109.1±3.2**
MOC, ml•min^{-1}	2348.6±67	3069.7±81**
MOC, ml•min^{-1}. kg^{-1}	35.2±1.1	38.6±1.4*

Notes: * – $p < 0.05$; ** – $p < 0.01$; T_{tot} – total time of work fulfillment; A_{tot} – total scope of fulfilled work; W_{rev} – load power at the moment of reverse; MOC – maximal oxygen consumption.

PWC_{170} indicator of girl-students-beginners was 109.2±4.4 W and boy students – by 42.9 W more (152.1±4.9 W). According to the offered in literature physical workability standards [9] the received data in the whole corresponded to average level. After recalculation of PWC_{170} indicator on 1 kg of body mass we can see that in girls it was less (1.64±0.08 W.kg^{-1}) comparing with boys (1.85±0.09 W•kg^{-1}). However, the difference between them was unconfident. Load power at the moment of reverse (W_{rev}): the data of girls were 82.4±2.5 W and boys – 109.1±3.2; difference was within 26.7 W (practically at level of standard deviation in both groups).

The leading indicator of physical workability is maximal oxygen consumption (MOC), which is determined by efficiency of cardio-respiratory system. PWC_{170} value and MOC level determine human physical workability. However, these indicators are directly interconnected. V.L. Karpman et al. [9] determined this connection by formula:

For not-trained:

$$MOC = 1.7 \cdot PWC_{170} + 1240, \text{ if } PWC170 < 900 \text{ kg} \cdot \text{m} \cdot \text{min}^{-1};$$

For trained:

$$MOC = 2.2 \cdot PWC_{170} + 1070, \text{ if } PWC170 \geq 900 \text{ kg} \cdot \text{m} \cdot \text{min}^{-1}.$$

The calculated MOC values have error up to ±15% from MOC value, received by direct method.

When fulfilling muscular work the girl-students' MOC was 2348.6±67 ml•min^{-1}. The boys' MOC was 3069.7±81 ml•min^{-1}. Relative MOC indicators and relative PWC_{170} values were at lower border of norm 9].

The data of physical fitness and physical workability correlation analysis are given in table 3.

Correlation analysis permitted to find numerous direct and reverse correlations between appropriate groups of indicators. For example in first years' students we found significant reverse correlations between most of physical workability parameters, such as: total time of work (T_{tot}), power of load at the moment of reverse W_{rev}), PWC_{170}, PWC_{170}/kg; total scope of fulfilled work (A_{tot})) and run tests, which give information about the whole spectrum of motor abilities (speed and speed-power qualities, dexterity, general endurance). We found weak negative correlation, first of all with short distances run (r = -0.22÷-0.44), moderate strength of correlations (r = -0.5÷-0.69) mainly with 1000meters' run and shuttle run (4×9 m), except some cases, where weak correlation prevailed (PWC_{170} – 'shuttle run (4×9m)" (r = -0.35), PWC_{170} – "1000 meters' run" (r = -0.44), PWC_{170}/kg – "1000 meters' run" (r = -0.38)) and strong correlation between control exercise for endurance and total scope of fulfilled work (r = -0.72).

Table 3. Correlation between physical workability and physical fitness indicators of 17-19 years' age students (n=150)

Indicators	T_{tot}, c	W_{prev}, W	PWC_{170}, W	$PWC_{170/kg}$, W•kg^{-1}	A_{tot}, kJ
30 meters' run	-03*	-0.26*	-	-0.36*	-0.39*
30 meters' run (from running), sec.	-	-0.24*	-	-0.22*	-
60 meters' run, sec.	-0.41**	-0.33*	-0.32*	-0.39**	-0.44**
Forward torso bending, in sitting position with feet apart, cm.	-	-	-	0.24*	-
Pressing ups in lying position, q-ty of times	0.48**	0.42**	0.39**	0.49**	0.57**
Legs' raising during 30 sec., q-ty of times	0.36**	0.31*	0.28*	-	0.39**
Long jump from the spot, cm	0.54**	0.45**	0.39**	-	0.59**
High jump from the spot, cm	0.44**	0.41**	0.35**	0.38**	0.45**
Triple jump from the spot, cm	0.66**	0.54**	0.48**	0.31*	0.69**
Throw of filled ball, cm	0.22*	-	-	-0.29*	-
Shuttle run (4×9 m), sec.	-0.58**	-0.5**	-0.35**	-	-0.63**
1000 meters' run, min., sec.	-0.69**	-0.52**	-0.44**	-0.38**	-0.72**

Notes: * – $p<0.05$; ** – $p<0.01$, confident correlation

Practically all parameters of physical workability had confident positive influence (r = 0.31÷0.69) on results of jump exercises. Exception was relative level of physical workability and long jump from the spot.

Much worse was influence of physical workability on results of pedagogic tests, which informed about backbone flexibility and about explosive power of arms and torso. It was witnessed by little quantity of weak correlations (1-2).

Discussion

In the sphere of physical culture and sports for monitoring students' physical workability there are widely used one-moment, two-moment and functional tests. Besides, methods of physical workability quantitative assessmentB were often used. Among them Ruffiet's test, Harvard step-test and test PWC_{170} are the most frequent [1, 4, 9]. However, the received by the mentioned above tests results give little information. The main reasons of it are: inaccuracy in receiving results; inaccuracy of approaches to finding appropriate indicators; they do not consider age changes in organisms of children and youth. Such researches were also accompanied by the absence of single approach and contradiction character of results. It is proved by our research. Some data confidently differ and exceed the compared figures nearly twice. The range of physical workability fluctuations is so wide that their practical usage is possible only with significance caution.

In our opinion method of physical workability testing with the help of physical load by closed cycle [5] complies with the most of known requirements. On the base of the received physical workability results we can assess health state as well as to correct physical education process in higher educational establishments.

This methodic did not get widespread use and was applied only in single studies of elite sportsmen functional reserves [5, 7]. Besides, it was implemented in physical education process of primary schools and some other educational establishments [12]. In available literature there are no complex studies of students' functional potentials, considering physical workability and physical fitness.

The received results of PWC_{170} and MOC are in good agreement with results of other researches [9]. It is worth to pay attention to the fact that fundamental researches of different age people's physical workability (including students) were conducted about 30 years ago. That is why fulfillment of mass studies for receiving up to date PWC model characteristics and other parameters is rather relevant. The presented new parameters of physical workability (T_{tot}, A_{tot}, W_{rev}) provide quite real opportunities to have widespread use in practice alongside with more known indicators of MOC, PWC_{150}, PWC_{170}. It proves relevance and promising potential of further researches.

Conclusions

Physical workability indicators were within age standards. These indicators were predicted better in boys than in girls. In most cases differences of the mentioned parameters between students by sex were confident.

Analysis of correlations showed that physical workability indicators substantially influence on physical fitness. The most intensively results of control exercises were influenced on (exercises, which assessed endurance, dexterity and legs' explosive power). It is expressed in maximal quantity of significant correlations and their strength. Physical workability moderately correlates with tests for speed power qualities at the account of weak correlation strength. Physical workability practically did not influence on development of flexibility and arms and torso explosive power. In total we registered only 3 significant weak correlations.

Acknowledgements

The research has been fulfilled according to topical plan of scientific-research works of biology and health principles department of South-Ukrainian national pedagogic university, named after K.D. Ushinskiy (Odessa) "Systemic adaptation to physical and mental loads at different stages of human ontogeny" state registration № 0109U000206).

Conflict of interests

The author declares that there is no conflict of interests.

References:

1. Aulik IV. *Opredelenie fizicheskoj rabotosposobnosti v klinike i sporte* [Determination of physical workability in clinic and sports], Moscow: Medicine; 1990. (in Russian)
2. Bosenko AI. *Sposib diagnostiki funkcional'nikh rezerviv liudini* [Method of diagnostic of human functional reserves]. Ukraine patent. 100860. 2003 Aug 1. (in Ukrainian)
3. Bosenko AI, Samokish II, Strashko SV, Orlik NA. Vikovi osoblivosti funkcional'nikh mozhlivostej studentok vishchikh navchal'nikh zakladiv [Age specificities of functional potentials of higher educational establishments' girl students]. *Visnik Chernigivs'kogo nacional'nogo pedagogichnogo universitetu*, 2013;107(2):132–135. (in Ukrainian)
4. Bosenko AI, Samokish II. Ociniuvannia navchal'nikh dosiagnen' z fizichnogo vikhovannia u vishchikh navchal'nikh zakladakh za dopomogoiu pokaznikiv veloergometrichnogo testuvannia [Assessment of educational progress in physical education at higher educational establishments by indicators of stationary bicycle testing]. *Nauka i osvita*, 2014;4:27–32. (in Ukrainian)
5. Davidenko DN, Andrianov VP, Iakovlev GM. Metodika ocenki funkcional'nykh rezervov organizma pri ispol'zovanii nagruzochnoj proby po zamknutomu ciklu izmeneniia moshchnosti [Methodic of organism's

functional reserves' assessment by closed cycle of power change]. *Puti mobilizacii funkcional'nykh rezervov sportsmena*, 1984;1:35–41. (in Russian)

6. Davidenko DN, Pasichnichenko VA. *Biologicheskie osnovy fizicheskoj kul'tury i sporta* [Biological principles of physical culture and sports], Sankt Petersburg: SPbSPU; 2008. (in Russian)
7. Davidenko DN, Filippov MM, Chistiakov VA. Gisterezisnyj metod ocenki adaptacionnykh rezervov organizma sportsmena [Hysteretic method of sportsman organism's adaptation reserves assessment]. *Mezhdunarodnaia nauchnaia konferenciia "Psikhologo-pedagogicheskie tekhnologii povysheniia umstvennoj i fizicheskoj rabotosposobnosti, snizheniia nervno-emocional'nogo napriazheniia u studentov v processe obrazovatel'noj deiatel'nosti", Belgorod, 2011* [International scientific conference "Psychological-pedagogic technologies of physical and mental workability improvement; weakening of students' nervous-emotional tension in their educational activity", Belgorod, 2011], Belgorod; 2011. P. 204–210. (in Russian)
8. Kornienko IA, Son'kin VD. «Biologicheskaia nadezhnost'», ontogenez i vozrastnaia dinamika myshechnoj rabotosposobnosti ["Biological reliability", ontogeny and age dynamic of muscular workability]. *Fiziologiia cheloveka*, 1999;1:98–108. (in Russian)
9. Karpman VL, Belocerkovskij ZB, Gudkov IA. *Testirovanie v sportivnoj medicine* [Testing in sport medicine], Moscow: Physical Culture and Sport; 1988. (in Russian)
10. Operajlo SI. Polozhennia pro organizaciiu fizichnogo vikhovannia i masovogo sportu u vishchikh navchal'nikh zakladakh [Instructions on organization of physical education and mass sports in higher educational establishments]. *Teoriia i metodika fizichnogo vikhovannia*, 2006;5:4–13. (in Ukrainian)
11. Samokish II. Novi pidkhodi do viiavlennia rivnia fizichnoi pracezdatnosti divchatok molodshogo shkil'nogo viku [New approaches to finding physical workability of junior school age girls]. *Pedagogics, psychology, medical-biological problems of physical training and sports*, 2005;3:41–46. (in Ukrainian)
12. Samokish II. *Metodika ociniuvannia navchal'nikh dosiagnen' divchatok molodshogo shkil'nogo viku v procesi zaniat' fizichnoiu kul'turoiu. Kand. Diss.* [Methodic of assessment of junior school age girls' educational progress in physical culture trainings. Cand. Diss.], Kiev; 2011. (in Ukrainian)
13. Samokih II. Hysteretic method of identifying features as a criterion for evaluating performance in physical education in higher education. *Physical Education of Students,* 2011;4:71–75.
14. Samokish II, Bosenko AI, Dishel' GO. Optimizaciia navchal'nogo procesu fizichnogo vikhovannia u vishchikh zakladakh osviti na osnovi monitoringu funkcional'nikh mozhlivostej studentiv [Optimization of physical education process in higher educational establishments on the base of monitoring of students' functional potentials]. *Nauka i osvita*, 2016;8:151–157. (in Ukrainian)
15. Samokish II. Monitoring fizichnoi pidgotovlenosti studentiv pershikh-drugikh kursiv shchodo stanu reguliatornikh mekhanizmiv sercevogo ritmu [Monitoring of 1st, 2nd year students' regulatory heart rate mechanisms]. *Naukovij visnik Pivdennoukrains'kogo nacional'nogo pedagogichnogo universitetu imeni K. D. Ushins'kogo*, 2016;2(109):74–78. (in Ukrainian)
16. Sukharev AG. *Zdorov'e i fizicheskoe vospitanie detej i podrostkov* [Health and physical education of children and adolescents], Moscow: Medicine; 1991. (in Russian)
17. Tikhvinskij SB, Aulik IV. *Opredelenie, metody i ocenka fizicheskoj rabotosposobnosti detej i podrostkov* [Determination, methods and assessment of children and adolescents' physical workability], Moscow; 1991. (in Russian)
18. Bondarenko SV, Darzinska NO, Sidilo LV. Formation of 17–18 yrs age girl students' visual performance by means of visual training at stage of adaptation to learning loads. *Pedagogics, psychology, medical-biological problems of physical training and sports*, 2015;4:10–15. doi:10.15561/18189172.2015.0402
19. Caldwell K, Harrison M, Adams M, Travis Triplett N. Effect of Pilates and taiji quan training on self-efficacy, sleep quality, mood, and physical performance of college students. *Journal of Bodywork and Movement Therapies.* 2009;13(2):155–163.
20. Fairclough SJ, Stratton G. Effects of a physical education intervention to improve student activity levels. *Physical Education and Sport Pedagogy*. 2006;11(1):29–44.

21. Ivashchenko OV. Methodic of pedagogic control of 16–17 years' age girls' motor fitness. *Pedagogics, psychology, medical-biological problems of physical training and sports*, 2016;5:26–32. doi:10.15561/18189172.2016.0504
22. Kopeikina EN, Drogomeretsky VV, Kondakov VL, Kovaleva MV, Iermakov SS. Modification of Harvard step-test for assessment of students' with health problems functional potentials. *Physical Education of Students*, 2016;4:44–50. doi:10.15561/20755279.2016.0405
23. Kozina ZL, Iermakov SS, Kadutskaya LA, Sobyanin FI, Krzeminski M, Sobko IN, Ryepko OA. Comparative characteristic of correlation between pulse subjective indicators of girl students' and school girls' reaction to physical load. *Physical Education of Students*, 2016;4:24–34. doi:10.15561/20755279.2016.0403
24. Kretschmann Rolf. Comparison of 9th grade students' physical activity levels during recess and regular class periods using objective measurement. *Pedagogics, psychology, medical-biological problems of physical training and sports*, 2016;4:59–63. doi:10.15561/18189172.2016.0409
25. Kudryavtsev MD, Kramida IE, Iermakov SS, Influence of studying in higher educational establishment on students' harmful computer habits. *Physical Education of Students*, 2016;5:17–23. doi:10.15561/20755279.2016.0503
26. Kudryavtsev MD, Kramida IE, Kuzmin VA, Iermakov SS, Cieslicka Miroslawa, Stankiewicz Blazej, Influence of study in hee on ubiquity and strength of students' computer gambling. *Physical Education of Students*, 2016;3:13–22. doi:10.15561/20755279.2016.0302
27. Lupu E. A Study Regarding the Impact of Motor Activities on the Students' Working Memory. *Procedia – Social and Behavioral Sciences.* 2015;187:514–519.
28. Mercier K, Doolittle S. Assessing Student Achievement in Physical Education for Teacher Evaluation. *Journal of Physical Education, Recreation & Dance*. 2013;84(3):38–42.
29. Proskurov EM. Dynamic of changes in health of 10–11 years old gymnasium boys under influence of comprehensive education's load. *Pedagogics, psychology, medical-biological problems of physical training and sports*, 2015;7:39–47. doi:10.15561/18189172.2015.0706
30. Pyatnychuk GO. Assessment of speed and power abilities of the students during the weekly training cycles. *Physical Education of Students*, 2014;1:39–43. doi:10.6084/m9.figshare.903692
31. Skurikhina NV, Kudryavtsev MD, Kuzmin VA, Iermakov SS. Fitness yoga as modern technology of special health groups' girl students' psycho-physical condition and psycho-social health strengthening. *Physical Education of Students*, 2016;20(2):24–31. doi:10.15561/20755279.2016.0204
32. Sobko IN, Ulaeva LA, Yakovenko YA. Factorial structure of physical rehabilitation group students' complex fitness. *Physical Education of Students*, 2016;20(2):32–37. doi:10.15561/20755279.2016.0205

31

SUPERSTITIOUS BEHAVIOR AMONG JUDO, TAEKWONDO AND BOXING PLAYERS

Gaurav Dureja, Gagandeep Singh
Department of Physical Education-TEL & R, Postgraduate Government College, Sector-11, Chandigarh (U.T.), India

Abstract. *Purpose:* The present study was designed to measure superstitious behavior among Judo, Taekwondo and Boxing players. *Material:* Thirty (N=30) male inter-college level players with the age group of 19-25 years were selected through purposive sampling technique to act as subjects from affiliated colleges of Panjab University, Chandigarh. They were further divided into three groups: Group-A [Judo (n=10)], Group-B [Taekwondo (n=10)] and Group-C [Boxing (n=10)]. One Way Analysis of Variance (ANOVA) was applied to find out the differences among judo, taekwondo and boxing players. Where 'F' values found significant, Least Significant Differences (LSD) Post-hoc test was applied to find out the direction and degree of difference. *Results:* The level of significance was set at 0.05. The result revealed significant differences among judo, taekwondo and boxing players on the sub parameters: clothing and appearance, preparation, team ritual and coach. However, no significant differences have been observed on the sub-parameters fetish, game/competition, prayer and parameter superstitious (Total). *Conclusions:* The obtained results showed significant differences on the sub-parameter Coach among Judo, Taekwondo and Boxing players. While calculating the mean values of entire groups, it has been observed that Boxing players demonstrate significantly better on the sub-parameter Coach. Therefore, it can be ascertained that Boxing players are more confident that coach bring a lucky charm to our game.
Keywords: Superstitious behavior, Judo, Taekwondo, Boxing, players.

Introduction

Superstitions are regarded as "a belief that one's fate is in the hands of unknown external powers governed by forces over which one has no control" [8]. Superstitions are irrational beliefs that influence the emotional states of people who hold them. They are learned forms of behavior, or dispositions about objects or situations, that direct the holder toward some preferred response [7]. Wann et al. [12] describe superstitious behavior as an action or series of actions believed to lead to or cause a specified, generally desirable, outcome. Brooks [3] explains that people engage in superstitious behaviors when they feel as if they are losing control over their own lives and their brains are searching for order and structure. Cultural and environmental factors also play a role. For example, it has been found that persons in high risk areas in the Middle East, currently in a state of disarray, are more likely to carry a lucky charm in hopes of regaining some order and structure and reducing some of their internal chaos [3].

Superstition in sports can be defined as "actions which are repetitive, formal, sequential, and distinct from technical performance and which the athlete believes to be powerful in controlling luck or other external factors" [2]. The repetitive nature of such events allows for the term 'ritual' to be used to describe these superstitious behaviors. A ritual in sport is usually defined as conscious activity involving heightened arousal with focused attention that provides a way of coping with a high stress situation [15].

Superstitious practices in sports have been linked to the theoretical perspectives of attribution [6], achievement motivation [13], reinforcement [9], and locus of control [16]. Attribution theory is based on individual perceptions about success and failure and relates to the need for achievement. Weiner [13] believed that when achievement is aroused, we tend to attribute our performance to a variety of possible causes or attribution elements, such as ability, effort, or luck. Athletes, competing under extreme conditions, may often feel that they don't have enough control over uncertainty, which affects their performance. Engaging in superstitious behavior can offer the assurance of illusory control in a high-stress or uncertain situation. If subsequent accidental connections are made between the ritual and favorable consequences, the behavior will be maintained as a superstition despite instances that go without such reinforcement. It is the chance element that is often present in sport, which contributes to the athlete's feelings of uncertainty and lack of control [11]. Therefore, the present study was designed with the purpose to investigate the superstitious behaviour among Judo, Taekwondo and Boxing players.

Method and material

Sample: Thirty (N=30) male inter-college level players with the age group of 19 to 25 years were selected through purposive sampling technique to act as subjects from, affiliated colleges of Panjab University, Chandigarh. They were further divided into three groups: Group-A [Judo (n=10)], Group-B [Taekwondo (n=10)] and Group-C [Boxing (n=10)].

Instrument:

The superstitious Questionnaire developed by Bleak and Frederick (1998) was administrated.

Statistical Techniques:

One Way Analysis of Variance (ANOVA) was employed to find out the differences among Judo, Taekwondo and Boxing players. Where 'F' values found significant, Least Significant Differences (LSD) Post-hoc test was applied to find out the direction and degree of difference. The level of significance was set at 0.05.

Results

Table 1. Descriptive analysis among Judo, Taekwondo and Boxing on the sub-parameter clothing and appearance

S. No.	Groups	N	Mean	Std. Deviation	Std. Error
1.	Judo	10	27.50	4.11	1.30
2.	Taekwondo	10	34.10	7.69	2.43
3.	Boxing	10	31.30	2.83	.89
	Total	30	30.96	5.80	1.05

Table 1 depicts the results Judo, Taekwondo and Boxing players on the sub-parameter Clothing and Appearance. The scores of Judo players showed the Mean and SD values as 27.50 and 4.11 respectively. The scores of Taekwondo players showed the Mean and SD values as 34.10 and 7.69 respectively. However, the scores of Boxing players showed had Mean and SD values as 31.30 and 2.83 respectively.

Table 2. One way analysis of variance (Anova) results among judo, taekwondo and boxing players with regard to the sub-parameter clothing and appearance

Source of Variation	Sum of Squares	Degree of Freedom	Mean Square	F-Value	P-Value (Sig.)
Between Groups	219.46	2	109.73		
Within Groups	757.50	27	28.05	3.91	.03*
Total	976.96	29			

* Confident at 0.05

It can be seen from table 2 that significant differences were found with regard to the sub-parameter Clothing and Appearance among Judo, Taekwondo and Boxing players as the P-value (Sig.) .03 was found smaller than 0.05 level of significance ($p<0.05$).

Since the obtained F-value was found significant, therefore, least significant difference (LSD) Post-hoc test was employed to study the direction and significance of difference between paired means among Judo, Taekwondo and Boxing players on the sub-parameter Clothing and Appearance. The results of LSD Post-hoc test have been presented in Table 3.

Table 3. Analysis of least significant difference (LSD) post-hoc test among judo, taekwondo and boxing players on the sub-parameter clothing and appearance

Means		Mean Difference	P-Value (Sig.)
Judo (27.50)	Taekwondo (34.10)	6.60	.01*
	Boxing (31.30)	3.80	.12
Taekwondo (34.10)	Judo (27.50)	6.60	.01*
	Boxing (31.30)	2.80	.24
Boxing (31.30)	Judo (27.50)	3.80	.12
	Taekwondo (34.10)	2.80	.24

* Confident at 0.05

It has been observed from the Table 3 that mean difference between judo and taekwondo players was found 6.60. The P-value (Sig.) .01 showed that taekwondo players had demonstrated significantly better clothing and appearance than their counterpart judo players.

The mean difference between judo and boxing players was found 3.80. The P-value (Sig.) .12 revealed that boxing players had exhibited better clothing and appearance though not significantly than their counterpart judo players.

The mean difference between taekwondo and boxing players was found 2.80. The P-value (Sig.) .24 revealed that taekwondo players had exhibited better clothing and appearance though not significantly than their counterpart boxing players. The graphical representation of means scores of clothing and appearance among Judo, Taekwondo and Boxing players has been exhibited in Figure 1.

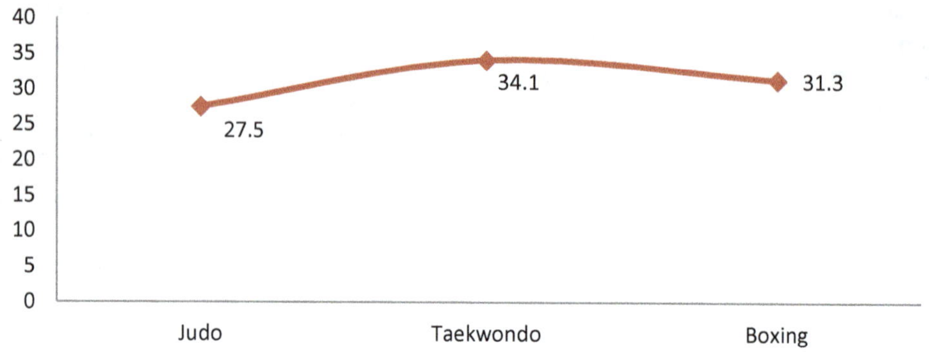

Figure 1. Graphical representation of mean scores with regard to judo, taekwondo and boxing players on the sub-parameter clothing and appearance

Table 4. Descriptive analysis among judo, taekwondo and boxing players on the sub-parameter fetish

S. No.	Groups	N	Mean	Std. Deviation	Std. Error
1.	Judo	10	14.90	7.20	2.27
2.	Taekwondo	10	13.30	4.92	1.55
3.	Boxing	10	17.00	4.24	1.34
	Total	30	15.06	5.61	1.02

Table 4 depicts the results among Judo, Taekwondo and Boxing players on the sub-parameter Fetish. The scores of judo players showed the Mean and SD values as 14.90 and 7.20 respectively. The scores of taekwondo players showed the Mean and SD values as 13.30 and 4.92 respectively. However, the scores of boxing players showed had Mean and SD values as 17.00 and 4.24 respectively.

Table 5. One way analysis of variance (Anova) results among judo, taekwondo and boxing players with regard to the sub-parameter fetish

Source of Variation	Sum of Squares	Degree of Freedom	Mean Square	F-Value	P-Value (Sig.)
Between Groups	68.86	2	34.43		
Within Groups	847.00	27	31.37	1.09	.34
Total	915.86	29			

* Confident at 0.05

It can be seen from Table 5 that insignificant differences were found with regard to the sub-parameter Fetish among Judo, Taekwondo and Boxing players as the P-value (Sig.) .34 was found higher than the 0.05 level of significance ($p>0.05$). Since F-value was found insignificant, therefore, there is no need to apply Post-hoc test.

Table 6. Descriptive analysis among judo, taekwondo and boxing players on the sub-parameter preparation

S. No.	Groups	N	Mean	Std. Deviation	Std. Error
1.	Judo	10	14.90	2.42	.76
2.	Taekwondo	10	21.50	4.62	1.46
3.	Boxing	10	17.20	3.39	1.07
	Total	30	17.86	4.44	.81

Table 6 depicts the results among Judo, Taekwondo and Boxing players on the sub-parameter Preparation. The scores of judo players showed the Mean and SD values as 14.90 and 2.42 respectively. The scores of taekwondo players showed the Mean and SD values as 21.50 and 4.62 respectively. However, the scores of boxing players showed had Mean and SD values as 17.20 and 3.39 respectively.

Table 7. One way analysis of variance (Anova) results among judo, taekwondo and boxing players with regard to the sub-parameter preparation

Source of Variation	Sum of Squares	Degree of freedom	Mean Square	F-Value	P-Value (Sig.)
Between Groups	224.46	2	112.23		
Within Groups	349.00	27	12.92	8.68	.00*
Total	573.46	29			

* Confident at 0.05

It can be seen from Table 7 that significant differences were found with regard to the sub-parameter Preparation among Judo, Taekwondo and Boxing players as the P-value (Sig.) .00 was found smaller than 0.05 level of significance ($p<0.05$).

Since the obtained F-value was found significant, therefore, least significant difference (LSD) Post-hoc test was employed to study the direction and significance of difference between paired means among Judo, Taekwondo and Boxing players on the sub-parameter preparation. The results of LSD Post-hoc test have been presented in Table 8.

Table 8. Analysis of least significant difference (LSD) post-hoc test among judo, taekwondo and boxing players on the sub-parameter preparation

Means		Mean Difference	P-Value (Sig.)
Judo (14.90)	Taekwondo (21.50)	6.60	.00*
	Boxing (17.20)	2.30	.16
Taekwondo (21.50)	Judo (14.90)	6.60	.00
	Boxing (17.20)	4.30*	.01*
Boxing (17.20)	Judo (14.90)	2.30	.16
	Taekwondo (21.50)	4.30*	.01*

* Confident at 0.05

It has been observed from the Table 8 that mean difference between judo and taekwondo players was found 6.60. The P-value (Sig.) .00 showed that taekwondo players had demonstrated significantly better preparation than their counterpart judo players.

The mean difference between judo and boxing players was found 2.30. The P-value (Sig.) .16 revealed that boxing players had exhibited better preparation though not significantly than their counterpart judo players.

It has been observed from the Table 8 that mean difference between judo and taekwondo players was found 4.30· The P-value (Sig.) .01 showed that taekwondo players had demonstrated significantly better preparation than their counterpart judo players. The graphical representation of means scores of preparation among Judo, Taekwondo and Boxing players has been exhibited in Figure 2.

Table 9. Descriptive analysis among judo, taekwondo and boxing players on the sub-parameter game/competition

S. No.	Groups	N	Mean	Std. Deviation	Std. Error
1.	Judo	10	13.50	3.20	1.01
2.	Taekwondo	10	12.30	4.24	1.34
3.	Boxing	10	11.70	3.71	1.17
	Total	30	12.50	3.69	.67

Table 9 depicts the results among Judo, Taekwondo and Boxing players on the sub-parameter Game/Competition. The scores of Judo players showed the Mean and SD values as 13.50 and 3.20 respectively. The scores of Taekwondo players showed the Mean and SD values as 12.30 and 4.24 respectively. However, the scores of Boxing players showed had Mean and SD values as 11.70 and 3.71 respectively.

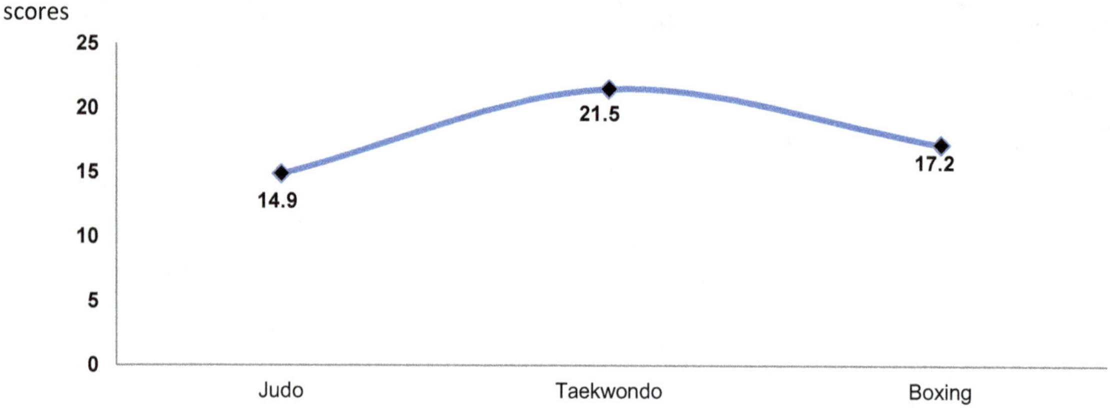

Figure 2. Graphical representation of mean scores with regard to judo, taekwondo and boxing players on the sub-parameter preparation

Table 10. One way analysis of variance (Anova) results among judo, taekwondo and boxing players with regard to the sub-parameter game/competition

Source of Variation	Sum of Squares	Degree of Freedom	Mean Square	F-Value	P-Value (Sig.)
Between Groups	16.80	2	8.40		
Within Groups	378.70	27	14.02	.59	.55
Total	395.50	29			

* Confident at 0.05

It can be seen from Table 10 that insignificant differences were found with regard to the sub-parameter Game/Competition among Judo, Taekwondo and Boxing players as the P-value (Sig.) .55 was found higher than the 0.05 level of significance (p>0.05). Since F-value was found insignificant, therefore, there is no need to apply Post-hoc test.

Table 11. Descriptive analysis among judo, taekwondo and boxing players on the sub-parameter team ritual

S. No.	Groups	N	Mean	Std. Deviation	Std. Error
1.	Judo	10	14.60	3.86	1.22
2.	Taekwondo	10	11.80	2.57	.81
3.	Boxing	10	9.90	3.60	1.13
	Total	30	12.10	3.81	.69

Table 11 depicts the results among Judo, Taekwondo and Boxing players on the sub-parameter Team Ritual. The scores of judo players showed the Mean and SD values as 14.60 and 3.86 respectively. The scores of taekwondo players showed the Mean and SD values as 11.80 and 2.57 respectively. However, the scores of boxing players showed had Mean and SD values as 9.90 and 3.60 respectively.

Table 12. One way analysis of variance (Anova) results among judo, taekwondo and boxing players with regard to the sub-parameter team ritual

Source of Variation	Sum of Squares	Degree of Freedom	Mean Square	F-Value	P-Value (Sig.)
Between Groups	111.80	2	55.90		
Within Groups	310.90	27	11.51	4.85	.01*
Total	422.70	29			

* Confident at 0.05

It can be seen from Table 12 that significant differences were found with regard to the sub-parameter Team Ritual among Judo, Taekwondo and Boxing players as the P-value (Sig.) .01 was found smaller than 0.05 level of significance ($p<0.05$).

Since the obtained F-value was found significant, therefore, least significant difference (LSD) Post-hoc test was employed to study the direction and significance of difference between paired means among Judo, Taekwondo and Boxing players on the sub-parameter Team Ritual. The results of LSD Post-hoc test have been presented in Table 13.

Table 13. Analysis of least significant difference (LSD) post-hoc test among judo, taekwondo and boxing players on the sub-parameter team ritual

Means		**Mean Difference**	**P-Value (Sig.)**
Judo (14.60)	Taekwondo (11.80)	2.80	.07
	Boxing (9.90)	4.70	.00*
Taekwondo (11.80)	Judo (14.60)	2.80	.07
	Boxing (9.90)	1.90	.22
Boxing (9.90)	Judo (14.60)	4.70	.00*
	Taekwondo (11.80)	1.90	.22

* Confident at 0.05

It has been observed from the Table 13 that mean difference between judo and taekwondo players was found 2.80. The P-value (Sig.) .07 showed that judo players had demonstrated significantly better Team Ritual than their counterpart taekwondo players.

It has been observed from the Table 13 that mean difference between judo and boxing players was found 4.70. The P-value (Sig.) .00 showed that judo players had demonstrated significantly better Team Ritual than their counterpart boxing players.

The mean difference between taekwondo and boxing players was found 1.90. The P-value (Sig.) .22 revealed that taekwondo players had exhibited better Team Ritual though not significantly than their counterpart boxing players. The graphical representation of means scores of Team Ritual among Judo, Taekwondo and Boxing players has been exhibited in Figure 3.

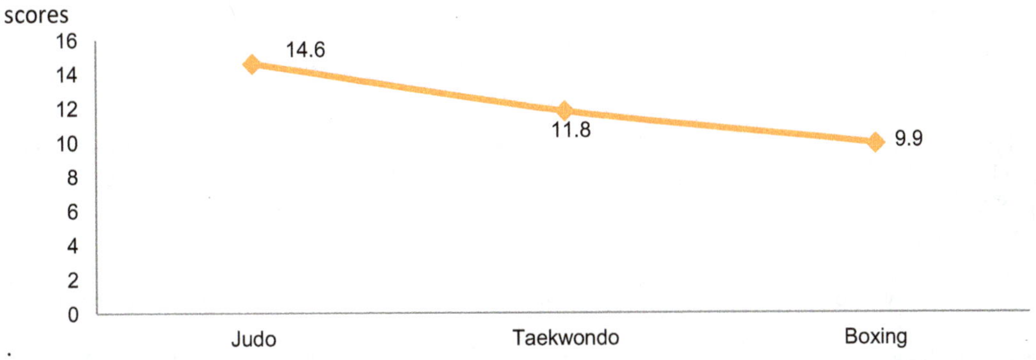

Figure 3. Graphical representation of mean scores with regard to judo, taekwondo and boxing players on the sub-parameter team ritual

Table 14. Descriptive analysis among judo, taekwondo and boxing players on the sub-parameter prayer

S. No.	**Groups**	**N**	**Mean**	**Std. Deviation**	**Std. Error**
1.	Judo	10	8.70	3.02	.95
2.	Taekwondo	10	8.40	3.02	.95
3.	Boxing	10	8.20	3.19	1.00
	Total	30	8.43	2.97	.54

Table 14 depicts the results among Judo, Taekwondo and Boxing players on the sub-parameter Prayer. The scores of judo players showed the Mean and SD values as 8.70 and 3.02 respectively. The scores of taekwondo players showed the Mean and SD values as 8.40 and 3.02 respectively. However, the scores of boxing players showed had Mean and SD values as 8.20 and 3.19 respectively.

Table 15. One way analysis of variance (Anova) results among judo, taekwondo and boxing players with regard to the sub-parameter prayer

Source of Variation	Sum of Squares	Degree of Freedom	Mean Square	F-Value	P-Value (Sig.)
Between Groups	1.26	2	.633		
Within Groups	256.10	27	9.48	.06	.93
Total	257.36	29			

* Confident at 0.05

It can be seen from Table 15 that insignificant differences were found with regard to the sub-parameter Prayer among Judo, Taekwondo and Boxing players as the P-value (Sig.) .93 was found higher than the 0.05 level of significance ($p>0.05$). Since F-value was found insignificant, therefore, there is no need to apply Post-hoc test.

Table 16. Descriptive analysis among judo, taekwondo and boxing players on the sub-parameter coach

S. No.	Groups	N	Mean	Std. Deviation	Std. Error
1.	Judo	10	5.20	2.04	.64
2.	Taekwondo	10	7.20	2.20	.69
3.	Boxing	10	8.60	2.87	.90
	Total	30	7.00	2.71	.49

Table 16 depicts the results among Judo, Taekwondo and Boxing players on the sub-parameter Coach. The scores of judo players showed the Mean and SD values as 5.20 and 2.04 respectively. The scores of taekwondo players showed the Mean and SD values as 7.20 and 2.20 respectively. However, the scores of boxing players showed had Mean and SD values as 8.60 and 2.87 respectively.

Table 17. One way analysis of variance (Anova) results among judo, taekwondo and boxing players with regard to the sub-parameter coach

Source of Variation	Sum of Squares	Degree of Freedom	Mean Square	F-Value	P-Value (Sig.)
Between Groups	58.40	2	29.20		
Within Groups	155.60	27	5.76	5.06	.01*
Total	214.00	29			

* Confident at 0.05

It can be seen from Table 17 that significant differences were found with regard to the sub-parameter Coach among Judo, Taekwondo and Boxing players as the P-value (Sig.) .01 was found smaller than 0.05 level of significance ($p<0.05$).

Since the obtained F-value was found significant, therefore, least significant difference (LSD) Post-hoc test was employed to study the direction and significance of difference between paired means among Judo, Taekwondo and Boxing players on the sub-parameter Coach. The results of LSD Post-hoc test have been presented in Table 18.

The mean difference between judo and taekwondo players was found 2.00. The P-value (Sig.) .07 revealed that taekwondo players had exhibited better Coach though not significantly than their counterpart judo players.

It has been observed from the Table 18 that mean difference between judo and boxing players was found 3.40. The P-value (Sig.) .00 showed that boxing players had demonstrated significantly better Coach than their counterpart judo players.

The mean difference between taekwondo and boxing players was found 1.40. The P-value (Sig.) .20 revealed that boxing players had exhibited better Coach though not significantly than their counterpart taekwondo players. The graphical representation of means scores of Coach among Judo, Taekwondo and Boxing players has been exhibited in Figure 4.

Table 18. Analysis of least significant difference (LSD) post-hoc test among judo, taekwondo and boxing players on the sub-parameter coach

Means		Mean Difference	P-Value (Sig.)
Judo (5.20)	Taekwondo (7.20)	2.00	.07
	Boxing (8.60)	3.40	.00*
Taekwondo (7.20)	Judo (5.20)	2.00	.07
	Boxing (8.60)	1.40	.20
Boxing (8.60)	Judo (5.20)	3.40	.00*
	Taekwondo (7.20)	1.40	.20

*Confident at 0.05

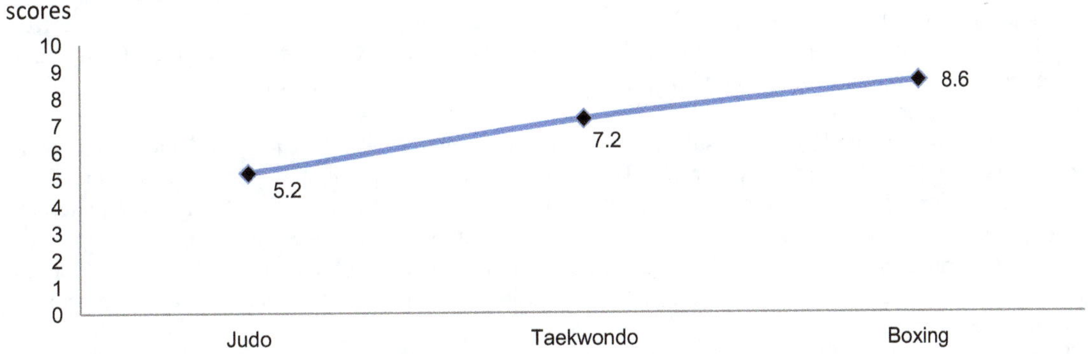

Figure 4. Graphical representation of mean scores with regard to judo, taekwondo and boxing players on the sub-parameter coach

Table 19. Descriptive analysis among judo, taekwondo and boxing players on the parameter superstitious (total)

S. No.	Groups	N	Mean	Std. Deviation	Std. Error
1.	Judo	10	99.30	13.67	4.32
2.	Taekwondo	10	108.60	19.02	6.01
3.	Boxing	10	102.60	18.91	5.97
	Total	30	103.50	17.22	3.14

Table 19 depicts the results among Judo, Taekwondo and Boxing players on the parameter Superstitious (Total). The scores of judo players showed the Mean and SD values as 99.30 and 13.67 respectively. The scores of taekwondo players showed the Mean and SD values as 108.60 and 19.02 respectively. However, the scores of boxing players showed had Mean and SD values as 102.60 and 18.91 respectively.

Table 20. One way analysis of variance (Anova) results among judo, taekwondo and boxing players with regard to the parameter superstitious (total)

Source of Variation	Sum of Squares	Degree of Freedom	Mean Square	F-Value	P-Value (Sig.)
Between Groups	444.60	2	222.30		
Within Groups	8160.90	27	302.25	.73	.48
Total	8605.50	29			

*Confident at 0.05

It can be seen from Table 20 that insignificant differences were found with regard to the parameter Superstitious (Total)among Judo, Taekwondo and Boxing players as the P-value (Sig.) .48 was found higher than the 0.05 level of significance (p>0.05). Since F-value was found insignificant, therefore, there is no need to apply Post-hoc test.

Discussion

It has been observed from the Table 1 to 3 that significant differences have been found among Judo, Taekwondo and Boxing players on the sub-parameter Clothing and Appearance. While calculating the mean values of all the groups, it was observed that taekwondo players had demonstrated significantly better clothing and appearance as compared to their counterpart Judo and Boxing players. The outcome of results might be due to the fact that taekwondo players to dress well to feel better prepared for game and also get hair cut on the day of game. It is clearly illustrated from the Table 4 to 5 that insignificant differences have been found among Judo, Taekwondo and Boxing players with regard to the sub-parameter Fetish. It can be safely summarized that individual players were equally developed on the above said sub-parameter. The results might be attributed to the fact that all the individual players(Judo, Taekwondo and Boxing) on the sub-parameter has think that team mascot and wear a lucky charm help on the day of competition. Wilson [14] examined that highly identified fans reported wanting to perform more superstitious behavior than low identified fans.

It has been observed from the results (Table 6 to 8) that significant differences were found on the sub-parameter Preparation. While comparing the mean values of the entire groups, it has been noticed that taekwondo players demonstrated significantly better Preparation than their counterpart Judo and Boxing players. It can be presumed that taekwondo players have the ability to prepare for competition to face any situation as compared to their counterpart Judo and Boxing players. However, no significant differences were noticed (Table 9 to 10) on the sub-parameter; Game/competition among Judo, Taekwondo and Boxing players. It can be safely summarized that judo, taekwondo and boxing players were equally developed on the above said sub-parameter. George and Sreedhar [5] concluded that significant effect with students coming from urban area believing more in superstitious than those coming from rural area.

It is evident from (Table 11 to 13) results that significant differences were found among judo, taekwondo and boxing players with regard to the sub-parameter Team Ritual. While comparing the mean values of the entire groups, it has been noticed that Judo players demonstrated significantly better Team Ritual than their counterpart taekwondo and boxing players. It shows that judo players are more determined to cheering during the competition which helps to perform as highest level. The insignificant differences were obtained (Table 14 to 15) judo, taekwondo and boxing players on the sub-parameter Prayer. It has been found that entire players exhibit prayer for success before each and every game.

The obtained results (Table 16 to 18) showed significant differences on the sub-parameter Coach among Judo, Taekwondo and Boxing players. While calculating the mean values of entire groups, it has been observed that Boxing players demonstrate significantly better on the sub-parameter Coach. Therefore, it can be ascertained that Boxing players are more confident that coach bring a lucky charm to our game. It is evident from (Table 19 to 20) results that insignificant differences were found among Judo, Taekwondo and Boxing players on the parameter Superstitious (Total). It has been observed that entire Individual players demonstrate were equally better on the parameter Superstitious (Total). Bal et al. [1] revealed significant intra-group differences among individual, dual and team sports on the variable superstitious behavior.

Conclusion

It is concluded that results revealed significant differences among Judo, Taekwondo and Boxing players on the sub parameters: clothing and appearance, preparation, team ritual and coach. However, no significant differences have been observed on the sub parameters fetish, game/competition, prayer and parameter superstitious (Total).

Conflict of interests

The authors declare that there is no conflict of interests.

References:

1. Bal BS, Singh D, Badwal KK, & Dhaliwal GS. Superstitions behaviour and decision making in collegiate athletes: An illogical phenomenon. *Advances in Physical Education*, 2014;4(1):1-5.
2. Bleak JL, & Frederick CM. Superstitious behavior in sport: levels of effectiveness and determinants of use in three collegiate sports. *Journal of Sport Behavior*, 1998;21:1-15.
3. Brooks M. Born believers: How your brain creates God. *New Scientist Magazine*, 2009;201:30-33.
4. Cicero H. *Pietas: selected studies in roman religion*. Leiden, Netherlands: Brill; 1980.
5. George S, & Sreedhar KP. Globalisation and the prevalence of superstitious beliefs. *Journal of the Indian Academy of Applied Psychology*, 2006;32(3):241-247.
6. Heider F. *The psychology of interpersonal relations*. New York: Wiley; 1958.
7. Hollander ED. *Principles and methods of social psychology.* 2nd Edition; New York: Oxford University Press; 1971.
8. Johada G. Superstition and emotional maladjustment. *Journal of Educational Research*, 1969;28(8):592-617.

9. Skinner BF. "Superstition" in the pigeon. *Journal of Experimental Psychology*, 1948;38:168-172.
10. Turcan R. *The Cults of the Roman Empire.* Nevill, Antonia (trans.).Oxford English Dictionary (Second ed.). Oxford University Press; 1996.
11. Van Raalte JL, Brewer BW, Neneroff CJ, & Linder DE. Chance orientation and superstitious behaviour on the putting green. *Journal of Sport Behavior*, 1991;14:41-50.
12. Wann DL, Grieve FG, End C, Zapalac RK, Lanter JR, Pease DG, & Wallace A. Examining the superstitious behaviors of sports fans: Types of superstitions, perceptions of impact, and relationship with team identification. *Athletic Insight,* 2010;***5:***21-44.
13. Weiner B. History of motivational research in education. *Journal of Educational Psychology*, 1990;82:616-622.
14. Wilson S. *The relationship between superstitious behaviours of sports*. (Unpublished Master's Dissertation). Western Kentucky University; 2011.
15. Womack M. Why athletes need ritual: A study of magic among professional athletes. In S.J. Hoffman (Ed.), *Sport and religion* (pp. 191–202). Champaign, IL: Human Kinetics; 1992.
16. Rotter Julian B. Generalized expectancies for internal versus external control of reinforcement. *Psychological Monographs: General and Applied*, 1966;80(1):1-28. http://dx.doi.org/10.1037/h0092976

32

STRUCTURAL-FUNCTIONAL MODEL OF MEDICAL STUDENTS' PROFESSIONAL-APPLIED PHYSICAL TRAINING

Petryshyn A.V.
Ukrainian Medical Dental Academy

Abstract. *Purpose:* to work out and experimentally prove model of professional-applied physical training of medical higher educational establishments' students. *Material:* in the research 80 students participated. In questioning physical education instructors of medical higher education establishments (n=20) participated. *Results:* influence of students' professionally important characteristics on general physical fitness indicators and functional state has been shown. Directions of students' physical fitness parameters' individual diagnostic and control over physical education effectiveness have been offered. Volumes of physical exercises in the structure of training have been found: special training (15-20%) and competition exercises (20-30%). *Conclusions:* the need in raising the level of professionally important for students' abilities has been noted: speed power, static power endurance, power endurance, coordination of arms' movements, static balance.
Key words: structural, functional, model, professional, academic process, students.

Introduction

In system of students' physical training there exist certain contradictions: between modern requirements to training of compatible workers and their insufficient professional competence; demand in students' readiness and their insufficient awareness of physical component's importance in the process of their training [4, 6, and 22]. Studies of these problems and practice of students' physical education expand ideas about significance and content of students' professional applied physical training (SPAPT), especially for specialists of medical profile [25, 26]. The authors note need in the following:

- Training of physical abilities, characterizing specialist's work in static position [25];
- Formation of future specialists' professional functional competences [26];
- Raising of girl-students' psycho-physical abilities [24];
- Professional formation; formation of professionally important qualities; finding of potential for self-realization in the future [21];
- Activation of personality's internal intentions; awakening of student's will to learning during all life [9];
- Promotion of student to higher level of poly-cultural competence [7].
  - Substantiation of SPAPT effectiveness criteria for future medical officers' professional functioning [20];
  - Training of kinesthetic, responsive and orientation coordinations. These coordination are important for quick and effective solution of professional tasks, connected with accuracy of perception in the shortest terms and keeping great scope of space information in memory [11, 32];
  - Effectively fulfill professional functioning in the aspect of health protection [14];
  - Psychological readiness of modern students to professional functioning by factor of resilience [19];

In he works, devoted to training of future medical workers, the need in the following is also noted:

- Introduction of martial arts elements in professional applied training of medical higher educational establishments' students. It permits to substantiate approaches to training of future medical workers' assertiveness by means of sambo or Judo [31];
- Creation of preconditions to increase of physical exercises' practicing effectiveness and strengthening od students' motivation for health strengthening [13];
- Training of general physical workability of medical colleges' girl students [28];

Separately it is necessary to mention the researches directed at increase of medical students' academic process quality [18, 28, and 31]. Such works are closely connected with the following: general structure of future medical specialist's fitness [35, 44]; methodology of teaching, which considers professional specific [36]; forms of distant teaching [42]. Raining of health criteria is of not less importance in such structure [34, 37; 39] as well as behavioral intentions of medical students [42].

Provisioning of conditions for realization of SPAPT program by students shall be considered an important direction. Such conditions include: students' attitude to physical loads [10, 17]; students' psycho-social health уровень [29]; possibility to choose the desired kind of sports [5, 20]; [17]; organization of sport trainings for disabled students [1]; proper pedagogic control [38, 40, 41].

Analysis of researches showed that SPAPT is not paid proper attention to. These aspects require systemizing and specifying in connection with modern technological progress and changes of specialists' functions. Such principle questions of SPAPT organization-pedagogic methodic for students (substantiation of its significance and effectiveness, didactic filling, organizational forms, control over realization) have been remaining insufficiently studied. It does not permit to simulate the system of SPAPT methodic in compliance with modern requirements [4, 27, and 33]. Besides, there are no researches, in which methodic of students' professional-applied physical training (SPAPT) would be systemically elucidated.

Hypothesis: we assumed that the worked out author's SPAPT for students will facilitate perfection of students' psycho-physical abilities, which influence on their readiness for future professional functioning.

The purpose of the research: is to scientifically substantiate, work out and experimentally prove the model of professional-applied qualities of medical higher educational establishments' students.

Material and methods

Participants: in the research 80 students participated. By testing results the students were divided into two groups: control (CG, n=40) and experimental (EG, n=40). Both groups' students were identical by physical condition and fitness. Their age was (17-20 years) and the level of psycho-physical state was approximately equal. Before experiment all students had equally low physical fitness. For determination of future medical workers' professionally oriented physical training we questioned physical education instructors of medical higher educational establishments (n=20).

Procedure (organization of the research): the research was being carried out during academic year (64 hours). Control group students were trained by traditional methodic. Experimental group students were trained by author's program. We studied influence of general physical fitness, functional state indicators on professionally important for medical workers criteria. Testing of indicators was fulfilled at the beginning and at the end of experiment. For this purpose we used standard tests [4, 11, and 18]. Diagnostic of medical students' professional-applied fitness by motivation-value criteria was realized with the help of questioning [3]. We used questionnaire for determination of criteria of professional self determination in HEE effectiveness [2].

The most adequate means of future medical workers' SPAPT diagnostic is quantitative-qualitative analysis of results of:

1) Morphological functional state: Ruffiet's test for cardio-vascular system, index of functional changers (IFC) – for determination of organism's adaptation level; Harvard step-test for physical workability [12].

2) Control testing of motor abilities' and physical condition formation [23]: test for quickness in exercise "100 meters' run"; "Shuttle run 4x9" for coordination of movements; 1000 meters' run for general endurance; test for power abilities; test for flexibility; test for balance; tests for coordination, for power endurance of legs' muscles; test for static power endurance; test "Throw of filled ball" for speed-power abilities.

Statistical analysis:

Statistical processing of testing final results was fulfilled with the help of Excel programs. We used factorial analysis.

Results

When choosing SPAPT criteria we took in consideration the content of its structure. We marked out the following criteria, which determine future medical worker's SPAPT effectiveness:

Motivation-value (firm cognitive interest, professional motivation for physical training);

Theoretical (conscious, systemic knowledge of SPAPT);

Gnostic – formation of theoretical knowledge system about SPAPT considering specificities of future professional functioning as well as completeness and consciousness in understanding of physical education role in human progress and specialist's training;

Reflexive - (readiness for independent SPAPT practicing: ability to independently organize and realize trainings, determine their effectiveness; knowledge and skills in self-diagnostic, self-control during trainings; ability to correct SPAPT process).

Analysis of higher educational students' SPAPT permitted to find the following: typical and variable physical education program has one serious disadvantage, i.e. normative orientation of training process. These programs also insufficiently consider formation influence of physical culture means with general and professional orientation complex usage. Analysis of existing physical education programs proves purposefulness of future medical workers' SPAPT perfection by introduction of special means and methods in trainings process, which would completely reproduce content and structure of professional training.

Questioning of physical education instructors pointed at need in introduction of specially worked out professionally oriented physical training programs, which would consider specificity of future professional functioning. Instructors (85.7%) think that it is necessary to form motor skills, considering specificity of future professional functioning. In opinion of 13 physical education instructors SPAPT shall be conducted not less than 4 hours a week and have orientation on formation of general endurance, special endurance, maximal strength, quickness of reaction, coordination, dexterity, flexibility, balance, decisiveness, communicability, emotional balance. More than half of instructors (8 persons, 61%) think that sport games and game exercises have the highest potential for formation of such abilities.

Common signs of physical education in the studied groups were: quantity of academic hours (64 in academic year); equal conditions of trainings (gym, facilities and etc.); system of assessment.

Distinctive signs:

1. Correlation of general physical training means (GTM) and SPAPT: in CG it was 85% : 15%.

2. In EG correlation of GTM and SPAPT varied depending on year of study (see fig. 1).

3. Variable component of EG program was based on usage of such kinds of sports as: mini-football, handball, baseball, swimming, ping-pong.

Basing on factorial analysis results we determined correlation and significance of every parameter of physical fitness (see fig.1).

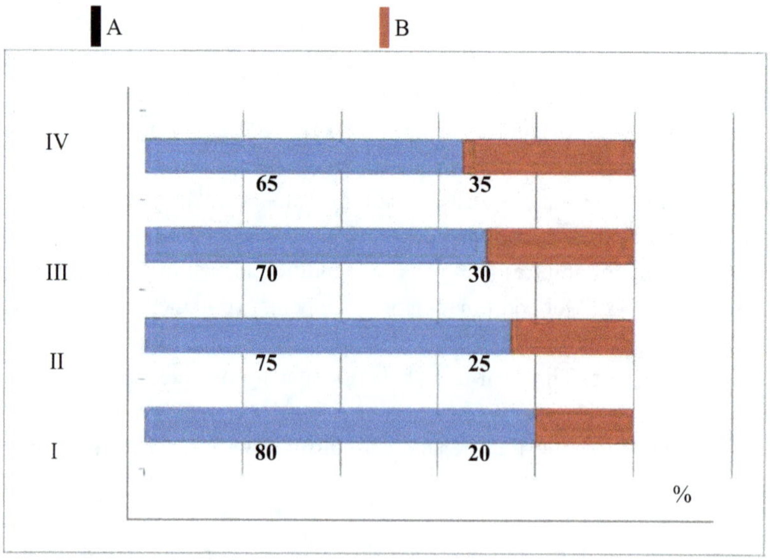

Fig.1. Correlation of GTM and SPAPT in author's program, %:
A –GTM; B – SPAPT; I – first semester; II – second semester; III – third semester; IV – fourth semester.

The content of author's differentiated program was directed at the following:

1. Development and perfection of main physical qualities at first year of study: strength, quickness, endurance, flexibility, coordination of movements. These qualities are the necessary basis for further development of special professionally important qualities.

2. Targeted training of professionally important qualities: static and dynamic power endurance, general endurance, coordination, coordination of arms' movements, balance in body static positions.

3. Training of professionally important neuro-dynamic functions: simple and complex visual-motor reactions.

4. Determination of technical sportsmanship in certain kind of sports and its further perfection.

5. Training of moral-will qualities: commitment, insistence, courage, decisiveness.

In the author's program specific means of SPAPT are physical exercises, which ensure training of general and special physical abilities. For this purpose we used general and special training methods, different training forms and SPAPT construction in compliance with tasks and purposes (in particular training system, their multiplicity, cyclicity, control and management).

The tasks of the author's programs were solved with the help of the following physical education and sports means:

1. General exercises were from 80% to 60% from general volume of exercises. They ensured comprehensive functional development of student's organism. Further, it permitted to specialize physical training on the base of high physical fitness. Such exercises completely corresponded to specificities of certain kind of sports. Though, to some extent they contradicted to them (in the aspect of comprehensive and harmonious physical development).

2. Auxiliary exercises, which corresponded to competition exercises by their content and structure. They created special base for further perfection in sport activity.

3. Special preparatory exercises were 15-20% from total volume of exercises in the structure of trainings. They took central place in system of sport training and embraced the circle of means, which, by their content and structure, are close to competition exercises. In author's program they are selected so that their content was maximally approached to professional movements of medical specialists.

4. Competition exercises were 20-30% from total volume of exercises, used in trainings, based on certain kind of sports. These exercises envisaged fulfillment of motor actions' complex, related to sport specialization.

In the author's program the following general exercises were used (see fig.2):

1. Exercises for insufficiently trained physical abilities - 60% from total volume of exercises.

2. Exercises for training other physical abilities - 40%.

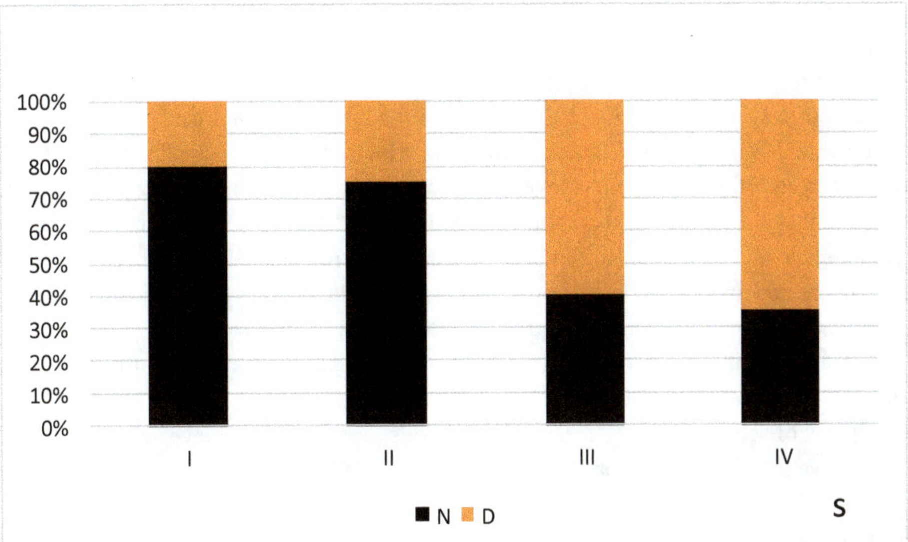

Fig.2. Structure and content of general exercises in the author's program: S – semester; N – exercises for insufficiently trained physical abilities; D – exercises for other physical abilities.

We marked out the system of SPAPT methods for higher educational establishments' students:

1) Cognitive (verbal, visual, diagnostic), which provide student with experience of SPAPT principles;

2) Organizational (practical, game, training, competition) – for practical realization of SPAPT program;

3) Control, owing to which it is possible to correct SPAPT methodic and stimulate further perfection (responsiveness, testing self-assessment).

Realization of the author's program took four stages. According to the worked out author's program physical education classes were conducted in the following directions:

1st semester – general physical training;

2nd semester – professionally oriented physical training;

3rd semester – professional-applied physical training;

4th semester – perfection of professional-applied physical training.

Improvement of indicators was regarded as positive result of author's SPAPT program realization.

By results of testing we found students' functional fitness. At the beginning of experiment by all tested functional parameters in EG and CG there were no any confident differences ($p < 0.05$) (see tables 1, 2).

Table 1. Indicators of EG and CG students' functional fitness at the beginning of experiment (n = 80)

Functional tests, indices	**EG (n=40)**	**CG (n=40)**	**Confidence, p**
	X±S	**X±S**	
Ruffiet's test (conv.un.)	10.1±0.92	10.7±1.04	>0.05
IFC (conv.un.)	3.1± 0.14	3..1± 0.12	>0.05
IHST(cov.un.)	61.3± 8.19	60.7± 8.91	>0.05

Note: IHST – index of Harvard step test.

Table 2. Indicators of EG and CG students' general physical fitness at the beginning of experiment (n = 80)

Physical abilities	**EG (n=40)**	**CG (n=40)**	**Confidence, p**
	X±S	X±S	
Endurance (sec.)	248.6±6.39	244.7±5.34	>0.05
Strength (times)	31.5±0.62	31.9±0.66	>0.05
Flexibility (cm)	15.7±0.71	15.4±0.61	>0.05
Coordination of movements (sec).	10.2±0.16	10.4±0.18	>0.05
Quickness (sec)	15.1±0.17	15.3±0.13	>0.05

Results of our research showed that the worked out SPAPT program causes more expressed positive changes in EG students' psycho-physical fitness, comparing with traditional. Its application in physical education process facilitates increase of physical fitness level and improvement of students' organism functional state.

It was found that in EG students there was confident ($p < 0.05$-< 0.001) improvement of a number of cardio vascular system's functional indicators. Ruffiet's test indicators increased by 25.1% at ($p < 0.01$). IFC (organism adaptation level) increased by 19.3% from initial value ($p < 0.01$) in EG. IFC indicators are determined by assessment scale as satisfactory adaptation. It witnesses about students' proper health.

We also found that in EG confidently ($p < 0.01$) indicator of physical workability improved 25.5%. By assessment scale such physical workability level is good.

The adequacy of selected SPAPT means and methods permitted to achieve substantial positive changes in dynamic of all above mentioned functional tests and indices in EG. By the end of experiment average indicator of these indices' increment was 23.3% in EG.

Analysis of testing results in respect to EG students' general physical fitness showed that there are positive changes in quantitative parameters of the indicators with confident difference at ($p < 0.05$-0.001) (see table 3).

Table 3. Indicators of EG and CG students' physical fitness before and after experiment

Physical abilities	Before experiment EG (n=40) X±S	CG (n=40) X±S	p	After experiment EG (n=40) X±S	CG (n=40) X±S	p
Endurance (sec.)	248.6±6.3	244.7±5.3	>0.05	201.4±6.72	233.7±5.35	<0.01
Coordination of movements (sec).	10.2±0.16	10.4±0.18	>0.05	8.4±0.14	9.2±0.15	<0.05
Quickness (sec)	15.1±0.17	15.3±0.13	>0.05	13.7±0.13	14.2±0.15	<0.05
Balance (sec.)	39.6±2.16	38.1±1.48	>0.05	54.8±1.78	41.1±2.23	<0.001
Coordination of arms' movements (sec).	10.7±0.54	10.8±0.88	>0.05	8.1±0.59	9.7±0.63	<0.05
Power endurance (sec.)	33.9±.84	34.7±1.39	>0.05	47.6±1.72	40.1±1.7	<0.001
Static power endurance (sec.)	32.6±1.40	32.3±1.64	>0.05	45.1±1.34	39.7±1.67	<0.001
Speed-power abilities (m)	6.0±0.36	6.1±0.35	>0.05	7.2±0.29	6.7±0.32	<0.05

Analysis of the received data proves effectiveness of the author's program SPAPT. It is also proved by statistically confident changes in EG students' functional fitness: Ruffiet's test – up to 25.1% ($p < 0.01$), IFC – up to 19.3% ($p < 0.01$), physical workability indicator – up to 25.5% ($p < 0.01$).

Discussion

In professional training student's general cultural level is determined by future professional functioning, by his/her specialization. It is proved in other works [8, 15, 16, and 18]. Besides, it is necessary to mention interconnection of professional and general culture; students' wider involvement in educational programs, in formation of individual-personality's culturelogic attitude to the world. Thus, modern medical worker shall have professionally important personality's qualities; basis of professionally necessary knowledge of medical sciences, clinical skills; certain behavioral strategies of professional duties' realization [30].

Methodological aspect of the studied problem has the following components: 1) professional training of medical profile students as scientific-pedagogic problem; 2) applied character of content and tasks of future medical workers' physical training; 3) organizational-pedagogic peculiarities of methodic of higher educational students' professional-applied physical training in modern conditions of higher education reformation [27]. It was also proved in our research.

Important element of our research is humanistic paradigm of future medical worker professional training. In this case organization of educational process is impossible without its appealing to personality: his/her age and individual features, qualities and abilities; value orientations, educational and spiritual-cultural demands and subjective experience. That is why study of SPAPT problem of future medical workers pre-conditions usage of personality's approach. It is also proved in other works [27, 30].

Labor conditions of medical workers are regarded as the most complex and tensed. This activity is characterized by significant mental and physical loads [33]. That is why it requires stable attention, quick reaction, coordination, endurance and high workability. In such case physical training is an important component of future medical workers' professional formation. It is directed at compulsory formation of medical students' professional motor skills and applied skills. Our research proves that perfection of students' physical fitness will facilitate effective mastering of chosen profession. It will ensure optimization of students' physical and psycho-physical state as well as health preservation and formation of comprehensively developed personality.

Our researches expanded ideas about content and importance of future medical specialists' SPAPT [25, 26]. The research's results showed that the worked out SPAPT program facilitates perfection of students' psycho-physical qualities; their readiness for future professional functioning.

Conclusions

1. Testing of the offered by us SPAPT methodic showed that application of the author's program ensured confident improvement of SPAPT every component's formation in experimental group.

2. Analysis of testing results in EG witnesses about positive changes in quantitative parameters. Besides, they prove and statistically confirmed the difference between final indicators of EG and CG students.

3.We confidently proved differences ($p < 0.05-0.001$) between initial and final indicators, which characterize professionally important for students abilities: speed-power skills, static power endurance, power endurance, arms' coordination, static balance.

Acknowledgements

The researches were conducted on the base of Poltava national pedagogic university, named after V.G. Korolenko in compliance with topic of scientific-research works of culturology and culturology teaching methodic department (state registration number 0116U002583).

Conflict of interests

The author declares that there is no conflict of interests.

References:

1. Adyrkhaev SG. Modern technology of physical education of disabled students in conditions of inclusive education. *Pedagogics, psychology, medical-biological problems of physical training and sports*, 2016;1:4-12. doi:10.15561/18189172.2016.0101
2. Aksenova NM. Osobennosti professional'nogo samoopredeleniia studentov [Peculiarities of students' professional self-determination]. *Sibirskaia psikhologiia segodnia*. 2003;2:190-199. (in Russian)
3. Alekseenko SN, Avdeeva MG, Drobot EV. *Cennostno-motivacionnye prioritety studentov medicinskogo vuza v otnoshenii zdorovogo obraza zhizni* [Value-motivation preferences of medical HEE students in respect to healthy life style]. Fundamental'nye issledovaniia, 2013;2 (1):16-19. (in Russian)
4. Bobyreva MM. *Sovershenstvovanie metodiki professional'no-prikladnoj fizicheskoj podgotovki studentov medicinskikh vuzov. Kand. Diss.* [Perfection of methodic of medical HEEs students'professional-applied physical training. Cand. Diss.], Almaty; 2008. (in Russian)
5. Gaskov AV, Kuzmin A.V., Kudryavtsev D.M., Iermakov S.S. Successfulness of general and special physical qualities' development on different stage of students-boxers' training. *Physical Education of Students*, 2016;1:4-11. doi:10.15561/20755279.2016.0101
6. Grigorchuk LI. *Gigiienichni aspekti profesijnoi adaptacii studentiv do umov navchannia u vishchikh medichnikh navchal'nikh zakladakh ta shliakhi ii optimizacii. Kand. Diss.* [Hygienic aspects of students' professional adaptation to conditions of medical educational establishments and ways of its optimization. Cand. Diss.], Kiev; 2000. (in Ukrainian)
7. Evseev Iu I. *Fizicheskaia kul'tura* [Physical culture], Rostov on Don; 2014. (in Russian)
8. Iermakov SS, Cieślicka Mirosława, Muszkieta Radosław. Physical culture in life of Eastern-European region students: modern state and prospects of development. *Physical Education of Students*, 2015;6:16-30. doi:10.15561/20755279.2015.0603
9. Ionova OM. Salutogenetic approach to professional training of future teachers. *Pedagogics, psychology, medical-biological problems of physical training and sports*, 2015;2:34-42. doi:10.15561/18189172.2015.0206
10. Kozina ZL, Iermakov SS, Kadutskaya LA, Sobyanin FI, Krzeminski M, Sobko IN, Ryepko OA. Comparative characteristic of correlation between pulse subjective indicators of girl students' and school girls' reaction to physical load. *Physical Education of Students*, 2016;4:24-34. doi:10.15561/20755279.2016.0403
11. Kolumbet AN. Methodic of girl students' professionally significant coordination qualities' perfection at physical education classes. *Physical Education of Students*, 2016;4:35-43. doi:10.15561/20755279.2016.0404
12. Kopeikina EN, Drogomeretsky VV, Kondakov VL, Kovaleva MV, Iermakov SS. Modification of Harvard step-test for assessment of students' with health problems functional potentials. *Physical Education of Students*, 2016;4:44-50. doi:10.15561/20755279.2016.0405
13. Kubaj GV. Position of medical colleges' students in respect to significance of physical exercises' practicing and resons, conditioning it. *Physical Education of Students*, 2015;6:38-42. doi:10.15561/20755279.2015.0605
14. Kudin SF. Formation of self-regulation culture of physical education faculty. *Physical Education of Students*, 2016;1:49-54. doi:10.15561/20755279.2016.0107
15. Kudryavtsev MD, Kopylov YuA, Kuzmin VA, Ionova OM, Yermakova TS. Personality oriented system of strengthening of students' physical, psychic and social-moral health. *Physical Education of Students*, 2016;3:58-64. doi:10.15561/20755279.2016.0308

16. Kudryavtsev MD, Kramida IE, Kuzmin VA, Iermakov SS, Cieslicka Miroslawa, Stankiewicz Blazej. Influence of study in hee on ubiquity and strength of students' computer gambling. *Physical Education of Students*, 2016;3:13-22. doi:10.15561/20755279.2016.0302
17. Kuzmin VA, Kopylov YuA, Kudryavtsev MD, Galimov GY, Iermakov SS. Substantiation of effectiveness of trainings on health related methodic for students with weakened motor fitness. *Physical Education of Students*, 2015;6:43-49. doi:10.15561/20755279.2015.0606
18. Pavlov VI. *Pedagogicheskaia sistema mnogourovnevoj fizicheskoj podgotovki vracha-stomatologa. Kand. Diss.* [Pedagogic system of multi-level physical training of dentist. Cand. Diss.], Saratov; 2000. (in Russian)
19. Pichurin VV. Resilience of students and their readiness for professional functioning. *Physical Education of Students*, 2015;3:38-43. doi:10.15561/20755279.2015.0305
20. Podrigalo LV, Iermakov SS, Alekseev AF, Rovnaya OA. Studying of interconnections of morphological functional indicators of students, who practice martial arts. *Physical Education of Students*, 2016;1:64-70. doi:10.15561/20755279.2016.0109
21. Radchenko AV. Professional self-assessment of future health basics teachers as professionally important quality. *Pedagogics, psychology, medical-biological problems of physical training and sports*, 2015;12:87-90. doi:10.15561/18189172.2015.12013
22. Raevskij RT. *Professional'no-prikladnaia fizicheskaia podgotovka studentov tekhnicheskikh vuzov* [Professional-applied physical training of technical; HEEs students], Moscow: High school; 1985. (in Russian)
23. Romanenko VA. *Diagnostika dvigatel'nykh sposobnostej* [Diagnostic of motor skills], Donetsk: DNU Publ.; 2005, (in Russian)
24. Salatenko IO, Dubinskaya OYa. Psycho-physical perfection of economic specialties' girl students under influence of sport-oriented technology, based on prevalence of volleyball practicing. *Pedagogics, psychology, medical-biological problems of physical training and sports*, 2015;12:103-108. doi:10.15561/18189172.2015.12016
25. Samsonova EA. Professional'no-prikladnaia fizicheskaia podgotovka sredi studentov medicinskogo universiteta [Professional-applied physical training of medical university students]. *Sci-article.ru*, [Internet]. 2014.;12. [cited 2016 Mar 16]; Available from: http://sci-article.ru/stat.php?i=1403452176 (in Russian)
26. Samsutina NM. Criteria, indicators and levels of formed professional functional competences of future teachers of physical culture. *Pedagogics, psychology, medical-biological problems of physical training and sports*, 2012;8:83-87.
27. Semenov B. Obgruntuvannia zmistu profesijno oriientovanoi fizichnoi pidgotovki studentiv fakul'tetu kharchovikh tekhnologij [Substantiation of professionally oriented physical training content for food technology students]. *Fizichne vikhovannia, sport i kul'tura zdorov'ia u suchasnomu suspil'stvi*, 2012;2(18):191-194. (in Ukrainian)
28. Semenova NV, Mahliovanyi AV. Dynamics of overall physical performance of the first year students of medical college under the influence of differentiate amount of physical activity. *Pedagogics, psychology, medical-biological problems of physical training and sports*, 2012;8:87-91.
29. Skurikhina NV, Kudryavtsev MD, Kuzmin VA, Iermakov SS. Fitness yoga as modern technology of special health groups' girl students' psycho-physical condition and psycho-social health strengthening. *Physical Education of Students*, 2016;20(2):24-31. doi:10.15561/20755279.2016.0204
30. Fotiniuk VG. Profesijno – prikladna fizichna pidgotovka iak efektivnij zasib gotovnosti studentiv do majbutn'oi diial'nosti za fakhom [Professional-applied physical training as effective mean of students' training for future professional activity]. *Vishcha osvita Ukraini*, 2012;1:436–442. (in Ukrainian)
31. Khripunova LD. To the question of the formation of personal qualities of future doctors by means of combat sports. *Physical Education of Students*, 2014;5:43-47. doi:10.15561/20755279.2014.0508
32. Chernovsky SM, Kolumbet AN. Determination of future designers' professionally important coordination qualities. *Physical Education of Students*, 2016;20(2):38-44. doi:10.15561/20755279.2016.0206
33. Shvidkij OV. *Gigiienichna optimizaciia navchannia i zakhodi shchodo okhoroni zdorov'ia studentiv medichnikh uchilishch v umovakh reformovanoi osviti. Kand. Diss.* [Hygienic optimization of learning and

health protection measures for medical colleges' students in conditions of reformed education. Cand. Diss.], Donetsk; 2003. (in Ukrainian)

34. Al-Hariri MT, Al-Hattami AA. Utilization of internet by health colleges students at the University of Dammam. *Journal of Taibah University Medical Sciences*. 2015;10(1):66–73.
35. East L, Hutchinson M. Evaluation of a filmed clinical scenario as a teaching resource for an introductory pharmacology unit for undergraduate health students: A pilot study. *Nurse Education Today,* 2015;35(12): 1252–1256).
36. Gherissi A, Tinsa F, Soussi S, Benzarti A. Teaching research methodology to student midwives through a socio-constructivist educational model: The experience of the high school for science and health techniques of Tunis. *Midwifery*. 2016;33:46–48.
37. Hadden KB. Health literacy training for health professions students. *Patient Education and Counseling*. 2015;98(7):918–920.
38. Ivashchenko O, Khudolii O, Yermakova T, Iermakov S, Nosko M, Nosko Y. Factorial and discriminant analysis as methodological basis of pedagogic control over motor and functional fitness of 14–16 year old girls. *Journal of Physical Education and Sport,* 2016. *16*(2), 442-451. doi:10.7752/jpes.2016.02068
39. Kara B, İşcan B. Predictors of Health Behaviors in Turkish Female Nursing Students. *Asian Nursing Research.* 2016;10(1):75–81.
40. Khudolii OM, Iermakov SS, Ananchenko KV. Factorial model of motor fitness of junior forms' boys. *Journal of Physical Education and Sport,* 2015. *15*(3), 585-591. doi:10.7752/jpes.2015.03088
41. Khudolii OM, Iermakov SS, Prusik K. Classification of motor fitness of 7-9 years old boys. *Journal of Physical Education and Sport,* 2015. *15*(2), 245-253. doi:10.7752/jpes.2015.02038
42. Lapkin S, Levett-Jones T, Gilligan C. Using the Theory of Planned Behaviour to examine health professional students' behavioural intentions in relation to medication safety and collaborative practice. *Nurse Education Today.* 2015;35(8):935–940.
43. Siri A, Rui M. Distance Education for Health Professions' Students. *Procedia - Social and Behavioral Sciences*. 2015;174(0):730–738.
44. Usher K, Woods C, Casella E, Glass N, Wilson R, Mayner L, et al. Australian health professions student use of social media. *Collegian*. 2014;21(2):95–101.

33

PERFECTION OF COORDINATION WITH THE HELP OF JUMP EXERCISES ON TRAMPOLINE

Boloban V.N., Tereshchenko I.A., Otsupok A.P., Krupenia S.V., Kovalenko Y.O., Otsupok An.P.
National University of Physical Education and Sport of Ukraine

Abstract. *Purpose:* to work out methodic of sportsmen's coordination perfection with the help of jumps on trampoline. *Material:* in the research 259 1st and 2nd year students (age 17-19 years) participated. The students were representatives of game and cyclic kinds of sports, sport gymnastic and martial arts. Among them there were 99 sportsmen with sport degrees. *Results:* we gave the definition of the term – coordination training. The students' sensor-motor coordination was confidently improved by means of the worked out methodic realization. The methodic included program of jump exercises on trampoline. We achieved positive dynamic of static-kinetic and static-dynamic balance as well as increased the quality of mastering of exercises with complex coordination. *Conclusions:* the methodic of sportsmen's coordination training with the help of jump exercises on trampoline was worked out, considering specificity of kinds of sports and sportsmen's qualification. This methodic improves sensor-motor coordination and is the basis of technical training and technical fitness.
Key words: sportsmen, sensor-motor abilities, methodic, coordination training, exercises, jumps on trampoline, testing, technical fitness.

Introduction

In kinds of sports with complex coordination structure competition exercises are fulfilled in difficult conditions of static-kinetic and static-dynamic balance [9, 11, 15]. Such kinds of sports include: sport kinds of gymnastic [1, 4, and 6], mountain skiing [11], sport wrestling [12], basketball [17], football [15] and other. Sportsmen have to solve motor tasks of body positions' control on supports and without support. They achieve coordination accuracy of motor actions in complex phase structure of sport exercises. Scientists conclude that decisive role in effective motor actions' control is played by sensor-motor coordination [2, 4, 18]. As it is shown by practice and experimental-methodic researches in some cases sensor-motor coordination is not sufficiently effective in demonstration of sports exercises. It is expressed in disordering of: body and bodies' system balance; space-time orientation of body on support and without support; temp-rhythm; differentiation of motor parameters. When fulfilling program reconstructions of competition exercises' motor structure, technical mistakes were found. Analysis of sport training modern state witnesses, that *coordination training* (CT) shall be an important direction. It shall be regarded as training process, directed at development and perfection of motor coordination with the help of special (specific) coordination exercises. Such exercises improve space, time and power indicators of systemic control over sportsman's movements. Coordination training is built, considering sportsman's indicators of special motor (physical) and special technical fitness. Besides, such training is built considering sensor-motor coordination (SMC), accumulated knowledge about level of perfection and individual sportsman's coordination abilities (CA); presence of valid means (coordination exercises) and methods of their realization in training and competition functioning. Coordination training is an element of system of sportsmen's many years' preparation.

Sensor motor coordination

In monograph by Prof. N.A. Bernstein [2] the following is written: "Coordination indeed is nothing but overcoming excessive degrees of freedom of our motor organs; i.e. transformation them into controlled systems". "We call introduction of continuous corrections in our movements on the base of sensor organs reports, principle of sensor corrections". "Sensor" (translated from Latin) means "related to sensitivity", "based on sensitivity" (p.54). Motor coordination (by N.A. Bernstein) ensures interaction of movements' construction levels at the account of sensor integration of Central nervous system (CNS) structures. Motor coordination abilities are understood as human abilities to quickly, accurately, bio-mechanically purposefully and inventively solve any motor tasks. Results of foreign scientists' works [14, 16, 17] also witness that sensor motor coordination is integral functioning of organism's sensor systems. Motor coordination is directed at development, control and correction of movements by means of sensor system's functioning: visual, tactile, proprioreceptive and interceptive sensor systems and olfaction sensor system.

Sensor motor coordination is rather a complex motor skill. This skill is in the base of control over sportsman's movements. It illustrates motor skills of elite sportsmen and sportsmen of low qualification. Sportsmen-beginners are separate category. At beginning stages of training – movements are included in sensor-motor coordination exercises. They can consist of a number of separate sensor-motor reactions, every of which has own beginning and end. In the process of training separate sensor-motor reactions are combine in flexible, plastic system of sensor-motor corrections of the fulfilled action – movement. Such approach is required for realization of generalized target (for example fulfillment of holistic sports exercise). Further complication of sensor-motor coordination takes place in case if it is necessary to control complex system. It is possible, when general and local coordination abilities are developed properly.

Coordination abilities

Multiple researchers of recent years showed that different manifestations of human coordination in physical education, sports, labor and military activity are rather specific. That is why instead of earlier term "dexterity" (which was rather multivalent) term "coordination abilities (CA) was introduced in theory and practice of sports. Besides, the system of such abilities and demand in differentiated approach to their development, have become relevant [3, 11, and 17]. Term "abilities" is regarded as manifestation of personality's individual qualities, which are subjective conditions of successful realization of motor functioning. They are not reduced to available knowledge, skills and abilities. Person's bents are their base. Abilities are detected by quickness, depth and strength of mastering motor actions' means and techniques. They are ordered psycho-physiological regulators, which condition possibilities of their acquiring and realization. Coordination abilities ensure economic and inventive, i.e. the most perfect, solution of motor tasks (especially difficult and sudden).

Professor Yu.K. Gaverdovskiy [6] regards these abilities as bents, developed by purposeful work. He points that there are the following abilities: to generalized or specialized types (equally important in any kind of activity); local abilities, which express the most brightly individual's bents to certain forms of activity. As a rule, full development of exactly such abilities plays decisive role in human self-realization (in particular sportsmen's).

Professor V.N. Platonov [11] writes: "Sportsman's coordination abilities are variable and specific for every kind of sport. However, they shall be differentiated into separate kinds by specific features of their manifestation, criteria of their assessment and factors, which condition them. Basing on results of special researches… one can mark out the following relatively independent kinds of coordination abilities: assessment and regulation of dynamic and movements' space-time parameters; keeping of balance and stability; sense of rhythm; orientation in space; inter and intra muscular coordination; ability for relaxation; coordination of movements. In actual training and competition functioning all mentioned abilities manifest not purely but in complex interaction. In definite situations some coordination abilities are leading and other are secondary. With it, instant change of different abilities' role is possible, caused by change of external circumstances. Especially noticeable it is in sport gymnastic, acrobatic, sport games, martial arts, mountain skiing: in all kinds of sports, in which result mainly depends on coordination abilities" (2015. – Vol. 2. – Pg.797).

Exercises of sport kinds of gymnastic were created artificially [1, 6]. They practically are not used in everyday life. At the same time, in the world unique competition exercises' systems with complex motor coordination exist and successfully develop. They are also successfully demonstrated in the form of compositions at sport competitions of different levels, Olympic Games including. In this connection requirements to physical, functional (sensor-motor) coordination and technical fitness of sportsmen are being worked out and perfected. Coordination complexity of competition programs remain the key tendency. Their difficulty (according to tables of difficulty of International gymnastic federation) shall be related to it also.

Professor V.N. Boloban [3] studied twelve coordination abilities, which correspond to specific of sport kinds of gymnastic. They characterize quality of sportsman's motor control. These abilities are realized in training and competition functioning differently. They are the basis of technical perfection and technical fitness. They are abilities for the following:

- Static and dynamic balance; balancing in system of interacting bodies;
- Assessment of proprioreceptive signals in orthgrade and reverse body positions;

- Vestibular balance and sensitivity;
- Assessment of time and space on support and without it;
- Differentiation of motor parameters;
- Assessment of motor stability and watching object (partner, opponent);
- Manifestation and change of motor rhythm-temp;
- Reactivity of movements by time of motor reaction;
- Movements frequency;
- Movements symmetry and asymmetry;
- Movements' concordance with music.

Many scientific works are devoted to study significant coordination abilities in many kinds of sports. Insignificant discrepancies, existing in them, only prove specific character of one or another ability manifestation and individual distinctions in its domination in relative kind of sports (or in separate kind of sports).

Development and perfection of coordination training programs

Recent years, in the world exercises' programs of general [11] and specific (local) influence on sportsman's motor coordination have been being worked out and perfected [5, 8, 12, 15].

General exercises' programs are directed at formation of solid foundation for motor skills in exercises' fulfillment. In this case, indicators of space, time and power motor parameters are considered. On the base of exercises' programs and algorithms of their realization basic fund of individual sportsman's movements – exercises is created. With it, sportsman's individual indicators of special fitness, specific of kind of sports, stages of training are considered. Exercises' programs with application of new technical means are used: SportKat (diagnostic-exercise); step-platforms Body – Balance (exercises on moving platforms); fit-ball; platforms – semi-spheres of type BOSU Balance Training; water slides with spring board of different height, which push sportsman in free flight with "landing" in water. They permit to develop body movements and perfect their control in space (usually used in freestyle). Means for training static-dynamic balance are used (for example ball throws in basket, standing on moving platform or semi-sphere) and etc. Different by structure exercises are fulfilled: turns, body twisting, forward and backward body bents with support on fit ball, with other subjects [11, 14, 15]. Sportsmen have opportunity to train surface and deeper muscles as well as to form muscular corset; to work at sensor systems' development and perfection of their integrative interaction in process of sports exercises' fulfillment. With it, improvement of vestibular sensor system's functioning, as the base of technical fitness, is accented [4, 13].

Programs of special exercises are worked out and realized for training local manifestation of specific coordination abilities; determination of their functioning characteristics and assessment criteria, as well as factors, which condition them. Such specific and locally manifested CA include: motor control in space; balance in reverse body position; balancing, juggling; temp-rhythm; feeling of time; feeling of sport apparatus; feeling of object; feeling of water; feeling of partner or opponent; muscular-joint feeling; vestibular sensitivity; balance in motion; fine motor abilities; balancing on narrow, mobile or high support; jumping; interaction of music and movements and so on. Special exercises' programs of specific impact actually have the same names in coordination training: program of positions; program of orientation; program of coordination; program of balance or stability; program of "light" acrobatic; program of rhythm; program of "sanging" [temp-rhythmic sportsman's boy interactions with support (hanging), without support and with turns around longitudinal axis]; program of mechanic interaction with support; program of landing; program for flexibility, mobility and other. For their realization physical and sport exercises of certain kind of sports are used as well as exercises of other (relative) kinds of sports and technical means [4,13]. *Alongside with it, it should be noted that there nearly no scientific-methodic materials, which would substantiate usage of trampoline jumps. Especially it concerns training and improvement sensor-motor coordination. In this case special importance is acquired by coordination training structure in different kinds of sports.*

Trampoline jumps is an Olympic kind of sports (since 2000). The prospects of this kind of sports are as follows: expansion of geography of countries, in which trampoline jumps are practiced; increase of quantity of trampoline jumpers; development of sport exercises of different groups of difficulty; perfection of sport technique; raising of sportsmanship level in individual and synchronous jumps.

Trampoline jumps exercises are used as mean of motor and functional-technical training in different kinds of sports, physical education and professional functioning (for example in vestibular analyzer training in mountain skiers, astronauts, sailors, drivers and so on). These exercises stimulate visual analyzer that facilitates motor control, avoiding air and sea sickness as well as activate breathing and improve blood circulation and result in positive psychological and emotional state. By effectiveness, trampoline jumps to large extent exceed usual cardio training. Scientists-physiologists from NASA found that usefulness of trampoline jumps significantly exceeds advantages of run (to be more exact by 68%). In contrast to track, trampoline springing jumps compensate up to 80% of loads on joints. By this reason 10 minutes of trampoline jumps have the same effectiveness as 30 minutes of jogging [19].

The purpose of the research: is to work out methodic of sportsmen's coordination training with application trampoline jumps.

The tasks of the research: 1. to study indicators of elite sportsmen's coordination indicators (in kinds of sports with complex motor coordination).
2. To work out coordination training methodic with application elite sportsmen's trampoline jumps as well as to test effectiveness of its application in practical trainings of 1st and 2nd year students of National university of physical education and sports of Ukraine (NUPESU).

Material and methods

Participants: in the research 1st and 2nd year students of NUPESU (n=238) participated. They were (142 boys and 96 girls of 17 – 18 years' age, who specialized in the following kinds of sports: games, cyclic, with complex coordination, martial arts. From them: masters and candidate master of sports – 78; 1st-2nd sports degrees sportsmen - 111 persons; without sport degrees - 49 persons. Besides 2nd year students of NUPESU n=21) (14 girls and 7 boys) of 18 – 19 years age, specializing in sport gymnastic, participated in the research. From them there were 15 masters of sports and 6 candidate masters of sports 13].

Organization of the research: the researches were conducted with 1st year students (September 2014 – May 2015 – 30 training sessions) and with 2nd year students (September 2015 – May 2016 – 30 training sessions). Sportsmen of sport gymnastic fulfilled coordination exercises during 30 sessions at 1st year and 60 training sessions at 2nd years (twice a week).

Statistical analysis: materials of the research were processed with the help of mathematical statistic methods (Excel, Statistika).

Results of the research

We have worked out methodic of sportsmen's coordination training with application of trampoline jumps (see fig. 1). Nine elements are in the base of it. The elements of priority are: individual indicators of students' technical fitness (sportsman, qualification) and program of trampoline jumps. The program included three blocks: elementary exercises on trampoline, combinations of elementary and basic exercises on trampoline.

Methodic and practical recommendations for mastering trampoline jumps' technique: the first practical steps of sportsmen in mastering trampoline jumps are connected with formation of "feeling" of sport apparatus, accurate body positions:

- Walking on trampoline network face or back toward direction of walk; rolls over on trampoline;
- Rocking and jumping on feet at little height on all surface of network (feet at shoulder width, feet apart (left leg, right leg));
- Rocking in the center of trampoline (on "cross", feet joined, arms downward, along torso) – "cross" is the main place of jumps on trampoline.

After acquiring self-confidence, jumps shall be fulfilled with arms raised upward [7, 10]. When training trampoline exercises, it is important to master required elements of *working carriage*. Working carriage permits to control feeling of body postures, body positions on support and without support. Specialists [1, 6, and 13] conventionally mark out the following types of working carriage: closed carriage, half-closed carriage, grouped carriage, half-grouped carriage, bent carriage, straight (arching) carriage. Working carriage is a multiplication of body postures and body positions in phase structure of sport exercise. For example, multiplication of posture "grouped" with back somersault is a working carriage. Actually working carriage is a signal position of movement – exercise [4]. It orients sportsman for fulfillment of exercise without extra motor reconstructions. It facilitates the trainee not to accumulate technical mistakes in exercise phases. Working carriage shall be stable motor skill.

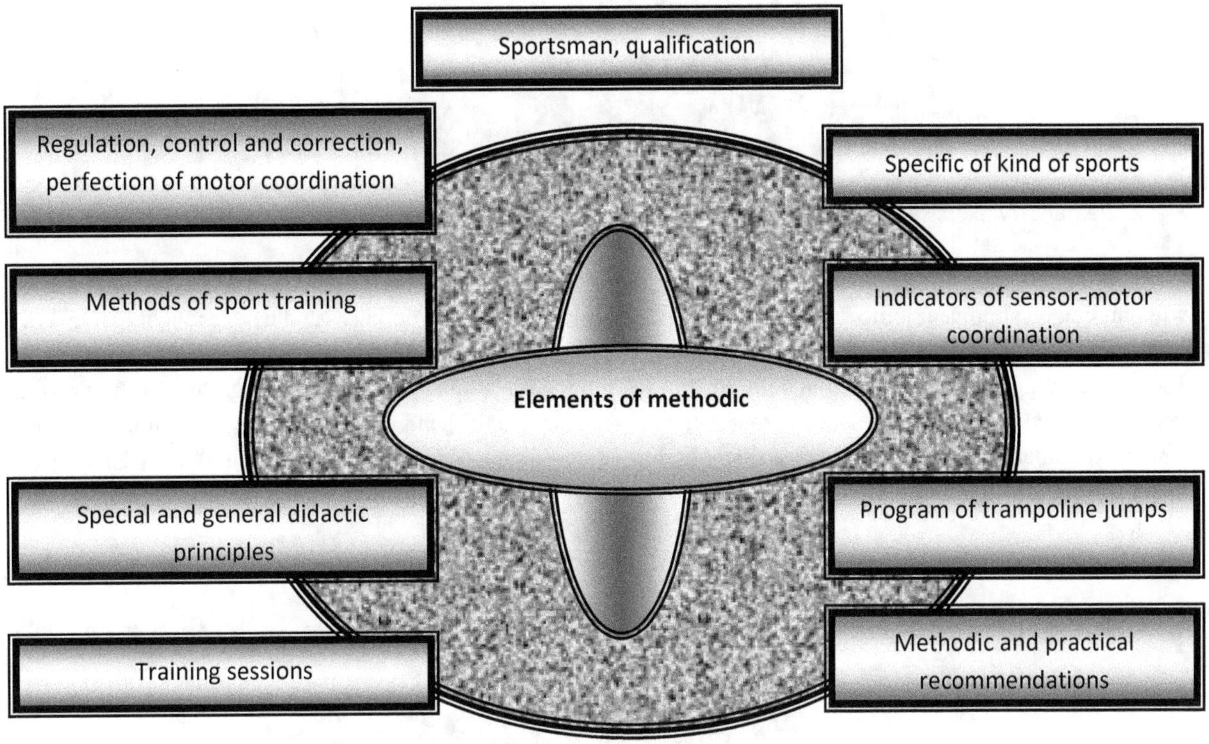

Fig.1. Elements of sportsmen's coordination training methodic with application of trampoline jumps

To achieve sufficient flight height after pushing off is possible only after 2-3 (sometimes 5-7), depending on exercise' complexity) jumps on the spot (in the center). In practice such jumps are called "temp jumps". This, at first sight simple exercise, shall be carefully mastered and perfected at all stages of sport exercises. In initial position legs are in narrow stance (for beginners it is possible to keep feet at shoulder width); torso is straight; arms – a little bit backward; eyes look forward. Pushing off is fulfilled at the account of ankle, knee joints' bending, agreed with elasticity of network; when legs are straightened and with pushing off arms are driven forward and upward. In flight hip, knee and ankle joints are straightened, toes – are also straitened and feet touch each other. From position arms upward (arms and body make one straight line): in the process of body descend arms move to horizontal position. Then arms start move a little back and downward. Just before touching the network, legs move to closed position (or at shoulder width) to increase stability; elite sportsmen usually keep feet close. *It is important to watch rhythm of arms' movement.* Jumps are fulfilled standing on legs, from sitting position,; from position on abdomen, on back; from position on knees; without rotation; with rotation forward and backward (around transapical axis) and around (together functioning) longitudinal and transapical axes (pirouettes). Exercises have different forms (compulsory body positions): grouped, half-grouped, bent, bent with feet apart; arching and straightened as well as additional body positions [for example jump "kazak", half-split, split, split with left (right) leg forward and other].

Helping plays important role in training of exercises of progressing difficulty. The most effective helping is with application of suspended turning belt. Besides, the following is used: manual belt (initial stages of training); helping with arms; foam mats in the place of sportsman's landing. Then it is possible to used built-in the floor trampoline; complex: trampoline and pit filled with foam polyurethane; in some cases all free trainees shall locate around trampoline for assistance, if required.

Program of jump exercises on trampoline

Block 1. Elementary exercises of trampoline jumps are: body in vertical sitting position; hands are on trampoline network with fingers pointed forward; stand on knees with arms dropped down; standing on knees with hands on network; grouping in lying on back position; lying position with arms pointed forward; body in lying on abdomen position with feet touching each other and bent arms with hands on network (see fig.2).

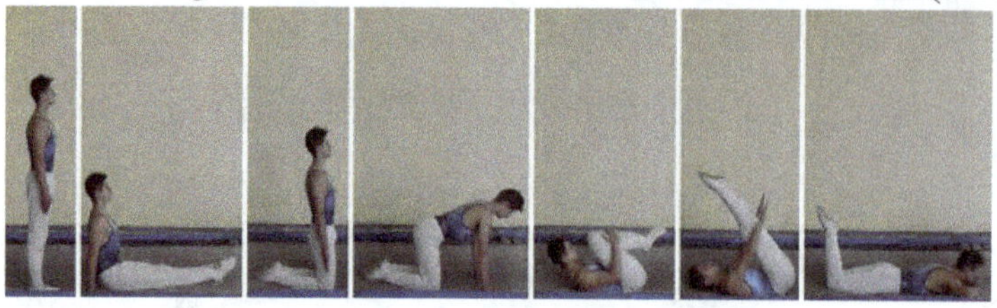

1 2 3 4 5 6 7

Fig. 2. Elementary exercises of trampoline jumps

Block 2. Basic exercises of trampoline jumps are: temp jumps; jump with landing in sitting position; jump with landing on abdomen; jump with landing on knees; jump with landing on knees and hands, touching network; jump with turn by 90° (4 x 90°) in both sides; jump with turn by 180° (2 x 180°) in both sides; jump with turn by 180° and landing in sitting position in both sides; back jump with landing on back, grouping; forward jump with landing on back; forward somersault, grouping; forward somersault, bending; backward somersault, grouping; backward somersault, bending; backward somersault in straightened position (¾ of rotation) with landing on abdomen; jump with turn by 360° in both sides; back somersault, bending, with turn by 360°.

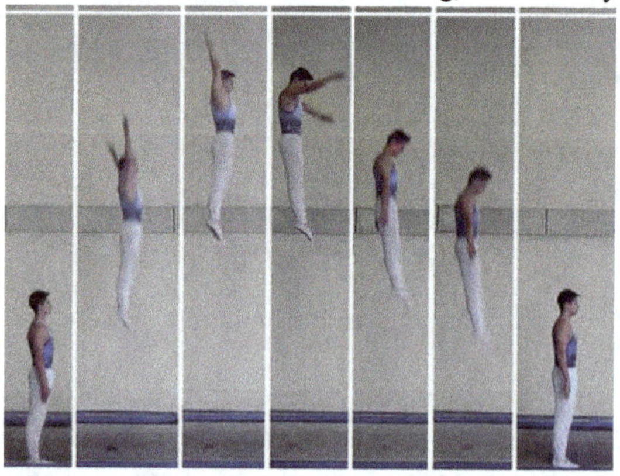

1 2 3 4 5 6 7

Fig.3. Temp jumps

Recommendations: keep vertical position (shots 1 – 3, half-closed working carriage) – head a little bent with chin touching chest and shoulder and hip joints bent (shots 4-5). It permits for sportsman to control straightness of body. Arms are waved from down to upward. Safety measures are: when landing with mestakes (absence of vertical position) it is necessary to relax legs and damp landing on network. Fulfill 5-7 repetitions in 4-5 attempts. In all next exercises technique of temp jumps is the same.

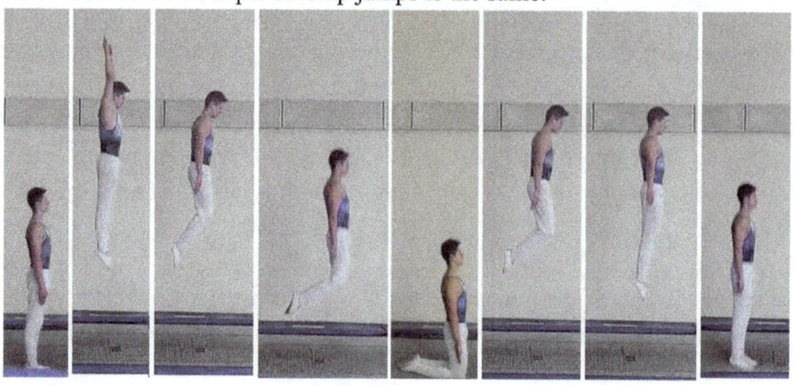

1 2 3 4 5 6 7 8

Fig.4. Jump with landing on knees

Recommendations: not high temp jumps (vertical position, shots 1-2); jump with landing on knees with straightened toes and arms dropped (shots 3-5); temp jumps with following stop (shots 6-8). Pay attention to absence of angle in hip joints; keep buttock muscles tensed with knees at the width of foot, when landing on knees. Repeat exrcise 2-4 times in 2-3 attempts.

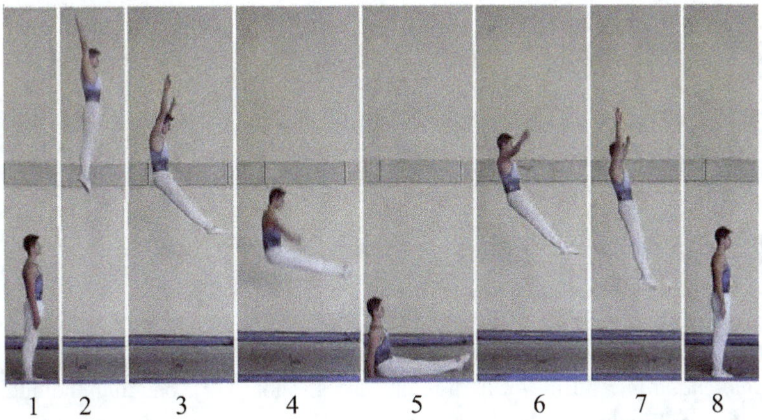

Fig. 5. Jump with landing in sitting position

Recommendations: fulfill temp jumps (vertical position, shots 1-2); whenn landing, raise legs forward and take sitting position with arms bent behind torson, on network and hands directed forward (shots 3-5); fulfil temp jump and stop (shots 6 – 8). Pay attention to simultaneous touching network with all back surface of legs and hands' position. Repeat exercise 2-4 times in 2-3 atempts.

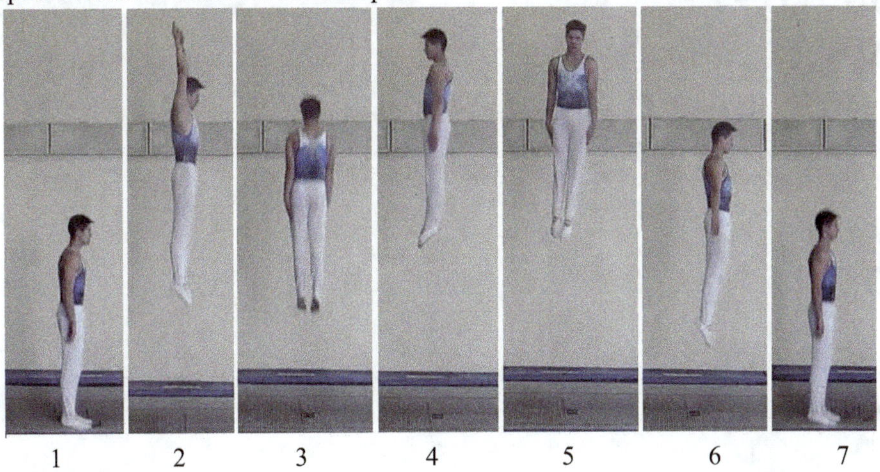

Fig.6. Jump with left turn by 360°

Recommendations: fulfill temp jumps (shots 1-2); then – upward jump with left turn by 360° (shots 3 – 6), with following temp jump and stoppage (shot 7). Turn shall be fulfilled in ascending part of jump in vertical position with arms pressed to torso. Fulfill exercise 2-4 times in 2-3 attempts.

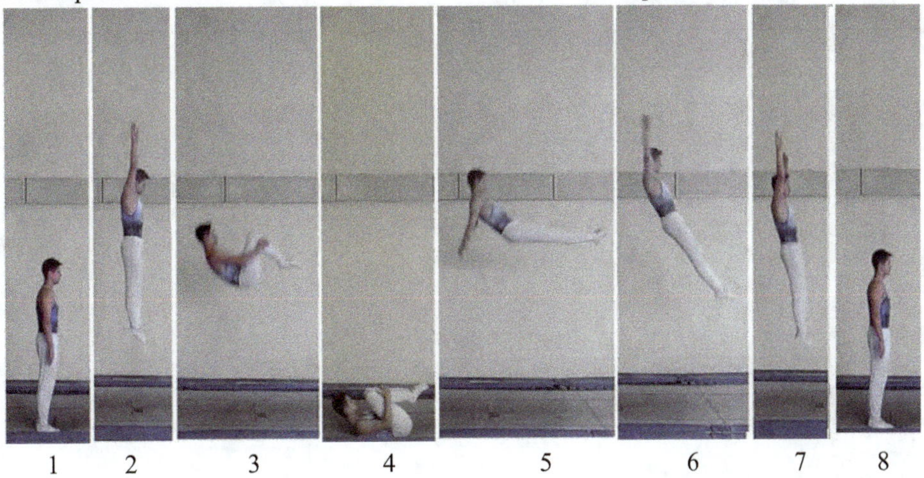

Fig.7. Backward jump with landing on back, grouping

Recommendations: fulfill not high temp jumps (shots 1-2); bending legs and grouping fulfill jump backard, landing on back, grouping (shots 3-4); unbending legs forward-upward land on network And stop (shots 5-8). Fulfill exercise 3-4 times in 2-3 attempts.

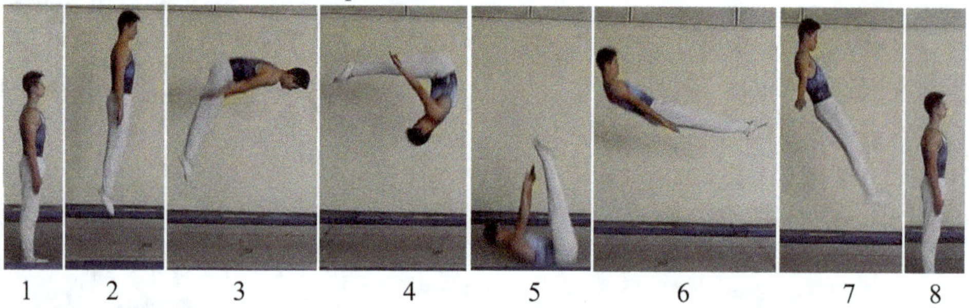

Fig.8. Forward jump with landing on back, bending with arms, directed forward

Recommendations: fulfill not high temp jumps (shots 1-2); bending shoulders forward and bnding in hip joints fulfill forward jump with landing on back in bent position with arms directed forward (shots 3 – 5); unbending elgs forward-upward, fulfill landing on network and stop (shots 6 – 8). Fulfill exercise 3-4 times in 2-3 attempts.

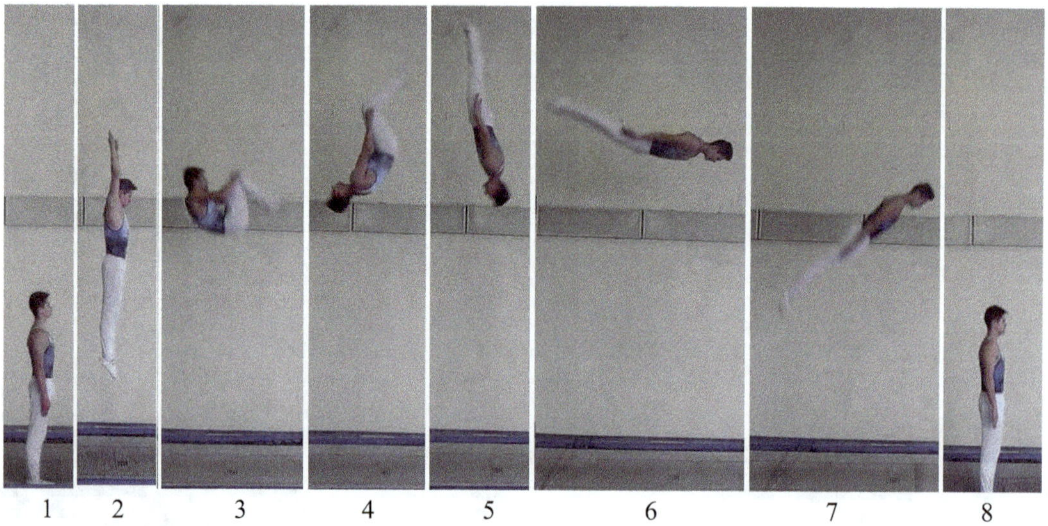

Fig.9. Back somersault

Recommendations: fulfill temp jumps (shots 1-2). In tep jumps create backward rotation and grpup body, bending legs with following quick ungrouping in ascending part of jump (shots 3-5). In descending part of jumps raise shoulders upward, taking vertical position with arms pressed to torso, land and stop (shots 6 – 8). Pay attention to tightness and quickness of grouping. Fulfill exercise 2-4 times in 2-3 attempts.

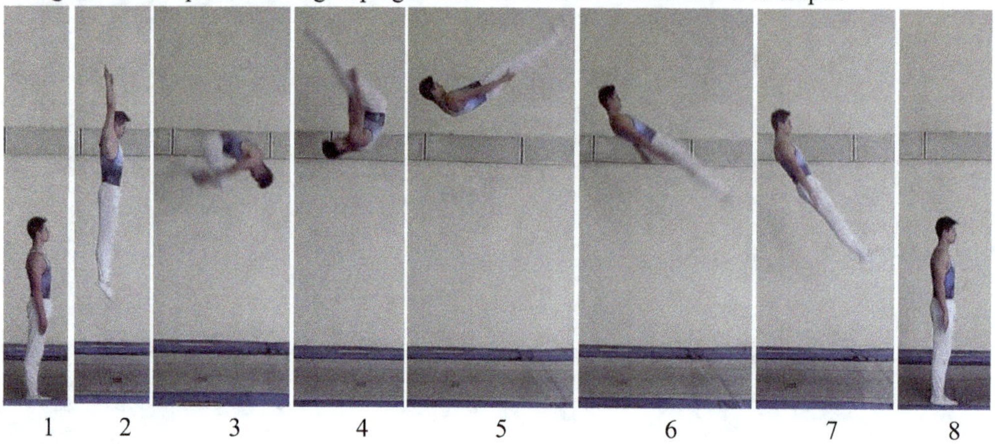

Fig.10. Forward somersault

Recommendations: fulfill temp jumps (shots 1-2); bending torso forward and legs, group body with following quick ungrouping in ascending part of jump (shots 3 – 5). In descending part of jump raise shoulders upward, taking vertical position with arms pressed to torso, then land and stop (shots 6 – 8). Pay attention to tightness and quickness of grouping. Fulfill exercise 2-4 times in 2-3 attempts.

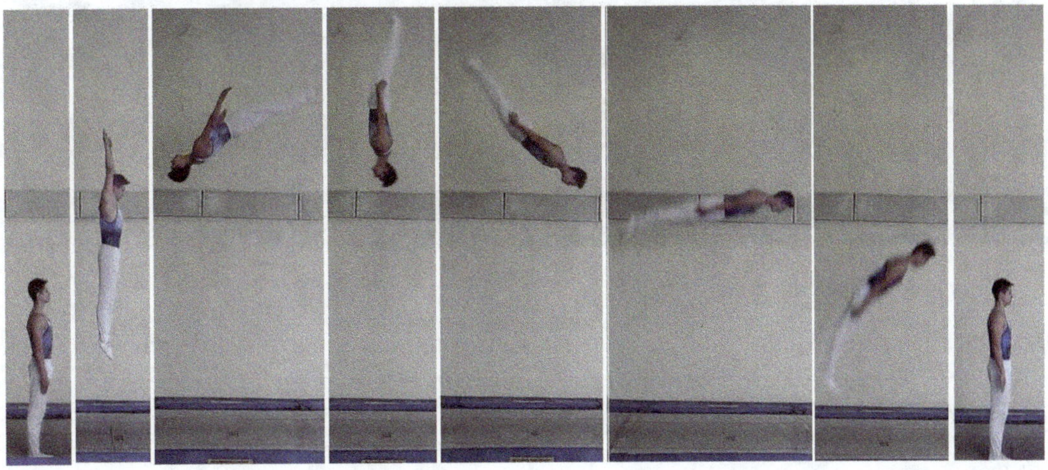

1 2 3 4 5 6 7 8

Fig.11. Back somersault, straightening

Recommendations: fulfill temp jumps (shots 1-2); in ascending part of jump, bending backward with insignificant arching raise straightened legs and press arms to torso (shots 3 – 5). In descendin part raise shoulder upward, taking vertical position, kand and stop (shots 6 – 8). Pay attention to straightness and tightness of body position in space. Fulfill exercise 2-4 times in 2-3 attempts.

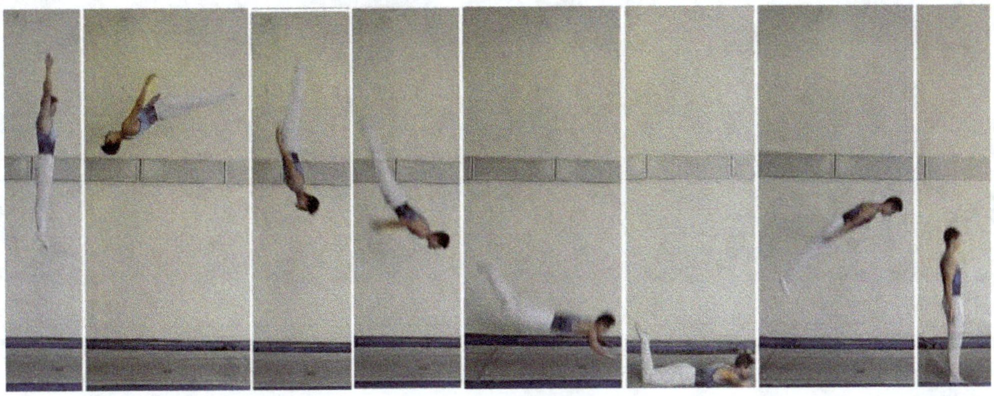

1 2 3 4 5 6 7 8

Fig.12. Back somersault, straightening with landing on abdomen

Recommendations: temp jumps (shot 1, three-four temp jumps are also possible); ¾ of back somersault straightening (shots 2 – 4)with landing on abdomen (shots 5 – 6) and coming upward to stop (shots 7 – 8).

Block 3. Examplary combinations of elementary and basic exercises of trampoline jumps program

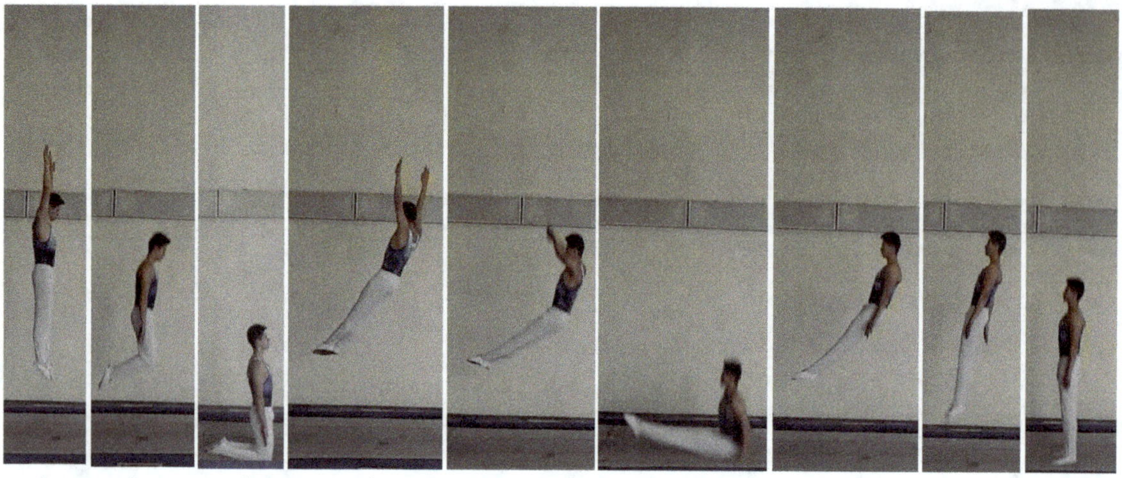
1 2 3 4 5 6 7 8 9

Fig. 13. Combination 1. Temp jumping (shot 1); jump in stance on knees (shots 2 – 3); jump upward with left turn by 180° and landing in sitting position (shots 4 – 6), then stop (shots 7 – 9).

Recommendations: in jump combination it is necessary to coordinate arms movements (in ascending part of trajectory arms go upward and in descending part – downward with accented arm moving to the side of turn (to the left or to the right)). Pay attention to accuracy of turn and taking sitting position with hands on network and fingers directed forward. Fulfill combination 2-4 times to each side.

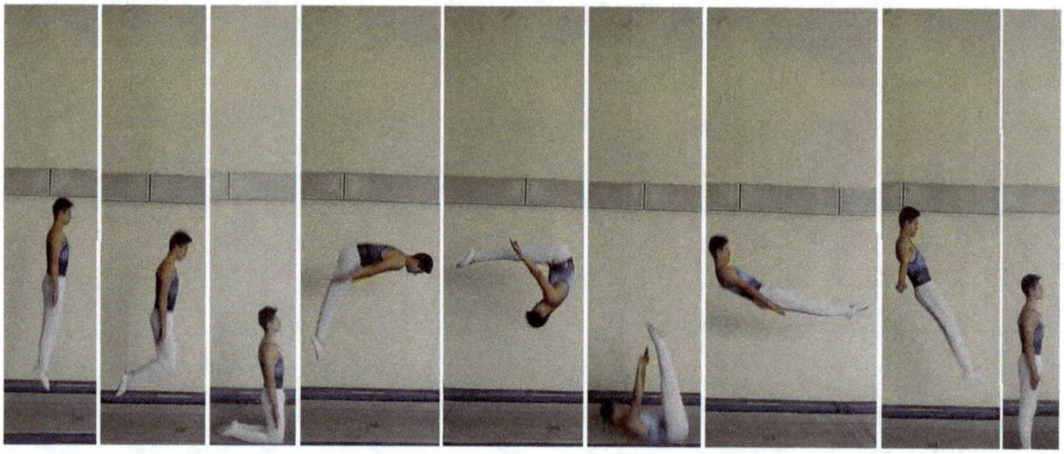
1 2 3 4 5 6 7 8 9

Fig.14. Combination 2. Temp jumping (shot 1); jump in stance on knees (shots 2 – 3); jump forward with landing in position lying on back, bending, arms are directed forward (shots 4 – 6); coming out of lying on back position and stoppage (shots 7 – 8).

Recommendations: Pay attention to creation of forward rotational movement with round back, head, bent on chest and to landing on network by all surface of back. Fulfill 2-3 times in 3-4 attempts.

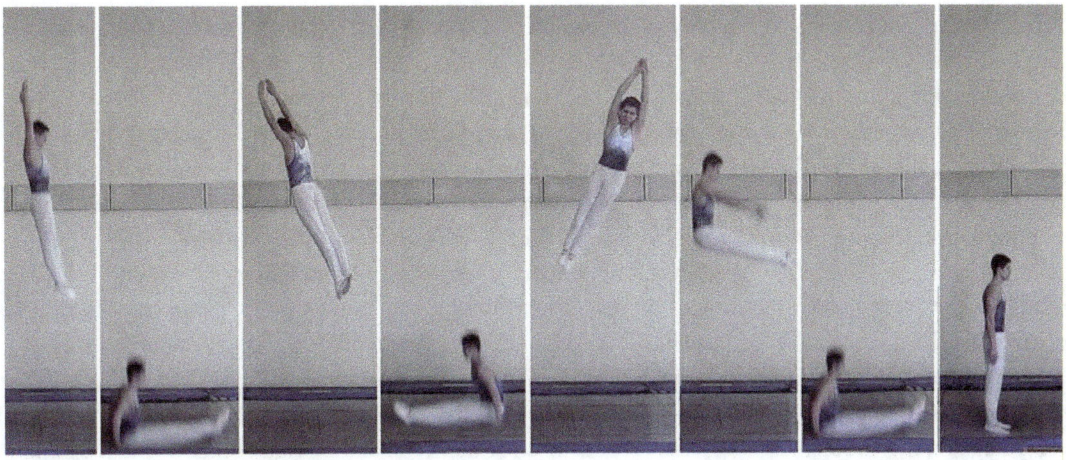

1 2 3 4 5 6 7 8

Fig.15. Combination 3. Temp jump (shot 1) and landing in sitting position (shot 2); jump upward with left turn by 180° andlanding in sitting position (shots 3 – 4); jump upward with right turn by 180° and landing in sitting position (shots 5 – 7); stoppage (shot 8).

Recommendations: when fulfilling right or left turns body shall be straightened with armes raised upward; landing shall be accurate. Fulfill 2 repetitions in 2-3 attempts.

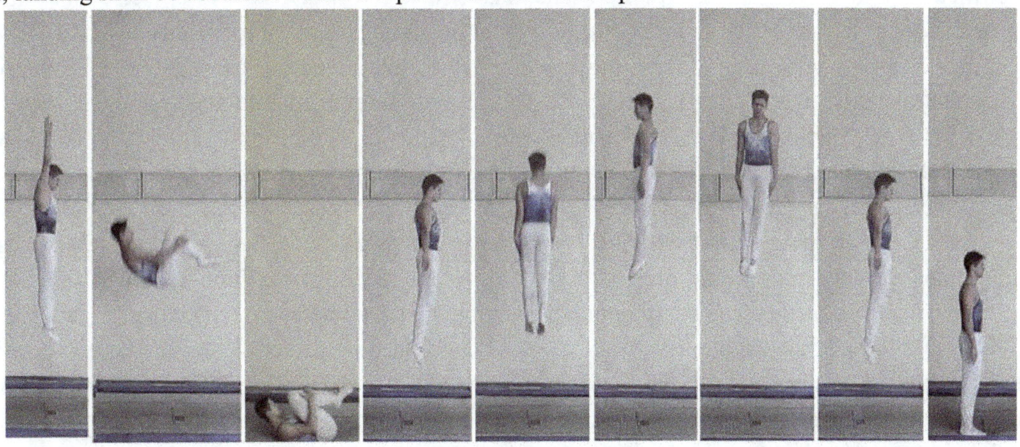

1 2 3 4 5 6 7 8 9

Fig 16. Combination 4. Temp jump (shot 1); jump backward, taking position landing on back and grouping (shots 2 – 3); jump forward and temp jump with turn by 360° (shots 4 – 8); stop (shot 9). 2 repetitions in every attempt, (2-3 attempts).

Recommendations: Pay attention to creation of back rotational movement with accent on taking lying on back position, groupoing. Left turn by 360° sall be fulfilled in ascending part of jump, in vertical position with arms, pressed to torso. Fulfill combination 2-4 times in 2-3 attempts to both sides.

The program exercises improved the quality of control over movements in space, regulation of body position on support, when fulfilling tests for static-kinetic and static-dynamic body stability; for coordination of symmetric and asymmetric limbs' movements. The confidentiality of results was at $p \leq 0.05$ (for sportsmen, specializing in game, cyclic sports and kinds of sports with complex coordination and in martial arts) and at $p \leq 0.01$ (sport gymnastic, calisthenics, sport acrobatic).

Discussion

"Coordination training" term in system of sportsmen's Olympic training has been becoming still more important by its efficiency in separate elements of motor functioning, resulted in appropriate sport results. Coordination training is one of modern training process components and important indicator of results, acieved by sportsmen in competition functioning. We worked at this article in period of Olypic games, 2016. Sportsmen demonstrated excellent results; they achieved impossible. Alongside with organism's high functional potentils, sportsmen demonstrated excellent motor control, static-dynamic balance and accurate regulation of body and bodies' system: triathlon – bicyclist; gymnast – apparatus; shooter – arm; female gymnast – object; horseman-horse; wrestler- opponent; rower – boat and etc. We are sure that for achievement of target sportsmen need to manifest high potentials of vestibular analyzer; ability to contract and relax activly working muscles; keep balance in orthograde and reverse body position; control and change temp-rhytm of movements – exercises; demonstrated proper coordination. Event at present time, Nikolay Alexandrovich Bernstein, at Olympic games 2016, would have stressed significance of perfection of sportsman's sensor systems, their functioning, depending on dynamic of motor and psycho-physiological tasks. Unfortunately not all Olympic games' participants had the best results. Specialists will have to analyze every separate case of failure; may be there will appear understanding of global work at development and perfection of sensor-motor coordination in coordination training structure in many years' sport training. There are examples to it. First of all they are the works of Professor V.N. Platonov [11], containing new knowledge on this problem as well as the works of other domestic and foreign authors c [4, 13, 17]. For this purpose exercises' programs with application of new technical means are used. It permits to train and perfection motor control in space, static-kinetic and static-dynamic balance. With the help of technical means different by structure exercises are fulfilled: turns, body twists, forwad-backward torso bents (for example with support on fit ball; with other objects designed for creation flexible-rigid but plastic muscular corset) [14, 15, 18]. The researches showed that in demonstration of training and competition programs sensor-motor coordination manifests weakly and is insufficient in motor, bio-mechanical and functional structuires of the fulfilled exercises. The following technical mistakes are registered: in motor control in space; in landing; in keeping balance of body and bodies' system; body stiffness in movements, requiring plasticity; inaccurate working carriage [4]. In our opinion, alongside with realization of traditional training and competition programs individual work with sportsman is required, which would be directed at sensor-motor coordination's training and perfection; at recognizing coordination abilities of first priority. Such abilities shall reflect specificity of a kind of sports, feeling of sport apparatus, partner, opponent. Besides, they shall be carefully considered by a coach.

Let us also note nearly complete absence of scientific-methodic materials, substantiating usage of trampoline jumps for development and perfection of sportsmen's sensor-motor coordination. One of the most important elements of the methodic is the program of trampoline jumps; methodic recommendations; regulation, control and correction of training process. With it, we found high role of factor "technique-coordination" in sportsmen's motor actions: technical level determines successfulness of control tests' fulfillment. In its turn, sensor-motor coordination is the base of technical fitness. Results of pedagogic experiment proved effectiveness of trampoline jumps exercises for perfection of motor coordination.

Conclusions

1. We registered no high level of sensor-motor coordination as the base of technical fitness of elite sportsmen, specializing in sports with complex coordination.

2. The worked out and implemented in training process methodic with application of trampoline jumps confidently improved sensor-motor coordination. It is the base of sportsmen's technical fitness and shall be of priority in system of sport training.

3. The methodic includes interconnected on the base of factor "technique-coordination" the following elements: sportsmen's technical fitness by individual indicators of sensor-motor coordination; specificity of kind of sports; program of trampoline jumps exercises, including three blocks of exercises: block of elementary trampoline jumps; block of basic trampoline jumps; block of elementary and basic exercises' combinations; methodic and practical recommendations; special and general-didactic principles; forms of trainings; elements of regulation, control and correction of motor actions.

Acknowledgements

The work has been fulfilled in compliance with combined plan of scientific-research works in sphere of physical culture and sports of Ukraine for 2011-2015. Code of topic is 2.15. The name of topic is "Control of static-dynamic stability of sportsman's body and bodies' system in kinds of sports with complex motor coordination", state registration № 0111U001726. Index UDK: 796.012.2. Scientific supervisor is doctor of pedagogical sciences Professor V.N. Boloban.

Conflict of interests

The author declares that there are no conflicts of interests.

References:

1. Arkaev LIa, Suchilin NG. *Kak gotovit' chempionov* [How to prepare champions], Moscow: Physical Culture and Sport; 2004. (in Russian)
2. Bernshtejn NA. *O lovkosti i ee razvitii* [On dexterity and its training], Moscow: Physical Culture and Sport; 1991. (in Russian)
3. Boloban VN. Elementy teorii i praktiki sportivnoj orientacii, otbora i komplektovaniia grupp v sportivnoj akrobatike [Elements of theory and practice of sport orientation, selection and completing of sport acrobatic groups]. *Pedagogics, psychology, medical-biological problems of physical training and sports*, 2009;2:21 – 31. (in Russian)
4. Boloban VN. Sensomotornaia koordinaciia kak osnova tekhnicheskoj podgotovki [Sensor-motor coordination as the base of technical fitness]. *Nauka v olimpijskom sporte*, 2015;2:73 – 80. (in Russian)
5. Borzov VF. Podgotovka legkoatleta – sprintera: strategiia, planirovanie, tekhnologii [Training of light athlete-sprinter: strategy, planning, technologies]. *Nauka v olimpijskom sporte*, 2013;4:71 – 82. (in Russian)
6. Gaverdovskij IuK. *Obuchenie sportivnym uprazhneniiam* [Training of sport exercises], Moscow: Physical Culture and Sport; 2007. (in Russian)
7. Danilov K, Nikolaev Iu. *Uprazhneniia na batute* [Exercises on trampoline], Moscow: Physical Culture and Sport; 1966. (in Russian)
8. Dobrynskaia N. Special'nye uprazhneniia v legkoatleticheskom mnogobor'e [Special exercises in light athletic multi-sport events]. *Nauka v olimpijskom sporte*, 2014;2:69 – 78. (in Russian)
9. Litvinenko YV, Sadowski Jerzy, Niznikowski Tomasz, Boloban VN. Static-dynamic stability of the body gymnasts qualifications. *Pedagogics, psychology, medical-biological problems of physical training and sports*, 2015;1:46-51. doi:10.15561/18189172.2015.0109
10. Ocupok A.P. *Metodika obucheniia uprazhneniiam sportivnykh vidov gimnastiki i pryzhkov na batute s uchetom fenomena funkcional'noj asimmetrii. Kand. Diss*. [Methodic of training to sport kinds of gymnastic exercises and trampoline jumps, considering functional asymmetry phenomenon. Cand. Diss.], Kiev; 1984. (in Russian)
11. Platonov VN. *Sistema podgotovki sportsmenov v olimpijskom sporte* [System of sportsmen training in Olympic sports], Kiev: Olympic Literature; 2015. (in Russian)
12. Sadovski E. *Osnovy trenirovki koordinacionnykh sposobnostej v vostochnykh iedinoborstvakh* [Principles of coordination abilities' training in oriental martial arts], Biala Podlaska: ZWWF; 2003. (in Russian)
13. Tereshchenko IA, Otsupok AP, Krupenya SV, Liauchuk TM, Boloban VN. Coordination training of sportsmen, specializing in sport kinds of gymnastic. *Physical Education of Students*, 2015;3:52-65. doi:10.15561/20755279.2015.0307
14. Hoffman Jay R. *NSCA/s Guide to Program Design*. Human Kinetics; 2012.
15. Hrysomallis C, McLaughlin P, Goodman C. Relationship between statics and dynamic balance test among elite Australian footballers. *J. Sci Med.Sport*, 2006;9(4):288 – 291.
16. Maas VF. *Uczenie sie przez zmuslu* [continuous training through feelings], Warsaw: WSIP; 1998. (in Polish)
17. Sadowski J, Wołosz P, Zieliński J. *Koordynacyjne zdolności motoryczne i umiejętności techniczne koszykarzy* [Coordination motor abilities and technical skills of basketball players], Biała Podlaska: WWFiS; 2012. (in Polish)
18. Sarabon N. Balance and Stability Training. *NSCA/s Guide to Program Design*. Editor Jay R. Hoffman. Human Kinetics; 2012.
19. *Luchshe, chem beg. 8 klassnykh argumentov v pol'zu pryzhkov na batute* [Better than run. 8 good arguments in favor of trampoline jumps]. [Internet] 2016 [cited 2016 Nov 22]. Available from: http://freshlover.ru/dvizhenie-i-sport/luchshe-chem-beg-8-krutyh-argumentov-v-polzu-pryzhkov-na-batute

34

METHODIC OF GIRL STUDENTS' PROFESSIONALLY SIGNIFICANT COORDINATION QUALITIES' PERFECTION AT PHYSICAL EDUCATION CLASSES

Kolumbet A.N.
Kiev National University of Technology and Design

Abstract. *Purpose:* implementation of new methodic of professionally significant coordination qualities' training in higher educational establishments' girl students at classes of physical education. *Material:* 204 girl students participated in the research. *Results:* in perfection of students' professionally significant coordination qualities it is important to observe certain correlation of exercises in every block of methodic. When planning exercises it is necessary to observe the following correlations: exercises for orientation in space – 32%; exercises for perfection of quickness – 19%; exercises for accuracy of movements and differentiation of muscular efforts – 16%; exercises for balance – 9%. *Conclusions:* in trainings of professionally significant coordination qualities it is necessary to use different forms of trainings' organization. In preparatory part it is desirable to apply frontal form; in main part – frontal and differentiated-group form.

Key words: physical education, coordination qualities.

Introduction

The realized reforms in modern system of Ukrainian higher education system started mechanisms, making increased requirements to student's personality, content of the mastered knowledge and skills, to student's adaptation to conditions of dynamically and suddenly changing life; to increase of health quality and achievement of high workability; to realization of constant motor rehabilitation [5, 11, 23, 29, and 33]. In these conditions it is important for a personality to understand importance of social cultural factors' influence, which could ensure maximal realization of interests for every person as well as realization of his (her) interests and abilities, realization of healthy life style.

One of factors of students' modern progressing ambiguous situation's solution is physical education. It is called for harmonization of body-spiritual potential; ensure formation of students' complete physical and mental health and achievement of high workability and creative longevity [2, 15, 21, 22, 40, 41]. Just this category of population shall accumulate the highest potential in the shortest time for further build up of society's and state welfare.

As many years' experience and results of scientific researches show [25, 28, 33, 39], during the whole period of study certain part of students have insufficient physical condition and physical fitness. For many times it was proved that existing organization and infrastructure of students' physical education in pedagogic educational establishments do not ensure solution of educational and health related tasks [5, 24, 33]. That is why demand in working out innovative physical education methodic of applied and health related orientation is increasing for them to facilitate increase of students' physical fitness and professional skillfulness.

It is necessary to note that girl students of pedagogic specialties do not practice sports regularly and do not have experience of enduring even easy physical loads. With it, they have problems with health. Many of them do not attend physical education classes regularly. That is why deficit of motor functioning, intrinsic to them, is increasing with every year [9, 11]. Besides, even physical and motor skills, which they had before entering higher educational establishment, are lost.

Till present time the problem of rising quality of pedagogic higher educational establishments' girl students' physical education has been being solved insufficiently both theoretically and practically. In conditions of traditional organization of physical education there is a contradictory situation, when coordination and professionally significant qualities are not paid attention to enough. In spite of rather significant quantity of scientific works, the desired result has not been achieved. One of variants of this problem's solution can be working out methodic of coordination qualities' training on the base of systemic-structural approach and its realization in physical education process of pedagogic higher educational establishments' girl students. Analysis of students' coordination and professionally important qualities showed that as on to day there are no works on formation of such abilities at physical education classes. There are also no appropriate methodic for perfection of professionally significant coordination qualities of students at physical education classes. In general only a few publications on this topic exist [1, 17, 18, 27].

High demand in theory and methodic of students' physical education in appropriate scientifically substantiated technologies determined the relevance of our researches.

Hypothesis: we assumed that working out and implementation of methodic of higher educational establishments' girl students' coordination qualities on the base of systemic-structural approach would facilitate improvement of professional indicators, characteristic for pedagogue specialty.

The purpose of the research: working out and implementation of new methodic of professionally significant coordination qualities' training in higher educational establishments' girl students at classes of physical education on the base of systemic-structural approach.

Material and methods

Participants: in the research 204 1st and 2nd year girl students (of 17-21 years' age) of Chernihiv National T.G. Shevchenko Pedagogical University, and Borys Grinchenko Kyiv University, participated. All girl students were related to main health group.

Organization of the research: the research was conducted during 2012-2013. The methodic included blocks, containing special exercises for formation and mastering professionally important coordination qualities.

Experiment was conducted in first and second semesters of academic year. In this period physical education program permits to distribute blocks of exercises for development of girl students' coordination qualities between light athletic trainings, sport games (basketball, volleyball), general physical training. Accordingly, duration of variable part of training session (within our experiment) took not more than 20% (18-20 minutes) from total time of training. Every group was trained twice a week with 90 minute duration of every class. The worked out by us methodic was designed for 34 weeks (68 classes, 136 hours) with fixed duration of every training.

The blocks of physical exercises for perfection of professionally significant qualities of girl students were used in preparatory and main parts of classes. Breathing and relaxation exercises, games and relay races were used at the end of main and in finalizing parts of trainings. Exercises in blocks were selected as per principle from simple to complex. Blocks with complex exercises lasted from 18 to 20 minutes. Simple exercises were practiced for 10-12 minutes. It permitted to use two blocks with different orientation on girl students' coordination qualities in one training session. Breathing and relaxation exercises were used in the following way: in simple blocks – 1-2 times; in complex blocks – after every exercise. Special attention was paid to breathing exercises with circle method of training and after work at every station. These exercises took 20 seconds.

In sports games we used physical exercises blocks, which were directed at perfection of girl students' accuracy in reproduction of actions; at response; at differentiation of power parameters. Complication of tasks was realized at the account of application of filled, basketball and volleyball balls, gymnastic sticks, skipping ropes, benches in blocks.

Statistical analysis: for every studied parameter we calculated mean value and mean square deviation. Assessment of confidence of differences was fulfilled by Student's t-criterion at 1% and 5% levels of significance.

When fulfilling complex pedagogic and biological examinations we observed Ukrainian legislation about health protection, Helsinki declaration 2000, directive №86/609 of European society about human participation in medical-biological researches.

Results

Results of study of girl students' coordination qualities showed that all their kinds have rather ambiguous dynamic within 1-4th years of study. With it, a number of indicators worsen significantly till the end of studying period [30-32]. Rather low was general level of girl students' health, their speed power indicators, physical endurance. Insufficient level of most of coordination qualities does not permit to completely form their professionally important qualities.

Correlation analysis showed the presence of close correlation of future pedagogues' professional and coordination qualities [32]. Strong correlation was found between pedagogues' readiness to professional functioning and kinesthetic qualities: accuracy of reproduction of pre-set amplitude of arms' movements; girl-students ability to hands' fine motor skills with basic coordination, which are covered by concept "Quickness of operative thinking". The most significant for students coordination qualities are: accuracy of reproduction, assessment of space, time and power parameters of movements; balance and quickness of responding; orientation in space; quick re-switching of motor functioning; vestibular stability.

We implemented special methodic, which considered correlation of different kinds of basic and professionally important girl students' qualities. The methodic is directed at correction and improvement of indicators. The methodic contains blocks of physical exercises, directed at perfection of the mentioned qualities. In the frames of variable part of general program on physical education the methodic included blocks, containing special exercises for formation and mastering of professionally important coordination qualities:

- Blocks of exercises for orientation in space (32%);
- Blocks of exercises for perfection of quickness 22%);
- Blocks of exercises for perfection of differentiated coordination qualities (19%);
- Blocks of exercises for accuracy of movements and differentiation of muscular efforts (16%);
- Blocks of exercises for balance (9%).

Each block included 4-5 exercises. All blocks were approximately equal by volume of load and time of fulfillment. Blocks' correlations were determined by quantity and level of their density (See fig. 1).

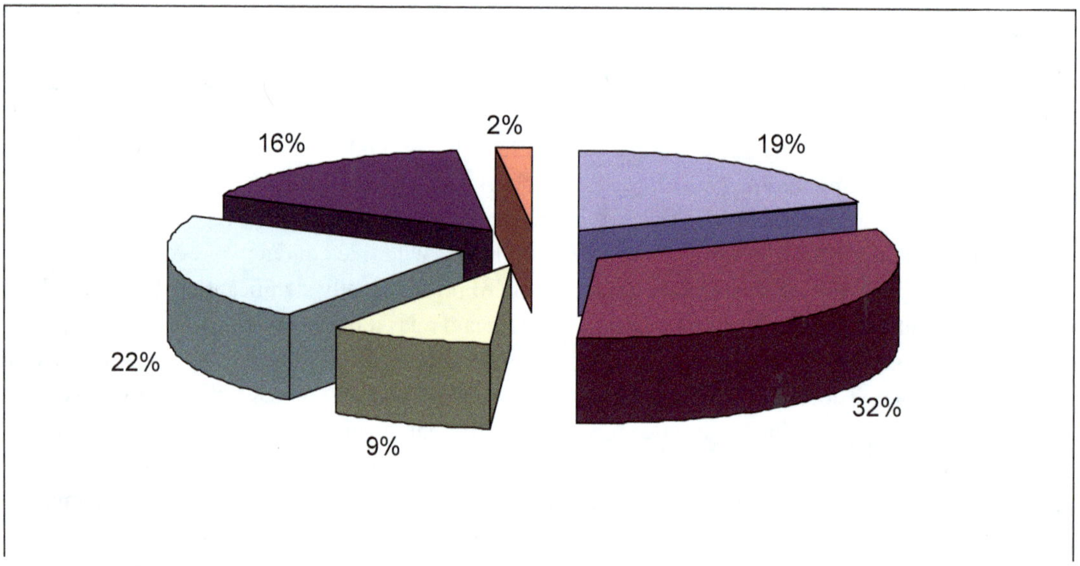

Fig. 1. Correlation of different orientation blocks in methodic of perfection of future specialists' professionally important coordination qualities.

Distinctive feature of the worked out by us methodic was differentiation approach. It permitted to create additional impact on weakly developed coordination abilities, depending on girl students' individual characteristics. When working out the methodic we also considered girl students' individual characteristics.

The main mean of coordination abilities' training were different exercises, which required correctness, speed, rational fulfillment of complex movements from a trainee. Besides, they required inventiveness for these actions' fulfillment in different conditions. We used new, unusual for girl students movements as well as exercises, which were fulfilled with changing either movements and motor actions or conditions of their executions.

For improvement of kinesthetic coordination qualities in experimental group we used tasks for accuracy of differentiation and reproduction of movement's space and power parameters. Exercises were complicated by exclusion of visual control, changing of fulfillment temp, introducing additional distracting movements. We used also "contrast tasks" and "approaching tasks".

For improvement of girl students' responding qualities we used the tasks, based on motion (run exercises, ball dribbling and movement with ball and so on). We used tasks for perfection of simple and complex reactions. The main part of the exercises was realized in section of sport games.

For perfection of static and dynamic balance we used exercises, in fulfillment of which keeping of balance was complicated:

- Keeping of different static postures;
- Keeping of balances, movements with small area of support;
- Keeping of movements with complex coordination, requiring efforts for maintaining certain body position;

For complicating different exercises and motor actions we used the following methodic techniques:

- Prolongation of time for keeping unstable position;
- Temporary exclusion or restriction of visual control;
- Reduction of support area;
- Introduction of previous or accompanying movements;
- Keeping balance against the background of vestibular apparatus irritation (after movements and turns) and in tired condition.

For improvement of ability to free muscular relaxation we selected exercises (change of free muscular relaxation and tension, breathing exercises, stretching exercises), which were fulfilled in the main part of training session (between main exercises and in finalizing part of training).

In trainings we used the method of strictly regulated exercise: the method of standard-repeated and variable (alternative) exercise; game and competition methods. The repeated method, in conditions of standard fulfillment, was used in the following way: for formation of new skill and mastering of space, time, dynamic and rhythmic characteristics of movement.

The method of variable exercise was used for improvement of already mastered motor skills. We used two variants of this method:

a) Strictly regulated varying (change of movement's direction, change of speed or temp, varying of initial or final positions, change of space restrictions);

b) Not strictly regulated varying (usual motor actions in unusual combinations: complicating of usual action by additional movements; combining of motor actions).

Competition method was used at separate trainings. Introduction of such elements increased motivation for maximally correct motor tasks' fulfillment. It increased efficiency of such trainings. More often this method was used for improvement of girl students' responding qualities.

Sport games were practiced both in control and experimental groups. In their application competition moment was considered. It positively reflected on fulfillment of separate elements by the participants of experimental group. Every game facilitated complex improvement of different coordination qualities of girl students. The program also included relay races [26, 33].

In trainings by the worked out by us methodic we used different forms of trainings' organization. In preparatory (warming up) part we used frontal form. In main part we used frontal and differentiated-group forms. Frontal form required girl students' building in 2-4 lines (instructor shall be in front of lines, in the center). When fulfilling tasks, instructor moves in the gym passing from one edge of line to the other and standing between lines. It facilitated quicker learning of the offered tasks. Besides, we used current method, when equal for all group exercises were fulfilled by the girls in motion following each other by 2-4 persons with definite rest intervals.

With differentiated-group form of trainings' organization, girls were divided into two-three departments. Every department was given task for perfection of physical condition and motor fitness. In every department leader was assigned (the girl with the highest physical fitness), who guided the work of girl students. Instructor watched over the work of all departments and directed, if it was necessary, any department.

When regulating load we considered the following components: load's duration and intensity, duration and character of intervals between exercises, quantity of exercises' repetitions. Duration and character of rest intervals between exercises depended on load. The quantity of repetitions varied depending of complexity of exercise from 4-6 to 10-12 times.

Discussion

Coordination qualities are the base of formation of many professionally significant qualities of future specialists. It witnesses about complex negative influence of weak motor functioning on youth [4, 7, 14, 35, 42-44].

Dependence of professionally important coordination qualities' development on professionalism of specialists in different spheres was noted in many scientific works [26, 30, 34, 36]. For professional progress in many professions good physical fitness and motor coordination are required. To large extent coordination determines the level of human motor potentials [1, 8, 10, 16, 20, 45, 46].

General principles of future pedagogic profile specialists' training for professional; functioning are reflected in some researches [3, 13, 32]. The authors determine purpose, content, forms and methods of professional-pedagogic and general humanitarian training of future pedagogue. However, the presented data are rather contradictory. It complicates their practical realization.

The techniques of improvement of some coordination qualities' kinds were realized by different researchers [1, 12, 18]. In particular, G.D. Oshchepkov and N.N. Guskova [19] found correlation of motor-coordination qualities with students' physical health and their general physical fitness: the higher physical fitness indicators are the better are coordination qualities. We determined that this correlation directly influences on specialist's professional qualities [14]. With it, this correlation was studied by S.A. Grigoryeva [6] in girl students of economic specialties. Questioning, conducted by the author, permitted to determine coordination qualities, required in active life activity of economic specialists: 1) kinesthetic; 2) responding; 3) rhythmic; 4) orientation. Results of such works correspond to our results. With it, for pedagogues professionally important are: differentiation, kinesthetic, orientation, responding qualities; static and dynamic balance [14]. Marking out of professionally important coordination qualities in specially worked out methodic permitted for us to achieve more progressive growth of pedagogic specialties' girl students' professionalism [31].

Complex approach in this aspect was realized, for the first time, in our works. The used by us methodic techniques of "contrast tasks" and "approaching tasks", for the first time were worked out by V.S. Farfel (1955-1976) and recommended for application by V.I. Liakh [17] and other specialists [7, 10, 20]. Exercises with simultaneous solution of several tasks improve coordination qualities. Exercises by rigid programs are considered to be less effective. It is connected with the fact that in case of other components' interference in motor system, its operation can significantly worsen [10; 12; 20]. It was proved in our researches [31]. Complex application of means in system of worked out physical education trainings perfects mechanism of coordination and compensation in controlling over movements as well as optimizes correlations of motor qualities, motor speed; improves motor-visual coordination, coordination re-constructions in motor re-switching, accuracy of muscular differentiation [12].

The worked out by us methodic was designed for 34 weeks (68 trainings, 136 hours). It corresponds to the data of other scientists. In opinion of other authors effective pedagogic influence in development and improvement of coordination qualities shall take not less than 20 classes [1, 12, and 17].

Conclusions

1. With improvement of professionally important coordination qualities of a pedagogue it is necessary to observe exercises' correlation in every block of the methodic.

2. When planning exercises in the methodic it is desirable to keep the following correlations: exercise for orientation in space – 32%; exercises for perfection of quickness – 22%; exercises for differential coordination qualities – 19%; exercises for accuracy of movements and differentiation of muscular efforts – 16%; exercises for balance – 9%.

3. When practicing perfection of professionally significant coordination qualities it is necessary to use different forms of trainings' organization. In preparatory part it is desirable to apply frontal from. In main part frontal and differentiated-group forms are desirable.

Acknowledgements

The researches were fulfilled in compliance with direction of scientific program of physical education faculty of Chernihiv National T.G. Shevchenko Pedagogical University, which is a part of university's topic

"Didactic principles of motor function's formation in persons, who practice physical education and sports" (state registration number

Conflict of interests

The author declares that there is no conflict of interests.

References:

1. Afanas'eva IV. Metodika sovershenstvovaniia professional'no znachimykh koordinacionnykh sposobnostej u budushchikh specialistov dizajnerov. Cand. Diss. [Methodic of improvement of professionally significant coordination abilities in future specialists-designers. Cand. Diss.], Omsk; 2008. (in Russian)
2. Bykov VA. Teoretiko-metodologicheskoe obosnovanie kompleksnoj sistemy sportivnoj podgotovki studentov vysshikh uchebnykh zavedenij fizicheskoj kul'tury [Theoretical-methodological substantiation of complex system of sports training of higher educational physical culture establishments' students]. Teoriia i praktika fizicheskoj kul'tury, 2004;2:50-54. (in Russian)
3. Vilenskij MIa, Safin MIa. Professional'naia napravlennost' fizicheskogo vospitaniia studentov pedagogicheskikh special'nostej [Professional orientation of pedagogic specialties' students' physical education]. Moscow: High school; 1989. (in Russian)
4. Gorskaia IIu, Suiangulova LA. Bazovye koordinacionnye sposobnosti shkol'nikov s razlichnym urovnem zdorov'ia [Basic coordination abilities of schoolchildren with different health level], Omsk: SibGUFK; 2000. (in Russian)
5. Grigor'ev VI. Krizis fizicheskoj kul'tury studentov i puti ego preodoleniia [Crisis of students' physical culture and ways of its overcoming], Teoriia i praktika fizicheskoj kul'tury, 2004;2:54-61. (in Russian)
6. Grigor'eva SA. Ekspertnaia ocenka koordinacionnykh sposobnostej, professional'no-znachimykh dlia bakalavrov ekonomicheskogo profilia [Expert assessment of coordination abilities, professionally significant for bachelors of economic profile]. Uchenye zapiski, 2011;5(75):47-50. (in Russian)
7. Zaporozhanov VA, Boraczynski T. Preparation of children with the limited possibilities to tutoring in a comprehensive school - a step to spirituality and humanism. *Pedagogics, psychology, medical-biological problems of physical training and sports,* 2009;9:52-55.
8. Il'inich VI. Professional'no-prikladnaia fizicheskaia podgotovka [Professional applied physical training], Moscow: High school; 1983. (in Russian)
9. Kabachkov VA, Polievskij SA. Razrabotka professional'no-prikladnoj fizicheskoj podgotovki i opyt ee vnedreniia v uchebnykh zavedeniiakh proftekhobrazovaniia [Development of professional-applied physical training and experience of its implementation in vocational educational establishments]. Teoriia i praktika fizicheskoj kul'tury, 1980;7;30-34. (in Russian)
10. Kirichenko SI. Professional'no-prikladnaia fizicheskaia podgotovka studentov ekonomicheskogo fakul'tet. Cand. Diss. [Professional-applied physical; training of economical faculty students. Cand. Diss.], Maikop; 1998. (in Russian)
11. Klimakova SN. Determinants of nonfixed locomotors system violations in preschool children. *Pedagogics, psychology, medical-biological problems of physical training and sports*, 2011;8:36-40.
12. Kogevnikova LK. Education of coordinating capabilities of students on exercises. *Physical Education of Students*, 2012;1:38-41.
13. Kolumbet AN. Influence of stimulated plasticity training method on coordination indicators of high pedagogic educational estableshments' girl students. *Physical Education of Students*, 2015;6:31-37. doi:10.15561/20755279.2015.0604
14. Kolumbet OM. *Rozvitok koordinacijnikh zdibnostej molodi* [Development of youth's coordination abilities], Kiev: Education Ukraine; 2014. (in Ukrainian)
15. Korobejnikov GV. Psikhofiziologicheskie mekhanizmy umstvennoj deiatel'nosti cheloveka [Psycho-physiological mechanisms of human mental activity], Kiev; 2002. (in Russian)
16. Korovin SS. Teoreticheskie i metodologicheskie osnovy professional'noj fizicheskoj kul'tury uchashchejsia molodezhi [Theoretical and methodological principles of students' professional physical culture], Moscow: VNIIFK; 1997. (in Russian)
17. Liakh VI. Koordinacionnye sposobnosti: diagnostika i razvitie [Coordination abilities: diagnostic and

training], Moscow: Division; 2006. (in Russian)

18. Nazarenko LD. Sredstva i metody razvitiia dvigatel'nykh koordinacij [Means and methods of motor coordination training], Moscow: Theory and Practice of Physical Culture; 2003. (in Russian)
19. Oshchepkov GD, Gus'kova NN. Koordinacionnye sposobnosti v pedagogicheskom processe na zaniatiiakh fizicheskoj kul'turoj [Coordination abilities in pedagogic process at physical culture classes]. Uchenye zapiski, 2008;6(40):82-86. (in Russian)
20. Raevskij RT. Professional'no-prikladnaia fizicheskaia podgotovka studentov tekhnicheskikh vuzov [Professional-applied physical training of technical HEEs' students], Moscow: High school; 1989. (in Russian)
21. Bazylyuk TA. Self-evaluation of health and interests of students of higher education institutions on course physical education. *Pedagogics, psychology, medical-biological problems of physical training and sports,* 2013;7:3-6. doi:10.6084/m9.figshare.735943
22. Beliak YI, Zinchenko NM. Dosing method of physical activity in aerobics classes for students. *Physical Education of Students*, 2014;5:8-13. doi:10.15561/20755279.2014.0502
23. Belykh SI. Structure of the concept of personality oriented physical education university students. *Physical Education of Students*, 2013;4:3-9. doi:10.6084/m9.figshare.669663
24. Bryukhanova NA, Bulgakova OV, Mokrova TI, Bogashchenko YA. Determination of possibilities of the use of high-intensive trainings facilities on lessons health aerobics. *Physical Education of Students,* 2013;2:25-29. doi:10.6084/m9.figshare.156376
25. Chernovsky SM, Kolumbet AN. Determination of future designers' professionally important coordination qualities. *Physical education of students*, 2016;2:38–44. doi:10.15561/20755279.2016.0206.
26. Gorelov AA, Kondakov VL, Usatov AN. To the question about the use of independent physical training in educational space of modern higher institute. *Physical education of students*, 2013;1:17–27. doi:10.6084/m9.figshare.156351
27. Hirtz P. *Coordinative abilities in school sports*. Berlin: Volk und Wissen, Volksseigener Verlag, 1985.
28. Iermakov SS, Apanasenko GL, Bondarenko TV, Prasol SD. Physical culture is a basic instrument of culture of health. *Pedagogics, psychology, medical-biological problems of physical training and sports*, 2010;11:31-33.
29. Iermakov SS, Ivashchenko PI, Guzov VV. Features of motivation of students to application of individual programs of physical self-preparation. *Physical Education of Students*, 2012;4:59-61.
30. Kolumbet AN. Physical education for the students of pedagogical specialities. *Science, Technology and Higher Education: III international research and practice conference*, Westwood, Canada, January 30, 2014. Westwood, Canada, 2014. P. 34-42.
31. Kolumbet AN. Development of coordination abilities of young people. *Science and Education: V international research and practice conference,* Munich, Germany, February 27-28, 2014. Munich, Germany, 2014. P. 54-62.
32. Kolumbet AN. Dynamic of girl students' psycho-physiological indicators in process of their study at pedagogical higher educational establishment. *Physical education of students*, 2016;1:29–36. doi:10.15561/20755279.2016.0104.
33. Kondakov VL, Kopeikina EN, Balysheva NV, Usatov AN, Skrug DA. Causes of declining interest of students to employment physical education and sports. *Physical education of students*, 2015;1:22–30. doi:10.15561/20755279.2015.0104.
34. Korobeynikov G. Psychophysiological Peculiarities of Sexual Dimorphism in Athletes. *Psychologe Research,* 2012;2(6):336-342.
35. Masliak IP. Physical health of young and middle age women under influence of step-aerobics exercises. *Pedagogics, psychology, medical-biological problems of physical training and sports*. 2015;10:45-50. doi:10.15561/18189172.2015.1007
36. Pogrebniak IM, Kudelko VE, Nagovitsina OP. Effect of improving aerobics classes at the level of flexibility of female students. *Pedagogics, psychology, medical-biological problems of physical training and sports*, 2013;5:49-52. doi:10.6084/m9.figshare.707099

37. Pop C, Ciomag V. The Influence of Aerobic Gymnastics on the Students' Body Image. *Procedia – Social and Behavioral Sciences,* 2014;117:129-135.
38. Prusik KK, Prusik K, Kozina ZL, Iermakov SS. Features of physical development, physical preparedness and functional state of boys and girls – students of Polish higher educational establishments. *Physical Education of Students*, 2013;1:54-61. doi:10.6084/m9.figshare.96415
39. Siri A, Rui M. Distance Education for Health Professions' Students. *Procedia - Social and Behavioral Sciences*. 2015;174:730–738.
40. Usher K, Woods C, Casella E, Glass N, Wilson R, Mayner L, et al. Australian health professions student use of social media. *Collegian*. 2014;21(2):95–101.
41. von Haaren B, Haertel S, Stumpp J, Hey S, Ebner-Priemer U. Reduced emotional stress reactivity to a real-life academic examination stressor in students participating in a 20-week aerobic exercise training: A randomised controlled trial using Ambulatory Assessment. *Psychology of Sport and Exercise*. 2015;20:67–75.
42. Williams B. Supporting Middle School Students Whose Parents Are Deployed: Challenges and Strategies for Schools. The Clearing House: *A Journal of Educational Strategies, Issues and Ideas*. 2013;86(4):128–135.
43. Wouters S, Duriez B, Luyckx K, Colpin H, Bijttebier P, Verschueren K. Parental goal promotion and college students' self-esteem level and contingency: The mediating role of need satisfaction. *Personality and Individual Differences*. 2014;66:140–145.
44. Wu H-Y, Wu H-S, Chen I-S, Chen H-C. Exploring the critical influential factors of creativity for college students: A multiple criteria decision-making approach. *Thinking Skills and Creativity*. 2014;11:1–21.
45. Yahyaei D, Foroushani ZJ, Mahini F. The School Role in Lively Education and Student's Mental Health. *Procedia - Social and Behavioral Sciences*. 2012;47:1408–1412.
46. Zepke N, Butler P, Leach L. Institutional research and improving the quality of student engagement. *Quality in Higher Education*. 2012;18(3):329–347.

DEVELOPMENT DYNAMIC OF HEALTHY LIFE STYLE PERSONALITY COMPONENT IN RELATIVELY HEALTHY STUDENTS

Kudryavtsev M.D. [1,2,5], Kramida I.E. [2], Iermakov S.S. [3], Osipov A.Yu. [1,4]
[1]Siberian Federal University, Russia
[2]Siberian State Aerospace University, Russia
[3]Kazimierz Wielki University in Bydgoszcz, Poland
[4]V.F. Voino-Yasenetsky Krasnoyarsk State Medical University, Russia
[5]Krasnoyarsk State Pedagogical University of V.P. Astafyev, Russia

Abstract. *Purpose:* to determine effectiveness of different physical culture trainings for development of students' healthy life style personality components. *Material:* 1st – 3rd year students, trained at physical culture lessons, participated in the research. All students related to main health group (students, having no health problems). In total 803 students participated in the research. The testing was conducted in periods from 2001 to 2005 and from 2010 to 2015. *Results:* positive changes of different personality's component of healthy life style were observed. Parameters of emotional stability and tolerance were found. Teaching in last years develops personality's components to less extent. The highest changes were determined in 3rd year students, independent on the program of their training. We did not find differences in degree of trainings' influence of specialized and typical classes. *Conclusions:* at trainings it is necessary to pay more attention to development personality's components of healthy life style, especially emotional stability and tolerance in respect to other people.
Key words: students, physical culture, specialization, healthy life style, personality.

Introduction

Specialists' training at high quality implies provisioning students with certain amount of knowledge, formation and development of workable personality. Personality's effective functioning is impossible without his/her healthy life style (HLS). The most frequent HLS is understood as healthy behavior: regular motor functioning; correct eating; useful habits, connected with correct day regime and alternation of work and rest; absence of harmful habits [8, 24, 32]. Such understanding of human HLS is restricted with by regarding human life as life of his physical body. However, human being is not only body. Human HLS shall include his healthy soul. Thus, human HLS includes: healthy behavior and thinking; healthy emotions; harmony in relations with surrounding world and own self [27]. That is why it is necessary to study behavioral base of human HLS; HLS of his/her mental component and personality's components. Especially it concerns the problems of formation and development of HLS personality components in the process of students' study at HEE.

Personality's components of HLS can be understood as human personality qualities, which characterize healthy thinking and harmony of human behavior and relations with surrounding world and him/her self *(positive state);* tolerant attitude to other people (*tolerance);* self-confidence, based on positive attitude towards hum/herself (*confidence);* ability to be in any situation emotionally positive that is an important factor of stress-resistance *(emotional stability)* [18]; vital activity, which characterizes personality's orientation on positive functioning (*activity).*

Each of enlisted five positive qualities of a student is integral one. It includes several particular characteristics – features of character or person's abilities. The list of particular characteristics of HLS every integral personality's component is give in [13, 14].

In the process of study at HEE personality components of students' HLS develop differently. It is necessary to regard as positive such changes, under which the enlisted above five qualities strengthen.

Recent years, in practice new principle of physical culture (PC) trainings' organization (in respect to relatively healthy students, MHG-main health group) has been being applied [13]. Students can choose typical physical culture trainings or one of specializations (power training, swimming, shaping or outdoor games) and attend classes as per schedule of the chosen direction. Such approach permitted to increase students' interest to trainings, their responsibility; decrease missing of classes. However the influence of such trainings' organization on development of relatively healthy students' HLS personality components still remains to be an open question.

Recent years rather a high number of scientific works on different kinds of sports and health related systems has appeared [6, 30, 39, 43]. Some works are devoted to training of physical [9, 31, 33] and psycho-physical [9, 38, 40, 41] abilities of different specialties students. But development of HLS personality components in the process of study at HEE is not regarded in these works. Some authors study formation of professionally significant qualities in different specialties' students by means of physical culture and sports (the works by N.A. Aleshev are the closest to us by topics) [2]). However, these authors do not study the problem of students' personality development (and more over – about development of their HLS personality components) in conditions of different PC organization: by typical program or by specializations.

In the course of our research we found the following *main contradictions:*

– Between active propaganda of healthy life style theory and practice and main directions of physical culture trainings' substantiation in modern society. It is connected with searching and opening new effective health related technologies and directions;

– Between theoretical substantiation of demand in strengthening students' motivation for healthy life style and actual situation as on to day. It is connected with insufficient quantity of physical culture motivated trainings;

– Between declaration healthy life style different elements' implementation in physical culture discipline and absence of specially worked out for students training programs. Such programs shall be based on application modern means for student' health improvement. Such programs shall facilitate actual increment of students, practicing healthy life style.

Recent years there have been observed unsubstantiated reduction of time for physical culture and quantity of youth, preferring sports or physical exercises to passive leisure [3, 35, 36, 42]. In this aspect we can mark out several works on the following problems: positive changes in students' personality [16, 17, 34]; HLS personality components in students of different health groups [14, 15, 37]. But some problems of dynamic of HLS personality components' development in students, trained by PC typical program and by specialization are being still unsolved. Besides, it is necessary to seek more effective variants of students' PC training.

The purpose of the work is to substantiate and perfect approaches to development of students' HLS personality components by means of physical culture trainings during three years of heir study.

The tasks of the research:

1. To fulfill comparative analysis of positive changes in HLS personality components of relatively healthy students, who are trained by at 1st-3rd years: a) by typical program (PC specialization); b) by specialization programs (PS (practicing sports) specialization).

2. To fulfill comparative analysis of HLS personality components' changes in relatively healthy students in periods from 2001-2005 and from 2010 to 2015.

Material and methods

Participants: 1st – 3rd year students, trained at physical culture lessons, participated in the research. All students related to main health group (students, having no health problems). For participation in the research we selected students, who actively attended physical culture classes. The students were combined in different groups: 2001–2005 and 2010–2015 years of study. These groups are marked in the following way (below, in brackets there are volumes of samples for groups of 2001–2005 and 2010–2015 accordingly): *1, 2, 3* – RHS (relatively healthy students) 1 (146 and 193 persons), 2 (163 and 83persons), 3 (46 and 50persons), who attended PC typical classes;) *1c, 2c, 3c* – RHS 1 (31persons), 2 (41persons), 3 (50 persons), who attended specialized trainings in 2010–2015.

Organization of the research:

The questioning was conducted in academic groups of 1st-3rd year students at the end of academic year. Questionnaires consisted of personality's main positive characteristics, located in free order. Students assessed (by scale from 0 to 10 points) the degree of every characteristic in them at the beginning and at the end of study period [19].

Statistical analysis: confidence of differences between values was assessed by Student's t-criterion (at significance level less than 0.05). The differences were interpreted as tendency at significance level more than 0.05, but less than 0.15 (in the table below such cases are marked with *). The received data were processed with the help of Microsoft Excel program.

Results of the research

The main results of students' questioning are given in summarizing table.

Table. Average increment of students' HLS personality componentsT for study period

Personality qualities		Years	Increment of marks +(0 –10) points						Important significant correlations	
			1	*1c*	*2*	*2c*	*3*	*3c*	For every period of years	In dynamic
Positive state	1	2001–2005	0.6		0.6		1.0		\`3\`>\`1\`, \`2\`	\`3$_1$\`* > \`3$_2$\`
	2	2010–2015	0.2	0.2	0.4	0.3	0.7	0.9	\`3, 3c\` > (other)	\`1$_1$\`>1$_2$\`, \`1c\`
Tolerance	1	2001–2005	0.2		0.2		0.6		\`3\`>\`1\`, \`2\`	\`3$_1$\` > \`3c\`
	2	2010–2015	0.1	0.0	0.1	0.1	0.4	0.2	\`3\` > (all, except \`3c\`)	
Self-confidence	1	2001–2005	0.6	–	0.7	–	1.0	–	\`3\`>\`1\`, \`2\`	\`1$_1$\` >\`1$_2$\` \`3$_1$\` > \`3$_2$\`
	2	2010–2015	0.3	0.5	0.8	0.5	0.7	0.8	\`2\`,\`3\`,\`3c\` > \`1\` \`2\` > \`2c\`*	
Activity	1	2001–2005	0.5	–	0.6	–	1.0	–	\`3\`>\`1\`, \`2\`	\`3$_1$\`>\`3$_2$\`,\`3c\`
	2	2010–2015	0.4	0.3	0.5	0.4	0.6	0.7	\`3c\`>\`1\`,\`1c\`	
Emotional stability	1	2001–2005	–0.1	–	–0.1	–	0.0	–	\`1\`= \`2\`=\`3\`	\`3$_1$\` > \`3c\`*
	2	2010–2015	–0.2	–0.2	–0.3	–0.3	–0.1	–0.3	\`1\`= \`1c\`; \`2\`=\`2c\`	

Notes: in the last two columns sign «\`» marks the data of average increment of points for personality qualities of appropriate year students. Indices«1» and «2» after main symbol of group mean accordingly 2001–2005» and «2010–2015».

Questioning of 1st-3rd year students about five personality components at the end of academic year showed the following:

1. Students had positive changes of HLS personality components (in both time ranges). For three personality components of all years' students (except emotional stability and tolerance of 1st and 2nd years students) final progress was significantly higher than initial. Final tolerance level of 1st and 2nd year students did not differ significantly from initial. Concerning 3rd year students of PC specialization, their final tolerance was significantly higher than initial (in both time ranges).

2. Positive changes of four HLS personality components (except self-confidence in 2010–2015) in all RHS groups of 1st and 2nd years differ insignificantly (in both time ranges). Positive change of self-confidence in RHS of 2nd year was significantly higher than in RHS of 1st year students. Further, these indicators did not change for students of PC specialization in 2010–2015. For 4 HLS personality components (except emotional stability) increment of personality components in 3rd year PHS of PS specialization (in both time ranges) was much higher than in 1st and 2nd year students. For students of PS specialization such correlation was observed for 3 HLS personality components: positive state, self-confidence and activity.

3. Two HLS personality components (emotional stability and tolerance in respect to other people) in PS specialization students do not change during all period of study. In students of PC specialization emotional stability also does not change during first three years of study. In this category of students significant increment is observed only after 3 years of study (only in growth of self-assessment for tolerance to other people).

4. For specializations PC and PS we did not find significant difference for 4 personality components. Concerning fifth HLS component (self-confidence) in students of PC specialization after 2nd year of study there

appears a tendency of higher assessment of its level. In the aspect of HLS personality components' development PC trainings does not differ from typical classes by effectiveness.

5. Comparing of 2001–2005 and 2010–2015 data points at negative dynamic of HLS personality components development: in 3rd year students – for all qualities of personality; in 1st year students – for positive state and self-confidence. To larger extent it concerns 3rd year students of specialization. It means that recent years training develops HLS personality components of most students less than 10 years ago. Besides, it was found that PC specialized trainings do not have advantages in development of student's personality in this direction.

Discussion

V.M. Rozin especially underlines: "Health can not be formed or built as a building. It can only grow but not without our efforts" [26].

At present time still more intensive application of health related technologies for students' HLS personality indicators prove the relevance of the present research. In this connection it is necessary to actualize solution of problems, hindering development of healthy life style personality components in students' education. Besides, it is necessary to take all measures for improvement of students' health components.

Students shall be offered clear steps to preservation optimal health; to keep positive mood [11]; to control the system of personal values; to creation of personal image, including physical, emotional and intellectual principles of young person's personality; to enrich practical philosophy of health, paying attention to mental and body development [8]. In every physical culture training it is necessary to strengthen students' motivation for healthy life style [28].

It is necessary to pay attention to the fact that physical culture and sports practicing are means of health improvement as well as physical perfection and rational leisure; mean of social activity rising. Such approach substantially influences on other sides of human activity: labor, moral and intellectual qualities.

Indeed, physical culture is one of main kinds of human culture. Its specificity is that this kind is profiled in direction of physical condition's optimization and individual's development in integrity with his/her psychic development. The basis of it are rational and effective usage of own motor functioning in combination with other cultural values [29].

The validity of the received results and approaches to creation of youth's healthy life style foundations is proved by works of other authors:

- About influence of sorts on personality's development [12];
- About morality, culture and youth's to-day's attitude to life problems' solution [4];
- About physical culture, as kind of human activity, specific features [1];
- Setting for creation of youth's healthy life style foundations [25].

Conception of human harmonious development shall also include unity, concordance and proportionality of "out-of-body", intrinsic only to human being qualities (will power, super-will power, morality, aesthetic, intellect) with all these in body and spirit integrity [12]. Modern students spend nearly all their time in virtual reality, where in different social sites they see ideal, handsome bodies of famous and ordinary people [4]. From this it follows that sport is now understood as fashion as compulsory component of healthy life style. As on to day sports have become one of fashionable directions of physical culture. However, it does not influence positively on students' attendance of learning and sport classes in higher educational establishments. Overloading with academic material requires significant strength, nervous and time losses from students. It forces students to neglect physical culture and sports as well as facilitates students' not seeing significance of physical development. In such cases students pay dominant attention to natural and humanitarian sciences. That is why the problem is to over-persuade students. It is necessary to prove that personality's development and directly human activity are impossible without successful physical development and physical fitness.

In context of the present work a relevant task is: formation of vitally important physical and motor qualities; perfection of psychic processes at levels: psycho-motor skills, thinking and imagination. It will be genuine care about youth; their personality's indictors, health and future professional workability.

The statement about possibility of students' character's development and hardening through physical culture and sports' practicing is undoubted. Such active position of sport-practicing and relatively healthy young people trains muscles and strengthens spirit. Comprehensively developed personality adapts to various modern conditions and successful future professional functioning quicker.

It is important to form attitude to sports [5, 7, and 22] as one of the main and integral values of young people's HLS. It will distract them from various harmful habits [19, 21]. Inculcation of such approach to youth's minds is important just at physical culture classes. [5, 20, 23]. It will result in active mastering personal values of physical culture practicing as well as facilitate practicing fashionable and useful healthy life style [10, 22, and 28].

Conclusions

1. In any variant of physical culture classes personality qualities of young people have tendency to certain development.

2. Correlation of HLS personality components with period of study is not linear. To larger extent their development is observed at first and third years of study. The highest changes of HLS personality components are observed in 3rd year students. These changes do not depend on the program of their training.

3. Trainings by specializations PC and PS influence approximately equally on development of students' HLS personality components.

4. At PC classes it is necessary to pay more attention to development of students' HLS personality components. Especially it concerns emotional stability and tolerance towards other people.

Conflict of interests

The authors declare that there is no conflict of interests.

References:

1. Aleksandrov SE. *Specifika fizicheskoj kul'tury kak vida chelovecheskoj deiatel'nosti. Kand. Diss*. [Specificity of physical culture as a kind of human activity. Cand. Diss.], Sankt Petersburg; 1993. (in Russian)
2. Aleshev NA. *Formirovanie professional'no znachimykh kachestv u budushchikh inzhenerov sredstvami fizkul'turno–sportivnoj deiatel'nosti. Kand. Diss.* [Formation of professionally important qualities in future engineers by means of physical culture-sports activity. Cand. Diss.], Cheboksary; 2007. (in Russian)
3. Anan'ev VA, Davidenko DN. *Etiudy valeologii* [Sketches on valueology], Sankt Petersburg: STU, BPA; 2001. (in Russian)
4. Bibler VS. *Nravstvennost'. Kul'tura. Sovremennost': Filosofskie razmyshleniia o zhiznennykh problemakh* [Morality. Culture. Nowadays: Philosophical speculations about life problems], Moscow: Knowledge; 1990. (in Russian)
5. Bliznevsky AA, Kudryavtsev MD, Iermakov SS, Jagiello W. Formation of active-effective attitude of 12-13 years' judo athletes to sports functioning in competition period. *Archives of Budo*, 2016; 12: 101-115.
6. Volozhanin SE. *Povyshenie urovnia fizicheskoj podgotovlennosti studentov vuza sredstvami atletizma. Kand. Diss*. [Increase of HEE students' physical fitness by means of athletics. Cand. Diss.], Ulan-Ude; 2007. (in Russian)
7. Gaskov AV, Kuzmin VA, Kudryavtsev MD, Iermakov SS. Successfulness of general and special physical qualities' development on different stage of students-boxers' training. *Physical Education of Students*, 2016;1:4-11. doi:10.15561/20755279.2016.0101
8. Diukov VM, Skurikhina NV. *VUZ zdorovogo obraza zhizni* [HEE of healthy life style], Lap Lambert Academic Publishing: Saarbrücken; 2013. (in Russian)
9. Kozina ZhL, Barybina LN, Kondak NN, Lisenko VV. Structure of complex preparedness of students - women's of higher technical institute of different sporting specializations. *Physical Education of Students*, 2010;6;29 – 32.
10. Kondakov VL, Kopeikina EN, Usatov AN. On purposefulness of application of physical culture-health related technology for prophylaxis of students' respiratory system disorders. *Physical Education of Students*, 2016;20(2):4-12. doi:10.15561/20755279.2016.0201

11. Kopylov YuA, Jackowska LN, Kudryavtsev MD, Kuzmin VA, Tolstopyatov IA, Iermakov SS. The concept of structure and content of health related trainings for higher educational establishments' students. *Physical Education of Students*, 2015;5:23-30. doi:10.15561/20755279.2015.0504
12. Korshunov IG. Vliianie sporta na razvitie lichnosti [Influence of sports on personality's development]. *SCI-ARTICLE.RU,* [Internet]. 2015 [cited 2016 Oct 29]; Available from: http://sci-article.ru/stat.php?i=1450014277 (in Russian)
13. Kramida IE, Maksimov IaA. Izmenenie lichnostnykh pokazatelej zdorovogo obraza zhizni studentov v period auditornogo obucheniia na fakul'tete fizicheskoj kul'tury i sporta SibGAU [Change of personalities' indicators of students' healthy life style in period of auditorium study at physical culture and sports faculty of SibGAU]. *Mezhdunarodnyj simpozium "Vostok – Rossiia – Zapad. Fizicheskaia kul'tura i sport, formirovanie zdorov'ia i zdorov'esberegaiushchie tekhnologii v sisteme obrazovaniia"* [International symposium "East-Russia-West. Physical culture and sports; formation of health and health related technologies in system of education"], Krasnoyarsk: RIO KSU; 2006. P. 280–285. (in Russian)
14. Kramida IE. Valeologicheskij praktikum na osnove gimnastiki cigun kak faktor razvitiia lichnostnykh komponentov zdorovogo obraza zhizni u studentov [Valueological practicum on the base of Tci-gun gymnastic as factor of development of students' healthy life style personality components' development]. *Vserossijskaia nauchno-prakticheskaia konferenciia "Aktual'nye problemy, mekhanizmy i perspektivy razvitiia fizicheskoj kul'tury i sporta v vysshikh uchebnykh zavedeniiakh Minsel'khoza Rossii"* [All Russian scientific-practical conference "Current problems and prospects of physical culture and sports in higher educational establishments of Ministry of agriculture of Russia], Irkutsk: IrGSKHA; 2011. P. 255-259. (in Russian)
15. Kramida IE. Ozdorovitel'nyj praktikum na osnove gimnastiki cigun kak faktor formirovaniia zdorovogo obraza zhizni u studentov [Health improvement practicum on the base of Tci-gun gymnastic as factor of development of students' healthy life style personality components' development]. *Vserossijskaia nauchno-prakticheskaia konferenciia "Optimizaciia uchebno-vospitatel'nogo i trenirovochnogo processa v uchebnykh zavedeniiakh vysshego professional'nogo obrazovaniia. Zdorovyj obraz zhizni, kak faktor profilaktiki narkomanii"* [All Russian scientific-practical conference "Optimization of educational and trainings processes in educational establishments of higher vocational training. Healthy life style as factor of drugs-taking prophylaxis"], Krasnoyarsk: Sibut; 2012. P. 353–356. (in Russian)
16. Kramida IE. Dynamics of personal development on healthy students. *Pedagogics, psychology, medical-biological problems of physical training and sports*, 2013;4: 30-34. doi:10.6084/m9.figshare.691013
17. Kramida IE. Training workshop on the basis of gymnastic qigoing as a factor of personal development of students with poor health. *Pedagogics, psychology, medical-biological problems of physical training and sports*, 2013;4: 35-40. doi:10.6084/m9.figshare.691014
18. Kudryavtsev MD, Galimov GIa, Gas'kov AV. Obosnovanie effektivnosti uchebnykh zaniatij po fizicheskoj kul'ture s ozdorovitel'noj i obrazovatel'noj napravlennost'iu na osnove ocenki pokazatelej ispol'zovaniia elementov zdorovogo obraza zhizni [Substantiation of physical culture trainings, oriented on health improvement and education, effectiveness on the base of healthy life style elements' assessment]. *Vestnik Buriatskogo gosudarstvennogo universiteta,* 2012;13:121-124. (in Russian)
19. Kudryavtsev MD, Kramida IE, Kuzmin VA, Iermakov SS. Cieslicka Miroslawa, Stankiewicz Blazej, Influence of study in hee on ubiquity and strength of students' computer gambling. *Physical Education of Students*, 2016;3:13-22. doi:10.15561/20755279.2016.0302
20. Kudryavtsev MD, Galimov GIa, Kuzmin VA, Kopylov YA, Gas'kov AV. Effektivnost' ispol'zovaniia v sisteme fizicheskogo vospitaniia studentov netradicionnykh sredstv na primere khatkha-jogi [Effectiveness of non traditional means' usage in physical education system on example of Hatha Yoga]. *Vestnik Buriatskogo gosudarstvennogo universiteta,* 2014;1:41-44. (in Russian)
21. Kudryavtsev MD, Kramida IE, Iermakov SS. Influence of studying in higher educational establishment on students' harmful computer habits. *Physical Education of Students*, 2016;5:17-23. doi:10.15561/20755279.2016.0503

22. Kuzmin VA, Kopylov YA, Kudryavtsev MD, Tolstopyatov IA, Galimov GY, Ionova OM. Formation of professionally important qualities of students with weakened motor fitness using a health related and sport-oriented training program. *Journal of Physical Education and Sport,* 2016;16(1):136-145. doi:10.7752/jpes.2016.01023
23. Kuzmin VA, Kopylov YuA, Kudryavtsev MD, Galimov GY, Iermakov SS. Substantiation of effectiveness of trainings on health related methodic for students with weakened motor fitness. *Physical Education of Students*, 2015;6:43-49. doi:10.15561/20755279.2015.0606
24. Lubysheva LI, Bal'sevich VK. Cennosti fizicheskoj kul'tury v zdorovom stile zhizni [Physical culture values in healthy life style] *Mezhdunarodnaia konferenciia "Sovremennye dostizheniia sportivnoj nauki"* [International conference "Modern achievements of sport science"], Sankt Petersburg; 1994. P. 124-125. (in Russian)
25. Nazarova EN, Zhilov IuD. *Osnovy zdorovogo obraza zhizni* [Principles of healthy life style], Moscow: Academy; 2013. (in Russian)
26. Rozin VM. *Koncepciia zdorov'ia* [Conception of health], MSMSU; 2011. (in Russian)
27. Seliutina GV, Diukov VM. *Prakticheskaia filosofiia zdorov'ia* [Practical philosophy of health], Lap Lambert Academic Publishing: Saarbrücken; 2013. (in Russian)
28. Skurikhina NV, Kudryavtsev MD, Kuzmin VA, Iermakov SS. Fitness yoga as modern technology of special health groups' girl students' psycho-physical condition and psycho-social health strengthening. *Physical Education of Students*, 2016;20(2):24-31. doi:10.15561/20755279.2016.0204
29. Geleckij VM. *Teoriia fizicheskoj kul'tury i sporta* [Theory of physical culture and sports]. Krasnoyarsk: IPK SFU; 2008. (in Russian)
30. Trofimova OV. *Sovershenstvovanie fizicheskogo vospitaniia studentok vuza na osnove uglublennogo izucheniia fitnes–aerobiki. Kand. Diss*. [Perfection of HEE girl students' physical education on the base of profound study of fitness-aerobic. Cand. Diss], Cheboksary; 2010. (in Russian)
31. Chernenko SA. Description of how the specialization influences the dynamics of the functional and motor abilities among the third to fifth year female students. *Physical Education of Students,* 2012;4: 130 – 134.
32. Golovina VA, Masliakova VA, Korobkova AV. *Fizicheskoe vospitanie* [Physical education]. Moscow: High school; 1983. (in Russian)
33. Bliznevsky AA, Kudryavtsev MD, Iermakov SS, Jagiello W. Formation of active-effective attitude of 12-13 years' judo athletes to sports functioning in competition period. *Archives of Budo,* 2016;12: 101-115.
34. Gaskov A.V., Kuzmin A. V., Kudryavtsev D. M., Iermakov S. S., Successfulness of general and special physical qualities' development on different stage of students-boxers' training. *Physical Education of Students*, 2016;1:4-11. doi:10.15561/20755279.2016.0101
35. Iermakov SS, Arziutov GN, Jagiello W. Quick training of students to judo techniques. *Archives of Budo,* 2016;12:15-24.
36. Iermakov SS, Podrigalo LV, Jagiełło W. Hand-grip strength as an indicator for predicting the success in martial arts athletes. *Archives of Budo,* 2016; 12: 179-186.
37. Kopeikina EN, Drogomeretsky VV, Kondakov VL, Kovaleva MV, Iermakov SS. Modification of Harvard step-test for assessment of students' with health problems functional potentials. *Physical Education of Students*, 2016;20(4):44-50. doi:10.15561/20755279.2016.0405
38. Kozina ZL, Iermakov SS, Kadutskaya LA, Sobyanin FI, Krzeminski M, Sobko IN, Ryepko OA. Comparative characteristic of correlation between pulse subjective indicators of girl students' and school girls' reaction to physical load. *Physical Education of Students*, 2016;20(4):24-34. doi:10.15561/20755279.2016.0403
39. Kudryavtsev MD, Kopylov YuA, Kuzmin VA, Ionova OM, Yermakova TS. Personality oriented system of strengthening of students' physical, psychic and social-moral health. *Physical Education of Students*, 2016;20(3):58-64. doi:10.15561/20755279.2016.0308
40. Kudryavtsev MD, Kramida IE, Iermakov SS. Influence of studying in higher educational establishment on students' harmful computer habits. *Physical Education of Students*, 2016;20(5):17-23. doi:10.15561/20755279.2016.0503
41. Kudryavtsev MD, Kramida IE, Kuzmin VA, Iermakov SS, Cieslicka Miroslawa., Stankiewicz Blazej. Influence of study in hee on ubiquity and strength of students' computer gambling. *Physical Education of Students*, 2016;20(3):13-22. doi:10.15561/20755279.2016.0302

42. Podrigalo LV, Iermakov SS, Alekseev AF, Rovnaya OA. Studying of interconnections of morphological functional indicators of students, who practice martial arts. *Physical Education of Students,* 2016;20(1):64-70. doi:10.15561/20755279.2016.0109
43. Skurikhina NV, Kudryavtsev MD, Kuzmin VA, Iermakov SS. Fitness yoga as modern technology of special health groups' girl students' psycho-physical condition and psycho-social health strengthening. *Physical Education of Students,* 2016;20(2):24-31. doi:10.15561/20755279.2016.0204.

SUBSTANTIATION OF EFFECTIVENESS OF TRAININGS ON HEALTH RELATED METHODIC FOR STUDENTS WITH WEAKENED MOTOR FITNESS

Kuzmin V.A.[1], Kopylov Yu.A.[2], Kudryavtsev M.D.[1], Galimov G.Y.[3], Iermakov S. S.[4]
[1]Siberian Federal University, Russia
[2]Institute of Developmental Physiology, Russia
[3]Buryat State University, Russia
[4]Kazimierz Wielki University in Bydgoszcz, Poland

Abstract. *Purpose:* to work out methodic, facilitating successful conduct of health related trainings of students withy weakened motor (physical) fitness. *Material:* in the research 47 students with weakened motor fitness participated. Analysis of indicators of morbidity frequency and duration was carried out on the base of medical records' studying during all academic year. Experimental methodic consisted of three chapters: execution of specifically selected Hatha yoga static postures, breathing exercises and boxing techniques. Breathing exercises were grouped in four complexes. Every complex was fulfilled during 6 trainings, after each of them the next followed. *Results:* it was found that frequency and duration of diseases statistically confidently decreased in academic year. It was shown that formation of healthy life style skills statistically confidently improved. *Conclusions:* we have determined: increased students' interest to physical culture practicing; reduction of frequency and duration of diseases; higher level of formation of healthy life style skills.
Key words: students, health improvement, methodic, diseases, fitness.

Introduction

Health related measures, reduced as usual to formation of body health – increase of functional fitness, resistance to colds, corrections of muscular skeletal apparatus and some other aspects,- were always paid rather close attention to [2]. Alongside with it there are the data, saying that it is practically impossible to selectively improve physiological aspects of health in isolation from psychic and social-moral health [21]. It complies with law of "relative independence of adaptation", which says: high adaptability to one factor does not result in the same adaptability to other factors (and on the contrary: such adaptability can restrict adaptation due to organism's physiological-morphological characteristics). Therefore, for motor, psychic and social-moral components of health it is necessary to build certain academic programs, which can critically differ from each other [20]. Up to the present time the law of "relatively independent adaptation" has not found its proper place in learning educational process of educational establishments. It is especially important to consider this law in educational system of higher educational establishments, where students already have serious deviations in health, acquired in school years [3].

Rising of students' motivation for physical culture – sport activity is regarded as one of priority directions of educational process perfection in HEE [5, 15, 24]. A number of factors, influencing on attitude to physical culture has been found. It was determined that the most significant for development of students and youth's physical culture were: rising of youth's interest to physical culture practicing [16, 22]; effective administrating of youth's physical education and physical training [14, 18]; orientation of students' physical education of formation of healthy life style [17, 23].

Purpose, tasks of the work, material and methods

The purpose of the work: is to work out methodic, facilitating successful conduct of health related trainings of students withy weakened motor (physical) fitness.

In the research 47 students of higher educational establishments with weakened motor fitness participated.

When planning academic program for experimental group we considered recommendations of methodic literature on formation of training process for students with weakened motor functioning.

Results of the research

The conducted by us complex researches on determination of students' social-moral health features revealed some important laws. We found correlation between the level of some motor qualities and socially significant features of students. Analysis of final results of students' fitness showed that the worked out experimental program facilitated more effective development of nearly all indicators.

Positive points of the experimental methodic is the fact that at the end of pedagogic experiment the students' studied indicators demonstrated statistically confident improvement: quantity and duration of diseases reduced; students' interest to physical culture practicing and level of healthy life style skills increased.

It can be explained by the fact that trainings with elements of boxing permits to make training of new motor skills more interesting, emotional; it shortens period of mastering of new material. Thus, it increases effectiveness of students' mastering discipline "Physical culture".

1. Determination of diseases' frequency and duration

Indicators of frequency and duration of diseases were studied on the base of medical records' analysis during academic year. We considered the quantity of diseases (see table 1) their duration (quantity of days – see table 2) during academic year.

Initial data of quantity and duration of diseases were taken by results of previous year.

Table 1. Quantity of diseases (M±m, %)

Testing		Differences	Confidence of differences	
Initial	Final		t	p
52.1 ± 3.8	41.8 ± 3.3	10.3	2.05	< 0.05

Quantity of diseases in academic year is statistically confident ($p<0.05$) below. Duration of diseases (in days) was as follows (see table 2).

Table 2. Duration of diseases (in days) (M±m, %)

Testing		Differences	Confidence of differences	
Initial	Final		t	p
113.2 ± 3.7	98.7 ± 4.8	14.5	2.39	< 0.05

Analysis of comparative data showed that students, who were trained by experimental methodic with application of boxing elements were more resistant to different diseases: by quantity of cases and by duration of diseases ($p<0.05$).

2. Formation of healthy life style skills

Final data (received in pedagogic experiment) showed statistically confident increase ($p<0.05$) of healthy life style skills' formation level (see table 3).

Table 3. Indicators of healthy life style skills' level, conv. units (M ± m)

Testing		Differences	Confidence of differences	
Initial	Final		t	p
40.3 ± 8.0	65.4 ± 8.2	25.1	2.19	<0.05

Analysis of the received data showed that application of health related methodic with boxing techniques permits to significantly increase level of healthy life style skills' formation in students with weakened motor fitness.

3. Assessment of interest to trainings

As our researches showed, initial interest of students with weakened motor fitness to physical culture and sports practicing did not exceed values, close to 3.77 points (by five-point scale).

After pedagogic experiment we found confident ($p<0.05$) data of interest increase in students with weakened motor fitness (see table 4).

Table 4. Indicators of level of interest (points) to trainings in students of control and experimental groups at the end of pedagogic experiment (M±m)

Testing		Differences	Confidence of differences	
Initial	Final		t	p
3.77 ± 0.1	4. 09 ± 0.1	0.32	2.26	< 0.05

Such positive results permit to state that interest of students to trainings can be formed for relatively short period of time (one academic year).

Discussion

At present the problem of physical education system's perfection, health strengthening and protection in period of students' studying in HEE is noticeably actualized. This system requires new scientific approaches and methodically substantiated solutions.

To day's attention of specialists to this problem to large extent is conditioned by intensive increasing of a number of negative tendencies, which accompany students' physical education. It is confirmed by the fact that the question about "aggressiveness of educational medium" has never been so acute; students' health indicators have never been so low; such low physical condition and motor fitness indicators have never been registered [10, 25–27].

Analysis of published literature showed that at present time individual features of students' physical condition, health, motor fitness, personality's characteristics (motives, strivings, self-confidence and so on) have been elucidated rather sparingly [13–17]. **The limit of such data seriously hinders the process of students' professional adaptation in educational medium.**

We assumed that the problems, which are faced by pedagogues and coaches in sphere of students' physical education, can be corrected with means and methods of boxing. As it was found traditional physical education system in state higher educational establishments can not realize to the fullest extent the tasks of students' motivation for physical culture activity. It is connected with absence of scientifically substantiated conception of physical education formation [11–13, 19].

The fulfilled in this direction scientific and methodic work permitted, in the whole, to rather effectively organize learning regime in higher school, to level the acuteness of problem of organism's overloading in conditions of educational process, to maintain students' workability in relatively optimal frames. The distinctive features of our research are the following:

1. We have developed the system of complex improvement of students' with weakened motor fitness indicators.

Experimental methodic consisted of three parts: execution of specially selected statics postures (asanas) of Hatha yoga system, breathing training and boxing techniques.

Breathing exercises were grouped in four complexes. Every complex was fulfilled during 6 trainings, after each of them the next followed.

Boxing part included main techniques: movements, straight and side punches, uppercuts, defenses.

2. We have worked out methodic of usage of complex system for improvement of students' with weakened motor fitness indicators.

All static exercises were fulfilled consequently one after other. After fulfillment of exercises students had passive rest in lying position.

Breathing exercises were fulfilled after Hatha yoga static postures in position sitting on heels.

Conclusions

Thus, content of auxiliary (health related) physical culture training implies some knowledge, skills and abilities, which should be mastered by students. Prevailing orientation of such trainings is orientation on health related, developing and general recreational tasks. With it formation of physical, psychic and social-moral health should be of preference as well as personality-oriented approach to system of individual choice of physical culture means. Application of non traditional health related means, like Hatha yoga, will be highly effective in system of students' physical education. It is also important to use the principle of versatility. It permits to use knowledge and means of auxiliary health related physical culture in different regions of country and for students with different levels of physical culture literacy and fitness [4, 6–10].

The conducted pedagogic experiment with students, who have weakened motor fitness, showed the following:

1. Frequency and duration of diseases during academic year confidently ($p<0.05$) reduced accordingly from 52.1 ± 3.8 to 41.8 ± 3.3; and from 113.2 ± 3.7 to 98.7 ± 4.8 days.

2. Formation of healthy life style skills statistically confidently ($p < 0.05$) increased from 40.3 ± 8.0 to 65.4 ± 8.2 convenient units.

3. After pedagogic experiment interest for physical culture trainings confidently increased ($p<0.05$) from 3.77 ± 0.1 to 4.09 ± 0.1 points.

4. The experimental methodic is effective and has specificity – increase of interest to physical; culture trainings by students on the base of the following: reduction of frequency and duration of diseases; conscious and firm skills of healthy life style.

Conflict of interests

The authors declare that there is no conflict of interests.

References:

1. Gruzhevsky VA. Appropriateness of the use of innovative technologies in the formation of personality oriented motivation of students to physical education. *Pedagogics, psychology, medical-biological problems of physical training and sports*, 2014;3:19–24. . http://dx.doi.org/10.6084/m9.figshare.936958
2. Zajcev GK. *Valeologo-pedagogicheskie osnovy obespecheniia zdorov'ia cheloveka v sisteme obrazovaniia. Doct. Diss.* [Valueological – pedagogic principles of ensuring of human health in educational system. Doct. Diss.], Sankt Petersburg; 1998. (in Russian)
3. Kopylov IuA, Kokova EI, Polianskaia NV. Razrabotka ozdorovitel'nogo bloka v sisteme fizicheskogo vospitaniia studentov vysshikh uchebnykh zavedenij [Development of health related block in system of higher educational establishment students' physical education]. *Vserossijskaia nauchno-prakticheskaia konferenciia «Optimizaciia uchebno-vospitatel'nogo i trenirovochnogo processa v uchebnykh zavedeniiakh vysshego professional'nogo obrazovaniia». 22 fevralia 2012 g. Krasnoiarsk* [All-Russian scientific-practical conference "Optimization of learning-educational and training process in educational establishments of higher vocational training" February 22nd, 2012, Krasnoyarsk], Krasnoyarsk; 2012. P. 374–379, (in Russian)
4. Kopylov YuA, Jackowska LN, Kudryavtsev MD, Kuzmin VA, Tolstopyatov IA, Iermakov SS. The concept of structure and content of health related trainings for higher educational establishments' students. *Physical Education of Students*, 2015;5:23–30. http://dx.doi.org/10.15561/20755279.2015.0504
5. Kosyns'kyi EO, Khodinov VM, Khrypliuk OP, Krot AS. Athletic and sporting interests of students in the physical education classes. *Pedagogics, psychology, medical-biological problems of physical training and sports*, 2013, vol.8, pp. 46–50. . http://dx.doi.org/10.6084/m9.figshare.745784
6. Kudriavcev MD, Galimov GIa, Gas'kov AV. Obosnovanie effektivnosti uchebnykh zaniatij po fizicheskoj kul'ture s ozdorovitel'noj i obrazovatel'noj napravlennost'iu na osnove ocenki pokazatelej ispol'zovaniia elementov zdorovogo obraza zhizni [Substantiation of effectiveness of health related and educational physical culture trainings on the base of assessment of healthy life style elements' usage]. *Vestnik Buriatskogo gosudarstvennogo universiteta.* 2012;13:121–124. (in Russian)
7. Kudriavcev MD, Galimov GIa, Strel'nikov VA. Organizaciia fizkul'turno-obrazovatel'noj deiatel'nosti v razvivaiushchem obuchenii [Organization of physical culture-educational activity in developing teaching]. *Vestnik Buriatskogo gosudarstvennogo universiteta.* 2012;1:97–105. (in Russian)
8. Kudriavcev MD, Konoshenko LA, Goncharova VG, Miadelec TN. Sociokul'turnaia reabilitaciia lic s ogranichennymi vozmozhnostiami zdorov'ia [Social-cultural rehabilitation of disabled persons]. *Zhurnal Sibirskogo Federal'nogo universiteta. Gumanitarnye nauki.* 2013;6(4):555–561. (in Russian);

9. Kudriavcev MD, Galimov GIa. Ozdorovitel'naia napravlennost' uchebnykh zaniatij po fizicheskoj kul'ture [Health related orientation of academic physical culture lessons]. *Vestnik Krasnoiarskogo gosudarstvennogo pedagogicheskogo universiteta.* 2013;2:118–121. (in Russian)
10. Kuz'min VA, Kudriavcev MD, Kopylov IuA, Galimov GIa, Strel'nikov VA. Konceptual'nye osnovy neobkhodimosti obnovleniia dopolnitel'nogo ozdorovitel'nogo fizicheskogo vospitaniia studentov [Conceptual principles of demand in students' health related physical education's renewal]. *Mezhdunarodnaia nauchno-prakticheskaia konferenciia "Molodaia sportivnaia nauka Belarusi", Minsk, 8–10 apr. 2014 g.* [International scientific-practical conference "Young sport science of Belarus", Minsk, April 8th- 10th, 2014], Minsk BGUFK; 2014;2. P. 162–165.]. (in Russian)
11. Kuz'min VA, Kudriavcev MD, Galimov GIa, Kopylov IuA, Gas'kov AV. Sovremennye podkhody k sozdaniiu koncepcii i obnovleniiu struktury i soderzhaniia ozdorovitel'nogo fizicheskogo vospitaniia studentov vuzov [Modern approaches to creation of conception and renewal the structure and content of health related physical education of HEE students]. *Vestnik Buriatskogo gosudarstvennogo universiteta.* 2014;13:34–41. (in Russian)
12. Kuz'min VA, Kudriavcev MD, Galimov GIa, Kopylov IuA, Gas'kov AV. Effektivnost' ispol'zovaniia v sisteme fizicheskogo vospitaniia studentov netradicionnykh sredstv na primere khatkha-jogi [Effectiveness of non-traditional means' application in system of students' physical education on example of Hat ha Yoga]. *Vestnik Buriatskogo gosudarstvennogo universiteta.* 2014;13:41–44. (in Russian)
13. Kuz'min VA, Kudriavcev MD, Galimov GIa, Kopylov IuA, Gas'kov AV, Strel'nikov VA. Osobennosti formirovaniia social'no znachimykh lichnostnykh kachestv studentov-bokserov kak osnovy budushchej professional'noj deiatel'nosti [Peculiarities of formation of students-boxers' socially significant qualities as the basis of their future professional functioning]. *Vestnik Buriatskogo gosudarstvennogo universiteta.* 2014;13:68–72. (in Russian)
14. Panachev VD. Upravliaiushchaia rol' kafedry v razvitii fizicheskoj kul'tury i sporta v vuze [Leading role of physical culture department in development of physical culture and sports in HEE]. *Teoriia i praktika fizicheskoj kul'tury* 2004;1:49–52. (in Russian)
15. Parkhomchik VI. Faktory, vliiaiushchie na razvitie motivacii v fizkul'turno-sportivnoj deiatel'nosti studencheskoj molodezhi [Factors, influencing on development of motivation in students' physical culture-sports activity]. *4 Respublikanskaia konferenciia "Tradicionnaia fizicheskaia kul'tura belorusov", 20 noiabria 2002 g.* [4th Republic conference "Traditional physical culture of Belarus people", November 20th, 2002], Minsk; 2002. P. 74–78 (in Russian)
16. Stoliarov VI, Kudriavcev NV. Novye formy fizkul'turno-sportivnoj raboty s uchashchejsia molodezh'iu [New forms of physical culture – sports work with students]. *Fizicheskaia kul'tura* 1998;1:21–26. (in Russian)
17. Shil'ko VG, Kapilevich LV, Guseva NL. Formirovanie zdorovogo obraza zhizni studentov cherez fizkul'turno-sportivnuiu deiatel'nost' [Formation of students' healthy life style through physical culture-sport functioning]. *Mezhdunarodnaia nauchno-prakticheskaia konferenciia "Aktual'nye problemy sokhraneniia i ukrepleniia zdorov'ia molodezhi Sibirskogo regiona", 18–25 iiunia 2006 g.* [International scientific-practical conference "Actual problems of health protection and strengthening of Siberian region youth", June 18th-25th, 2006], Irkutsk; 2006. P 69. (in Russian)
18. Yurchyshyn YV. Modern information tools: their place in students' extra-curriculum and involvement of them in motor activity of health related orientation. *Physical Education of Students*, 2015;4:44–50. http://dx.doi.org/10.15561/20755279.2015.0407
19. Adashevskiy VM, Iermakov SS, Firsova IuIu. Physical mathematical modelling of difficult elements of acrobatic rock-and-roll. *Physical Education of Students*, 2013;3:3–10. doi:10.6084/m9.figshare.662463
20. Bar-or O. Health benefits of physical activity during childhood and adolescents. *President's Council on Physical Fitness and Sports Physical Activity and Fitness Research Digest.* 1995;2:1–8.
21. Bohm D. A New theory of the relationship of mind and body. *J. Amer. Soc. Psych. Research.* 1986;80(2):113–135.
22. Iermakova TS. Forming of healthylife style of pupils via prism of physical culture outside of school (historical aspect). *Pedagogics, psychology, medical-biological problems of physical training and sports* 2011;6:50–56.

23. Iermakova TS. The peculiarities of work of the European network of health promoting schools (comparative analysis). *Pedagogics, psychology, medical-biological problems of physical training and sports*, 2013;10:87–90. doi:10.6084/m9.figshare.775339
24. Iermakova TS. The usage by the modern school an experience of high school pupils' healthy life style forming (the second part of XX century). *Pedagogics, Psychology, Medical-Biological Problems of Physical Training and Sports*. 2010;11:34 – 37.
25. Podrigalo LV, Iermakov SS, Nosko MO, Galashko MN, Galashko NI. Study and analysis of armwrestlers' forearm muscles' strength. *Journal of Physical Education and Sport*, 2015;15(3):531–537. http://dx.doi.org/10.7752/jpes.2015.03080
26. Prusik Krzysztof, Prusik Katarzyna, Kozina ZhL, Iermakov SS. Features of physical development, physical preparedness and functional state of boys and girls – students of Polish higher educational establishments. *Physical Education of Students*, 2013;1:54–61. http://dx.doi.org/10.6084/m9.figshare.96415
27. Żukowska Hanna, Szark-Eckardt Mirosława, Muszkieta Radosław, Iermakova TS. Characteristics of body posture in the sagittal plane and fitness of first-form pupils from rural areas. *Pedagogics, psychology, medical-biological problems of physical training and sports*, 2014;7:50–60. http://dx.doi.org/10.6084/m9.figshare.1015583

INVESTIGATION OF EGO AND TASK ORIENTATION AMONG INTERNATIONAL WRESTLING REFEREES

Barbas I.[1], Bebetsos E.[1], Christos K.[2], Curby D.[3], Mirzaei B.[4]
[1]Democritus University of Thrace, School of Physical Education & Sport Science, Komotini, Greece
[2]University of Athens, School of Physical Education & Sport Science, Athens, Greece
[3]International Network of Wrestling Researchers (INWR), USA
[4]University of Guilan, Rasht, Iran

Abstract. *Aim:* study was to investigate any possible effect(s) of experiences from active membership and participation in task or ego orientations among referees in the sport of wrestling. *Material:* The sample consisted of 213 international referees from 30 countries (Greece, Turkey, Bulgaria, France, Italy, Germany, Sweden, Finland, Switzerland, Russia, Poland, Hungary, U.S.A, Ukraine, Armenia, Azerbaijan, Iran, Japan, Korea, Mongolia, Kazakhstan, Egypt, Canada, Georgia, Croatia, Uzbekistan, Norway, Cuba, Belarus, & Tunisia). Their age ranged from 26 to 60 yrs. old (*M*=43, *SD*=8.6). During the procedure, the participants were asked to fill a specific questionnaire, the «Task and Ego Orientation in Sport Questionnaire» (Duda & Nicholls, 1992). Results: Results showed that the referees from elite wrestling level' countries (Russia, Azerbaijan, Iran, Turkey, Georgia, Armenia, Bulgaria, Ukraine, U.S.A., Korea, Japan, Kazakhstan, & Cuba) are more task oriented than those from the non-elite wrestling level' countries. Researchers believe that this occurred because referees from non-elite wrestling level' countries might have less game-sport experience and more specifically in high level games. At the same time, the Olympic experience referees were more task oriented than the non-Olympic experienced. *Conclusion:* Referee's decisions are an important issue in the sport milieu. The investigations in decision-making by referees and factors that affect it are rather scarce and research should focus on such topics. Improvement of decision-making by referees, would lead to safer and better performance. Thus, better understanding of referees' behavior, through identification and operationalization of the factors affecting it, might lead to more effective selection, training and performance.
Key words: task orientations, referees, decision-making, wrestling.

Introduction

One of the factors which could assist in better comprehending referees' decisions is achievement orientation. In achievement motivation in sport, goals have been perceived as being related to the way individuals believe, feel or regulate their abilities [1, 8, 11-13]. Nicholls [14] claimed that goal orientation is related to a number of attitudes, convictions and values. In his theory he postulated the existence of two main goal orientations, task and ego, which are independent of each other but differ among individuals and across environments. Research has showed that a person with an ego orientation is more likely to approve improper sport behaviors and accept athletic aggression, while this does not hold true for persons with task orientation [5, 6]. Individuals with task orientation are more likely to choose moral than non-moral values when there is a conflict [4, 5] and to respect social conventions, personal commitment, the rules and officials [7].

Cross-sectional studies in the USA [3] and Greece [16] have indicated positive relationship between participation in sport and goal orientations, but it is still unclear whether this is the cause or effect of youngsters' involvement in sport. According to social learning theory [2], participation in sport is expected to cultivate youngsters' goals to further improve and demonstrate their sport abilities. Hence, the positive relationship between goal orientations and participation in sport, found in cross-sectional studies, could be ascribed to social learning effects of sport involvement on goal orientations, rather than the opposite. In addition, given the different opinions about the role of ego orientation in sport achievement [4, 9], the interactive effects of task and ego orientation should be also reported. One could possibly assume that the positive effects of task orientation on sport involvement are even stronger when they are accompanied by high ego orientation but they are undermined when they are joined by low ego orientation [9], although some authors suggest that ego orientation has no benefits in youth sports [10].

Internationally minimal attempts were made in order to investigate any relations between goal orientation and any sport officials. As a result of that, the significant aspect of this study is the first attempt to investigate levels of goal orientation among international wrestling referees.

Hypothesis: The task orientations among international referees of wrestling depend on the development of the struggle in a particular country.

Aim: the study was to investigate any possible effect(s) of experiences from active membership and participation in task or ego orientations among referees in the sport of wrestling.

Materials and Methods

Participants

The sample consisted of 213 international referees from 30 countries (Greece, Turkey, Bulgaria, France, Italy, Germany, Sweden, Finland, Switzerland, Russia, Poland, Hungary, U.S.A, Ukraine, Armenia, Azerbaijan, Iran, Japan, Korea, Mongolia, Kazakhstan, Egypt, Canada, Georgia, Croatia, Uzbekistan, Norway, Cuba, Belarus, & Tunisia). Their age ranged from 26 to 60 yrs. old (M=43, SD=8.6).

Research Design

During the procedure, the participants were asked to fill a specific questionnaire, the "Task and Ego Orientation in Sport Questionnaire" (Duda & Nicholls, 1992). This questionnaire was translated into Greek with the use of the back-translation technique [15]. Apart from, this questionnaire was adapted from to Greek mentality and modified for referees [17]. There are two independent scales related to either Task or Ego Orientation. In its present form, each statement begins with "I feel more successful as a referee when ..." followed by 13 different endings. For example, the endings related to Task Orientation include "I learn to apply the rules correctly", "something I learn makes me want to referee even more", "learn something that helps me referee better by trying harder", "try really hard to referee well". For Ego Orientation, examples are "I am the only one who can referee a hard game", "I can do better than other referees", " other referees cannot do as well as I can", "other referees mess up while I do not", "my decisions are better than those of other referees". The respondent was asked to indicate how much he agreed with each of the 13 statements (7 of which relate to Task Orientation and 6 to Ego). Responses are given on a 5-point Likert scale with anchors of 5: strongly agree and 1: strongly disagree.

Statistical Analysis

Statistical analysis was performed with the help of programming package Statgraphics 5.1 (Manugistics, Inc.). The methods of parametric statistics of t-criterion of Student were applied.

Results

The results showed that using the Cronbach's coefficient α internal consistency for "Task" was .80 and for "Ego" .84.

Although the analyses revealed no statistical significant differences among the sample, crosstabs indicated significant results. More specifically, the sample divided into 2 groups. Group 1, referees of Elite wrestling level' countries (N=70), and Group 2, Non-elite (N=40). Results showed that the referees from Elite wrestling level' countries (Russia, Azerbaijan, Iran, Turkey, Georgia, Armenia, Bulgaria, Ukraine, U.S.A., Korea, Japan, Kazakhstan, & Cuba) are more task oriented, than those from Non-elite wrestling level' countries. Researchers believe that this occurred because referees from non-elite wrestling level' countries might have less game-sport experience and more specifically in high level games (Fig. 1).

Also, the sample divided into 3 groups, according to their referring experience. Group 1 was referees with experience up to 11 yrs. (N=33), Group 2 from 12 up to 19 yrs. (N=34), and Group 3 from 20 yrs. and on (N=43). The results showed that referees with more experience are more Task oriented than the other 2 groups. Researchers believe that referees with more yrs. of experience are more into the "personal commitment" idea than less experienced ones (Figure 2).

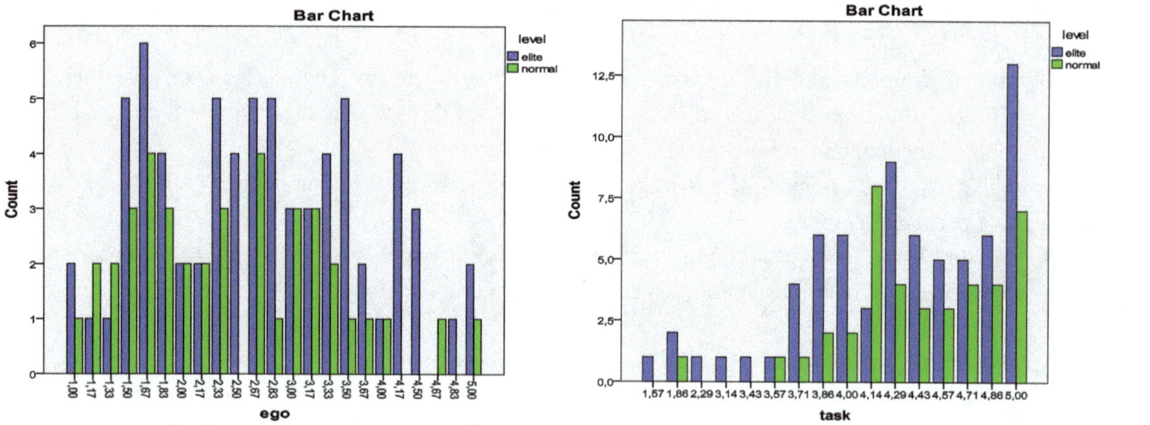

Figure 1. Elite and non-elite referees.

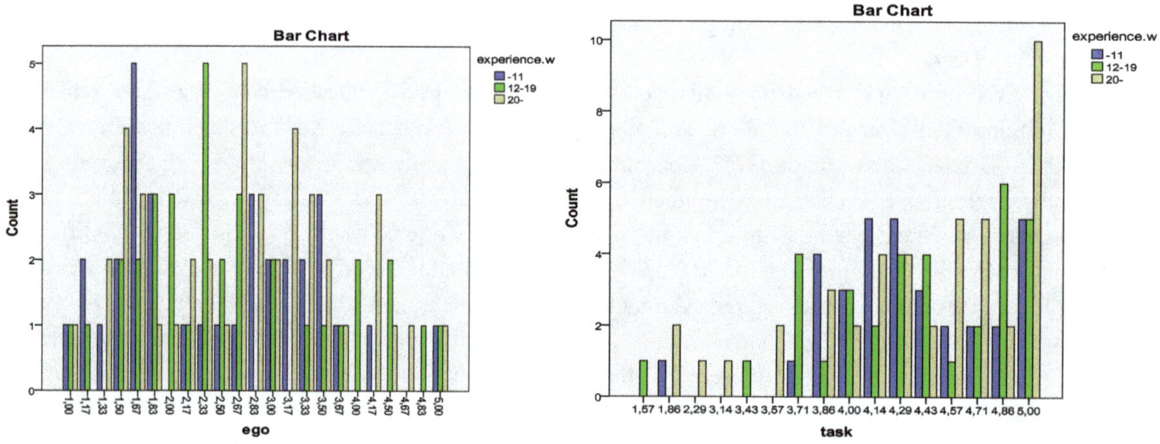

Figure 2. Levels of experience.

Finally, the sample divided into 2 groups according their Olympic Games' experience. Group 1, the Olympic referees (N=32), and Group 2 the Non-Olympic (N=78). The results showed that the Olympic experience referees were more Task oriented than the Non-Olympic experienced. These results are consistent with the previous ones (Figure 3).

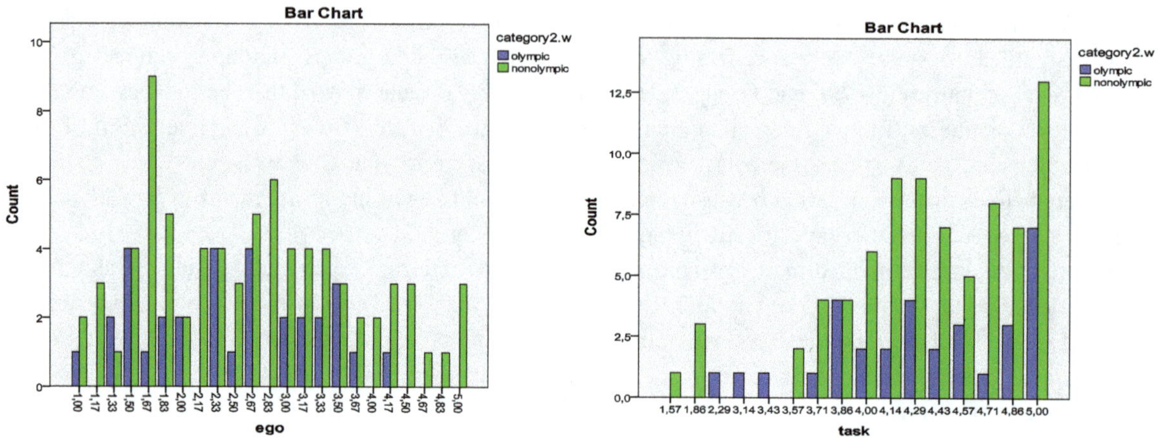

Figure 3. Olympic and Non-Olympic experience referees.

Discussion

The results of this study support the positive role of perceived athletic competence, task orientation and intrinsic motivation in sport and exercise involvement. Further studies examining the mediator variables between sport and exercise involvement and task orientation, perceived competence and intrinsic motivation are called for [8, 12, 13]. It is important to understand the self regulation strategies trigger port and exercise behaviour [2, 4, 5]. Referee's decisions are an important issue in the sport milieu [3, 16]. The investigations in decision-making by referees and factors that affect it are rather scarce and research should focus on such topics. Improvement of decision-making by referees, would lead to safer and better performance [10,14]. Finally, a better understanding of referees' behavior, through identification and operationalization of the factors affecting it, might lead to more effective selection, training and performance.

Finally, the causal relationship of sport and exercise involvement with goal orientations, perceived competence and intrinsic motivation must be investigated in different cultures to determine whether these social-cognitive variables have universal importance. Future research should be focused on comparison between referees (i.e. background difference, level difference, stress & anxiety, attention, self-confidence) on different exercise levels and settings.

Conclusions

Referee's decisions are an important issue in the sport milieu. The investigations in decision-making by referees and factors that affect it are rather scarce and research should focus on such topics. Improvement of decision-making by referees, would lead to safer and better performance. Thus, better understanding of referees' behavior, through identification and operationalization of the factors affecting it, might lead to more effective selection, training and performance.

Conflict of interests

The authors declare that there is no conflict of interests.

References:

1. Competitive, cooperative, and individualistic goal structures: A cognitive-motivational analysis. In: R. E. Ames y C. Ames (Eds.). *Research on motivation in education*, Nueva York: Academic; 1984.
2. Press.Bandura A. *Social foundations of thought and action: A social cognitive theory.* Englewood Cliffs, NJ: Prentice-Hall; 1986.
3. Duda JL. Goal perspectives, participation and persistence in sport. *International Journal of Sport Psychology.* 1989;20:42-56.
4. Duda JL. Perpetuating myths: A response to Hardy's 1996 Coleman Griffith Address. *Journal of Applied Sport Psychology.* 1997;9:307-313.
5. Duda JL, Olson LK, Templin TJ. The relationship of task and ego orientation to sportsmanship attitudes and the perceived legitimacy of injurious acts. *Research Quarterly for Exercise and Sport.* 1991; 62: 79-87.
6. Duda JL, Nicholls JG. Dimensions of achievement motivation in schoolwork and sport. *Journal of Educational Psychology.*1992; 84: 290-299.
7. Dunn JGH, Dunn JC. Goal orientation, perceptions of aggression, and sportspersonship in elite male youth ice hockey players. *The Sport Psychologist.* 1999; 13: 183-200.
8. Dweck CS, Elliott E. Achievement motivation. In: E. Hetherington, (Ed.), *Socialisation, personality, and social development.* New York; 1983.
9. Hardy L. Three myths about applied consultancy work. *Journal of Applied Sport Psychology.* 1997; 9: 277-294.
10. Liukkonen J, Telama R, Biddle S. Enjoyment in youth sports: A goal perspectives approach. *European Yearbook of Sport Psychology.* 1998; 2: 55-75.
11. Maehr M, Braskamp L. The motivation factor: a theory of personal investment. Lexington, MA: Lexington; 1986.
12. Nicholls JG. Achievement motivation: conceptions of ability, subjective experiences, task choice, and performance. *Psychological Review.* 1984; 91: 328-346.

13. Nicholls JG. Conceptions of ability and achievement motivation. *Research on motivation in education: student motivation.* 1984; 1: 39-73.
14. Nicholls JG. *The competitive ethos and democratic education*. Cambridge, Mass: Harvard University Press; 1989.
15. Papaioannou A, McDonald A. I. Goals perspectives and purposes of physical education as perceived by Greek adolescents. *Physical Education Review.* 1993; 16: 41-48.
16. Papaioannou A. "I agree with the referee's abuse, that's how I also beat.. .": Prediction of sport violence and attitudes towards sport violence. *European Yearbook of Sport Psycholog.* 1997; 1: 113 - 129.
17. Proios M, Doganis G, Athanailidis I. Moral development and form of participation, type of sport, and sport experience. *Perceptual and motor skills.* 2004; 99(2): 633-642.

Permissions

All chapters in this book were first published in PES, by Ukrainian Academy of Sciences/H.S. Skovoroda Kharkov National Pedagogical University; hereby published with permission under the Creative Commons Attribution License or equivalent. Every chapter published in this book has been scrutinized by our experts. Their significance has been extensively debated. The topics covered herein carry significant findings which will fuel the growth of the discipline. They may even be implemented as practical applications or may be referred to as a beginning point for another development.

The contributors of this book come from diverse backgrounds, making this book a truly international effort. This book will bring forth new frontiers with its revolutionizing research information and detailed analysis of the nascent developments around the world.

We would like to thank all the contributing authors for lending their expertise to make the book truly unique. They have played a crucial role in the development of this book. Without their invaluable contributions this book wouldn't have been possible. They have made vital efforts to compile up to date information on the varied aspects of this subject to make this book a valuable addition to the collection of many professionals and students.

This book was conceptualized with the vision of imparting up-to-date information and advanced data in this field. To ensure the same, a matchless editorial board was set up. Every individual on the board went through rigorous rounds of assessment to prove their worth. After which they invested a large part of their time researching and compiling the most relevant data for our readers.

The editorial board has been involved in producing this book since its inception. They have spent rigorous hours researching and exploring the diverse topics which have resulted in the successful publishing of this book. They have passed on their knowledge of decades through this book. To expedite this challenging task, the publisher supported the team at every step. A small team of assistant editors was also appointed to further simplify the editing procedure and attain best results for the readers.

Apart from the editorial board, the designing team has also invested a significant amount of their time in understanding the subject and creating the most relevant covers. They scrutinized every image to scout for the most suitable representation of the subject and create an appropriate cover for the book.

The publishing team has been an ardent support to the editorial, designing and production team. Their endless efforts to recruit the best for this project, has resulted in the accomplishment of this book. They are a veteran in the field of academics and their pool of knowledge is as vast as their experience in printing. Their expertise and guidance has proved useful at every step. Their uncompromising quality standards have made this book an exceptional effort. Their encouragement from time to time has been an inspiration for everyone.

The publisher and the editorial board hope that this book will prove to be a valuable piece of knowledge for researchers, students, practitioners and scholars across the globe.

List of Contributors

Anikieiev D. M.
Institute of Penal Service

Kenioua Mouloud
Institute of physical education and sport, Ouargla University, Algeria

Boumasjed Abd Elkader
Institute of physical education and sport, Mostaganem University, Algeria

Jagiello W and Jagiello Marina
University of Physical Education and Sport, Gdansk, Poland

Kozina Zh. L
Kharkov National Pedagogical University, Ukraine

Hossein Soltani
Young Researchers and Elite Club, Torbat-e Heydarieh Branch, Islamic Azad University, Torbat-e Heydarieh, Iran

Zahra Hojati
Department of Physical Education and Sport Sciences, Birjand Branch, Islamic Azad University, Birjand, Iran

Seyed Reza Attarzadeh Hossini
Sport Physiology Faculty of Physical Education and Sport Sciences, Ferdowsi University of Mashhad, Mashhad, IR Iran

Rovniy A. S. and Lastochkin V. M.
Kharkov State Academy of Physical Culture Sumy State A.S.Makarenko Pedagogical University

Ramin Shabani, Roya Rahmatian and Fatemeh Izaddoust
Department of Exercise Physiology, Rasht Branch, Islamic Azad University, Rasht, Iran

Kravchenko O. V.
National University of Physical Education and Sport of Ukraine

Sobko I. N., Ulaeva L. A. and Yakovenko Y. A.
Simon Kuznets Kharkov National Economic University

Korobeynikov G. V. and Korobeynikova L. G.
National University of Physical Education and Sport of Ukraine

Latyshev S. V.
Rostov State University of Civil Engineering

Latyshev N. V.
Donetsk National University

Goraschenko A. U.
State University of Physical Education and Sport the Republic of Moldova

Gant H. Y. and Orlenko O. M.
Kharkov State Academy of Physical Culture

Kudin S. F.
Chernigov National Pedagogical University

Kuzmin V. A.
Siberian Federal University, Russia

Osipov A. Yu.
Siberian Federal University, Russia
V.F. Voino-Yasenetsky Krasnoyarsk State Medical University, Russia

Kudryavtsev M. D.
Siberian Federal University, Russia
Siberian State Aerospace University, Russia
Krasnoyarsk State Pedagogical University of V.P. Astafyev, Russia

Kramida I. E.
Siberian State Aerospace University, Russia

Iermakov S. S.
Kazimierz Wielki University, Poland

Sidorov L. K.
Krasnoyarsk State Pedagogical University of V.P. Astafyev, Russia

Dereka T. Hr.
Borys Grinchenko Kyiv University

Bezkorovainyi D. A.
Kharkiv National University of Municipal Economy

Fatemeh Balbasi, Ramin Shabani and Marzieh Nazari
Department of exercise physiology, Rasht Branch, Islamic Azad University, Rasht, Iran

Mayevsky M. I.
Pavlo Tychyna Uman State Pedagogical University

Gordienko Y. V.
Poltava National Technical Yuri Kondratyuk University

Shafiee Shahram, Rahim Ramezaninezhad and Hakime Afrouzeh
University of Guilan, Iran

Vahid Rabbani
Allameh Tabataba'i University, Tehran, Iran

Chernovsky S. M. and Kolumbet A. N.
Kiev National University of Technology and Design

Benar Noshin
Associate Professor at University of Guilan, Iran

Emami Mina
Master in Sport Management, University of Guilan, Iran

Eftekhari Ozra
Master in Sport Management, University of Shomal, Iran

Yeganeh Far Nastaran
Lecturer at Islamic Azad University Bandar Anzali Branch, Iran

Khan Mohammadi Ali Mohammad
Master in Sport Management, University of Guilan, Iran

Rahmat Ali Jafari, Arsalan Damirchi and Bahman Mirzaei
Department of Exercise Physiology, Faculty of Sport Sciences, University of Guilan, Iran

Hadi Nobari
PhD student of Biochemistry and Exercise Metabolism, University of Isfahan, Iran

Liashenko V. N., Tumanova V. N. and Hatsko E. V.
Kiev University Boris Grinchenko

Pyatnickaya D. V.
Kharkov Humanitarian Pedagogical Academy

Hamidreza Goharrostami
Assistant Professor, Faculty of Physical Education, University of Guilan, Iran

Mustafa Mollaei Nejad
M.A. Strategic Management of Sport Organizations at the University of Guilan, Iran

Rahim Ramezani Nejad
Professor, Faculty of Physical Education, University of Guilan, Iran

Azam Abdollahi
M. A. Strategic Management of Sport Organizations at the University of Guilan, Iran

Kozina Zh. L.
H.S. Skovoroda Kharkiv National Pedagogical University

Ol'khovyj O. M. and Temchenko V. A.
Kharkov National University

Kolumbet A. N. and Dudorova L. Yu.
Kiev National University of Technology and Design

Romanov Y. N., Isaev A. P. and Romanova L. A.
South Ural State University Institute of Sport, Tourism and Service, Chelyabinsk, Russia

Shevtsov A.V.
Lesgaft National State University of Physical Education, Sport and Health, St.-Petersburg, Russia

Cieslicka M. and Muszkieta R.
Kazimierz Wielki University in Bydgoszcz, Poland

Masliak I. P. and Krivoruchko N. V.
Kharkov State Academy of Physical Culture

Samokih I. I.
Odessa National O. S. Popov Academy of Telecommunications

Gaurav Dureja and Gagandeep Singh
Department of Physical Education-TEL & R, Postgraduate Government College, Sector-11, Chandigarh (U.T.), India

Petryshyn A. V.
Ukrainian Medical Dental Academy

Boloban V. N., Tereshchenko I. A., Otsupok A. P., Krupenia S. V. and Kovalenko Y. O.
National University of Physical Education and Sport of Ukraine

Kolumbet A. N.
Kiev National University of Technology and Design

Kudryavtsev M. D.
Siberian Federal University, Russia
Siberian State Aerospace University, Russia
Krasnoyarsk State Pedagogical University of V.P. Astafyev, Russia

Kramida I. E.
Siberian State Aerospace University, Russia

Iermakov S. S.
Kazimierz Wielki University in Bydgoszcz, Poland

Osipov A. Yu.
Siberian Federal University, Russia
V.F. Voino-Yasenetsky Krasnoyarsk State Medical University, Russia

Kuzmin V. A. and Kudryavtsev M.D.
1Siberian Federal University, Russia

Kopylov Yu. A.
Institute of Developmental Physiology, Russia

Galimov G. Y.
Buryat State University, Russia

Iermakov S. S.
Kazimierz Wielki University in Bydgoszcz, Poland

Barbas I. and Bebetsos E.
Democritus University of Thrace, School of Physical Education & Sport Science, Komotini, Greece

Christos K.
University of Athens, School of Physical Education & Sport Science, Athens, Greece

Curby D.
International Network of Wrestling Researchers (INWR), USA

Mirzaei B.
University of Guilan, Rasht, Iran

Index

www.ingramcontent.com/pod-product-compliance
Lightning Source LLC
LaVergne TN
LVHW080928210926
848485LV00004B/750
* 9 7 8 1 6 4 1 1 6 6 3 4 8 *